# SACRIFICE

## The True Story of
## Courage over Chernobyl

*by*
*Cap Parlier*

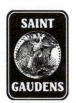

### SAINT GAUDENS PRESS
Prescott, Arizona & Ventura, California

**Books by Cap Parlier:**
The Phoenix Seduction
Sacrifice

**and with Kevin E. Ready:**
TWA 800 - Accident or Incident?

These and other great books available from Saint Gaudens Press
http://www.saintgaudenspress.com  or call  toll-free 1-(800) 281-5170
Visit Cap Parlier's Web Site at http://www.parlier.com

**Saint Gaudens Press**
Post Office Box 2646
Ventura, CA 93002-2646

Saint Gaudens, Saint Gaudens Press and the Winged Liberty colophon
are trademarks of Saint Gaudens Press

ISBN: 0-943039-02-9
Library of Congress Card Number: 00-108409
Printed in the United States of America

### PUBLISHER'S NOTE:

The author was a participant in the events depicted.  For numerous reasons, including  the death or infirmity of some participants and the difficulty of obtaining certain records of the Soviet actions in the events depicted, the author and publisher have chosen  to fictionalize certain personal events and private conversations  that  the  author  was  not  a  party  to.  However,  the  story,  the sacrifices by the heroic people involved, the historical events and all events and conversations in which the author was a party are entirely true.

### COVER ART

A reproduction of an original oil painting by Captain-Navigator Valerie O. Shmakova,  Soviet Air Force, and Chernobyl navigator.  The artist gave the painting  to  the  author  during  his  visit  to  their  base  at  Torzhuk.  Captain Shmakova's handwritten inscription on the back of the painting:

> *To Test Pilot*
> *Cap Parlier*
> *A symbol of our friendship, from the pilots who*
> *worked on the aftermath of the Chernobyl disaster.*
> *Given in the City of Torzhuk*
> *01 August 1991*

## DEDICATION

### Anatoly Demjanovich Grishchenko

This book is dedicated to a husband, father, experimental test pilot, friend and hero. He lost his last, most valiant struggle against radiation-induced leukemia on 2.July.1990. Our prayers and best wishes must go to his widow, Galina, and their sons.

Chernobyl released 30 to 40 times the radioactivity of the bombs dropped on Hiroshima and Nagasaki.

This book is also dedicated to all those who worked so hard to contain the aftermath of the tragic explosion of Reactor No.4 at Chernobyl, Ukraine, Union of Soviet Socialist Republics, on 26.April.1986, and especially to the many pilots who flew in the face of enormous risk.

Nuclear medical experts indicate the majority of high dosage exposures will become symptomatic within 20 years of exposure. Anatoly Grishchenko may have been the first of the pilots to lose his life as a result of his exposure. He will most certainly not be the last. The sacrifice of the pilots kept the disaster from becoming far worse for the people of Earth.

The author would like to pay special tribute to a good friend who took a risk to make a connection and assist his comrade. Gourgen Rubenovich Karapetyan, Hero of the Soviet Union, continues to work tirelessly to find help for the pilots of Chernobyl. Gourgen is one of those unique souls on this planet that finds no limits to his generosity, humanity and friendship. Gourgen established The Grishchenko Foundation in Moscow, Russia, as a companion to The Grishchenko Fund in the United States of America. The sole purpose of both the Grishchenko Foundation in Russia and the Grishchenko Fund in America is to raise money for the medical treatment of the Chernobyl pilots.

### Admiral Elmo Russell Zumwalt, Jr. USN (Ret.)

A great man who gave back far more than he received from his country. While all can say he was controversial, none can deny his courage, confidence, compassion and the love he displayed in so many ways and on so many occasions to his friends and to all the world. He gave selflessly of himself to all those who needed him. This Earth and its society are diminished with his passing.

## NOTICE

The publisher and author will contribute a portion of all profits from this book to The Grishchenko Fund to assist in the medical treatment of Chernobyl pilots in the West.

If you would like to make a contribution to The Grishchenko Fund, send to:
**The Grishchenko Fund**
c/o The Marrow Foundation
Or, if you would prefer to contribute to the general fund of The Marrow Foundation to assist anyone in need of a bone marrow transplant, please contact:
**The Marrow Foundation**

400 Seventh Street, NW, Telephone:  (202) 638-6601
Suite 206  Fax:  (202) 638-0641
Washington, DC  20004  eMail:  tmf@nmdp.org
USA  http://www.themarrowfoundation.org

To become a voluntary bone marrow donor, as the author is, or to obtain useful information for potential volunteer donors, including health-screening questions and connections to local donor centers.
Readers in the United States of America should contact:
**National Marrow Donor Program**

Telephone:  (800) MARROW2
Fax:  (202) 627-7692
http://www.marrow.org

Readers outside the United States should contact the bone marrow donor program in their country.

## ACKNOWLEDGMENTS

Special gratitude must go to John Richard, Leta Buresh, Dale Johnson, John Schmidt, Kevin & Olga Ready, Fred Peck, and the author's parents for their constructive criticism . . . without them, this effort would be diminished. It must be understood, any errors in language or science belong to the author, *in toto*.

There are many people whose personal, selfless contributions made this effort possible. The late Dr. Bob Graves, DVM, Colorado rancher and founder of the Laura Graves Foundation, the predecessor of the National Marrow Donor Program, made the connections and linkages work. Dr. John Hansen, MD, soft tissue oncologist and former chief of the bone marrow transplantation unit at the Fred Hutchinson Cancer Research Center, was and still is a true friend and teacher. His generous and patient tutelage on the rudiments of leukemia, human immunogenetics and bone marrow transplantation have been a bountiful and boundless gold mine. Dr. Pat Beatty, MD, now chief of the bone marrow transplant unit at the University of Utah, went far beyond the call of duty.

Unique and special appreciation must go to Susan Summers, former nurse at the US Embassy in Moscow; Carol Eberhart, US State Department; and John Pekkanen, author of the May 1991 Reader's Digest article, *"The Man Who Flew into Hell."* Last, but by no means least, a heartfelt recognition of the physicians, nurses and support personnel of the Fred Hutchinson Cancer Research Center, Seattle, Washington, USA, past, present and future, for the enormous extra care they give each and every patient, and the additional support and patience they offer to the families and friends of their patients.

The author must recognize the late Mark Vineberg, General Designer, Mil Design Bureau; Marat Tishchenko, retired General Designer, Mil Design Bureau; and without question, Anatoly Kovatchur, test pilot *extraordinaire*. These men helped the author see that we are all the same. While governments may differ, lovers of aviation share a common bond the world over, regardless of language.

# 1

"That . . . is impressive," Gourgen Karapetyan whispered to himself beneath the deafening roar of the powerful fighter engines less than a kilometer from him. He smiled as he watched the airplane leap off the runway immediately into the gyrations of the airshow rehearsal.

The air was still damp from the several previous days of low, thick overcast and incessant rain. This was the first day in many the sun actually poked through the broken clouds, and the cloud base had risen sufficiently for the aggressive, airshow flying. While it was not perfect weather, barely marginal actually, it was acceptable for his friend's fair weather routine.

For Gourgen Rubenovich Karapetyan, the senior and most experienced, experimental test pilot at the Mil Design Bureau, the day's practice was complete. The engineers had some concern about his tail rotor gearbox, but Gourgen knew with an inner confidence the rugged Mi-28 prototype attack helicopter could take the aggressive airshow demonstration he performed. He now enjoyed the benefit of flying early in the sequence, watching his friend Anatoly do his routine for the approval judges.

The smooth, blended body, contours and sleek lines of the MiG-29 fighter with its distinctive underwing, canted, sharp, rectangular intakes and twin vertical tails offered elegance and grace in the skies immediately above the famous airfield. Gourgen could sense the movements of Anatoly Kovatchur, the Mikoyan-Gurevich show pilot for the last few years. Gourgen gripped the imaginary stick in his hands, making almost imperceptible control inputs to make the agile fighter dance in the sky. The anticipation always mounted for Gourgen as the nose of the fighter rose sharply until it was pointed precisely 90° straight up.  With the afterburners lit and both engines developing their full, 18,250 pounds thrust each, the aircraft accelerated like a powerful rocket.  As it passed 1,000 meters altitude, the engines throttled back to idle.  The machine decelerated rapidly.  As the airspeed decayed and the fighter appeared to hang for a moment, motionless in the air, Gourgen watched the large tailplanes move smartly to the full nose down position, which meant Anatoly had his stick full aft in his lap.  The airplane began to fall backward in what pilots called a classic hammerhead stall, a popular maneuver for the venerable propeller fighters of World War II, but virtually unheard of among turbojet or turbofan aircraft.

Gourgen's heart skipped a beat every time he watched Anatoly perform that maneuver. Conventional jet engines did not appreciate the added backpressure or reverse flow into the exhaust.  Jet engines usually coughed in protest.  However, the Soviet designers were justly proud of the robust design of the Isotov RD-33, low-bypass, turbofan engine with its automatic restart feature, should the back pressure cause an engine flameout.  The hammerhead stall provided a very public demonstration of how rugged their engines were.

As the fighter fell on its tail, the force of the reverse airstream on the large tailplanes, now fully deflected, functioned in the opposite direction pushing the tail back and the nose down.  The nose fell gracefully, but sharply forward.  The aircraft was now pointed 90° straight down.  Gourgen could see the minute corrections as Anatoly quickly adjusted his position on the far side of the show line and away from the myriad of blue and white stripped tents, or chalets as they called them, and the gathered crowd of professionals watching his rehearsal routine.  The nose of the fighter rose smoothly, Gourgen subconsciously gripped the imaginary throttles in his left hand pushing the levers forward to the full throttle gate, actually a noticeable notch, the pilot's called a detent, that helped them feel the full throttle position just short of lighting the spray rings of the afterburners at the exhaust end of the engines.  As the nose reached the horizon, Gourgen pushed the imaginary throttles through the detent, lighting the afterburners.  A smile washed across his face as he remembered the kick in the backside the afterburners had given him when he had flown the two-seat, MiG-29UB trainer version with Anatoly. Despite the many times he had seen or flown Anatoly's routine with him in the two seat version, Gourgen watched with abject fascination as the aircraft rolled to 90° right and turned hard. Gourgen groaned sympathetically against the g-forces. The aircraft turned through 450° in a level, high energy, short radius turn, so that the orange glow of engine exhausts pointed toward the crowd. The wings leveled, then rolled back in the opposite direction and turned hard again. Gourgen could see the orange eyes disappear as Anatoly pulled the throttles back, to decelerate and prepare for the next maneuver of his routine.

The aircraft slowed. Gourgen could barely see the small adjustments in the fighter's altitude, attitude and the tightness of the turn to place the machine directly above the show line at 200 meters altitude. The fighter's wings level on a path parallel to the main runway. As the airspeed decayed, the airplane's nose slowly rose and continued well past the landing attitude. Gourgen could hear the engines gradually increasing thrust. The aircraft soon stabilized at 27° nose up, in level flight with an airspeed just above 140 kilometers per hour. This was the segment of Anatoly's routine the pilot's called a high alpha demonstration, to show the very slow speed handling qualities, clean aerodynamics and substantial excess power from the engines. The nose was now so high Anatoly could not see in front of him and where he was going. Gourgen knew Anatoly would be rapidly scanning his instruments to ensure the proper attitude and altitude as well as his checkpoints on either side of the aircraft to ensure his flight path was correct. Gourgen loved to tease Anatoly since helicopter pilots routinely used the offset track technique during external-load lift operations.

The aircraft settled perfectly into the abnormal, but stable, slow flight condition as it seemed to inch along the show line parallel to the main runway. In several hundred meters, at the intersection of the runways, Anatoly would firmly push the throttles through the gate detent, lighting both afterburners again and climbing like a missile with big wings. The impressive maneuver would not happen this day.

Gourgen saw the burst of ragged orange flame flash behind what looked like the right engine. This is not good, he thought instantly. Then, he heard the dull thud, or perhaps a hesitation in the fighter's engine sounds. He could see the rudders and ailerons deflecting rapidly to their travel limits. "This is really not good," he muttered. Like an agonizing, Hollywood death scene from some old American Western movie, the aircraft's nose began to slide to the right toward the crowd. He could see that Anatoly was fighting with the wounded fighter.

As the nose started to drop, there was no control left. The machine now began to veer off more rapidly. The nose moved right and down, then the left wing rose sharply. "Eject," Gourgen said, more to himself.

The aircraft continued to roll over on its back as the nose fell toward the ground. The dying fighter quickly went into a vertical descend like an arrow about to impact the earth. "Eject! Eject!" shouted Gourgen, nearly screaming, as if to command his friend to pull the red and white stripped loops between his legs.

At something like 100 meters above the ground and certain death, Gourgen saw the canopy blasted away from the fighter. Bright yellowish orange flames rocketed Anatoly's seat away from the stricken aircraft. The hemispherical parachute canopy opened sharply, but only just a few instants before Anatoly hit the ground. The menacing orange flames and ugly black smoke exploded and billowed instantly as the MiG-29 buried itself in the ground and broke apart. Gourgen could no longer see his friend. He scrambled up his Mi-28 attack helicopter parked behind him.

Sitting on top of the rotor hub, Gourgen could see the impact point. The orange and black of the fire occupied the majority of the scene, but he caught glimpses of Anatoly's parachute canopy fluttering on the ground just behind the fire. He stood several times, attempting to get a better view, but to no avail.

The large red trucks with their flashing lights surrounded the burning remains of whatever was left of the once elegant MiG-29 fighter. The smoke quickly turned from black to gray, then to a dirty light grayish-white color as the firefighters performed their miracles of professional efficiency. He still could not see Anatoly. As the firefighters gained the upper hand on the fire, he could see the smaller trucks behind the impact crater. By the time he could see clearly, men were lifting a stretcher device with a man strapped to it, into the ambulance. The men moved quickly and with precision. Gourgen felt like that was a good sign. That man had to be Anatoly. From the movements of the emergency crew, Anatoly was still alive, and they were trying to keep him that way.

"What happened?" shouted Mark Vineberg from the ground.

Gourgen looked down to his colleague. Vineberg was the senior Mil engineer with the airshow group. "Anatoly has crashed."

"Did he get out?"

"Yes, but only barely." He saw Mark glance back toward the crash site although Gourgen was certain he could not see much. "I think he is alive. They have taken him away in the ambulance."

The wail of sirens beyond the nervous murmur of the mesmerized crowd occupied the atmosphere around them. The heap of what was once an awesome fighter now lay smoldering in a patch of burnt grass between the main runway and the parallel taxiway. The firefighters completed their somber work. Others, not part of the fire crew, began to gather around the pile. They were undoubtedly security agents to protect the site, and others were airport management.

The loudspeakers announced in French, then in English, that flight operations had been suspended, and conveyed the admonition to remain clear of roadways and taxiways to allow emergency and official vehicles to perform their duties. Gourgen continued to sit on the rotor hub taking in the activity around the crash site.

"Are you coming down?" asked Mark.

Gourgen looked down at Vineberg, again. His mind wanted to think of other things. "No, not yet." The senior engineer nodded his head and walked toward the Il-96, wide-body, civil transport aircraft that was the *de facto* meeting room for the Soviet airshow team.

A fairly large crowd remained gathered at the barrier line nearest the impact site. Gourgen thought about moving closer himself, but the urge passed quickly. Fragments of the crowd began to dissipate either from an inability to see anything of substance or because more pressing business commanded their attention. Sitting on the rotor hub of his helicopter, not quite three meters above the ground, Gourgen had the best vantage point.

As he stared off into the distance, the scene began to blur as his mind drifted off to other thoughts. What if Anatoly died? Anatoly was a critical link in the chain of events he had set in motion to aid one of their colleagues and seek help in curing the blight Chernobyl had caused. Would Anatoly's death or injury change the events already set in motion? Gourgen had known Anatoly Kovatchur only seven years when the veteran fighter pilot finished his combat tour in Afghanistan and left the Air Force to join the elite flight test establishment at Zhukovsky, the center of Soviet aviation research and testing, south-southeast of Moscow.

Gourgen's mind wandered further back in time to the moment their lives began to change, although none of them had recognized it. It had started as such a routine mission, like so many other special projects they were asked to perform. So much had happened since the early spring of 1986, and yet there was so much left to be done if they were going to help Tolya. The spring of 1986 . . . "Dear God," he whispered to himself, as his mother had taught him all those years ago, "how much has happened."

Mark Vineberg walked beside a tall slender man in a royal blue, flight suit and a brown leather jacket with a fur collar. The distinctive red, white and blue of the American flag on his left shoulder marked the man's nationality. "Gourgen, this is Cap Parlier," he said in English.

Gourgen recognized the name instantly. This was the American Anatoly met at the Farnborough Airshow a year ago, and the man they all hoped would help them gain the specialized treatment Tolya, the familiar name for their colleague, Anatoly Demjanovich Grishchenko, and undoubtedly other of the Chernobyl pilots, needed in the West. Gourgen nodded his head.

"This is Gourgen Karapetyan, the chief pilot for Mil," continued Mark.

Parlier extended his hand. The two pilots grasped each other firmly in the traditional Western greeting. "It is an honor to meet you," said the American.

Gourgen nodded his head, again.

Now, they reached critical mass. Put two pilots together and even add a design engineer and the talk will inevitably and inexorably run to aircraft and the art of flying. Gourgen and Mark were justly proud of their Mi-28 attack helicopter, and they needed to convey that pride to their American guest.

Like some bizarre courtship, the two pilots – one Soviet and the other American – traded experiences. They began to laugh at shared moments despite Gourgen's halting English and Parlier's brutally rudimentary Russian. So many terms of aviation made direct translation without the need for query.

By the time they retired to the small travel trailer the Mil team used as a work center for a sharing of black bread, they had become friends. The talk of aviation continued.

Parlier's expression turned serious. "May I ask about Anatoly Kovatchur?"

"Yes, certainly. You do know he crashed four days ago?" Parlier nodded his head and held is worried expression. "He is recovering at the ambassador's residence."

"So, he will be OK?"

"Yes. He came so close."

"I saw the news in the United States before I left for Paris. He is a very good man."

"Yes, as you say."

"Did you see the crash?"

"Yes. I watched every move. Anatoly ejected just before hitting the ground.  He was worried about the airplane going into the crowd."

"Thank God, he got out OK."

"Yes."

"Can I see him?"

"He is confined, I guess you say, for a few more days.  I know he wants to see you, so perhaps a little later."

"Excellent.  Well, if you see him, please convey my best wishes for his speedy recovery."

"Yes.  I will do that."

Several mechanics in light blue, oil stained, work overalls came into the trailer.  Gourgen introduced them to his American guest.  They asked several questions about the aircraft that Gourgen promptly answered.  In a few minutes, they returned to their bench seats across the small, fold down table that occupied the front half of the trailer.

"Anatoly told me you flew at Chernobyl," said Parlier with concerned seriousness.

Gourgen nodded his head.  "Only a little, but enough."

"Is everyone all right?"

"Many pilots flew at that place.  Terrible tragedy.  All pilots sick."

"Radiation poisoning is very serious."

"Yes, so the doctors say."

"You appear healthy."

"I am OK, as you say."

"How about the others?"

"The doctors say all will recover.  Only one is having trouble."

"What happened there?" Parlier asked with genuine curiosity.

Mark Vineberg leaned into the trailer and spoke in Russian.  It was time for the bus to take them to their hotel.

Gourgen nodded his head and looked back to his new friend.  "We must go.  Perhaps, I can tell you about this another day."

"At your pleasure," said Parlier as he extended his hand to

Gourgen. "Thank you for everything. I look forward to tomorrow."

"Yes."

The airshow began as scheduled on Monday for the business of international aviation. Cap Parlier reciprocated with a tour for Gourgen, Mark and several others of the American Army's AH-64A Apache attack helicopter. The talk of aviation continued unabated. Three days passed before the two pilots found time to be alone to continue their previous exchange.

Gourgen could feel his expression turn serious as they sat across the fold-down table in the small trailer. He knew it was time for him to get a feel for this American. Was he really the one to help them? "You said you want to know about flying at Chernobyl," he said, late Thursday evening.

"Yes, if you don't mind."

"No, I do not mind." Gourgen looked deep in the hazel eyes of the tall American. He knew there was genuine concern and care, like a brother waiting anxiously for what he knew would be bad news. He would tell Parlier as much as he knew. Gourgen took a bite of black bread, chewed and swallowed, then took a long drink of French, sparkling, bottled water. "Our connection to that disaster place began on a nice spring day in 1986." And so, Gourgen returned to that time to recount the story to Cap Parlier.

# 2

*13:30, Thursday, 10.April.1986*
*60 km south of Kiev, Ukraine, USSR*

"Spring has come early this year," said Anatoly Demjanovich Grishchenko as he stared out the right window of the world's largest helicopter.

There was only a nod of the pilot's head as he concentrated on the slight, precise control inputs to move the Mil Type 26 heavy lift helicopter, the most capable, as well as the largest, vertical lifter in the world. The light blue-on-white *Aeroflot* markings told everyone this was a civilian job. The large, nine metric ton, bridge sections had to be positioned within a few centimeters, so the construction workers could complete the fine alignment and secure them in place. The secret, Karapetyan knew, was very slow, precise movements. Gourgen watched his positioning cues on the ground as well as the signal guide on the completed portion of the bridge.

"Four meters, no swing," came the intercom announcement from the loadmaster watching through an observation window in the belly of the aircraft at the bridge section suspended by a heavy cable.

"Looking good," Grishchenko added as he watched the other completed section of the bridge move across the chin windows in the nose of the huge helicopter.

"Three meters, no swing. The ground crew has the corner lines."

Karapetyan did not have to see the rectangular bridge section nor the nearly two-dozen men slowly pulling on the ropes attached to each corner of the fabricated, replacement bridge span to know exactly what was happening beneath him. The announcement from the loadmaster meant that the lives of the ground crew were now at risk, and soon, a few key workers would be in grave danger until the alignment pins could be driven home and the weight of the load was completely carried by the bridge supports.

Gourgen could feel the rivulets of sweat descending his chest, arms and legs. The cool, conditioned temperature of the spacious cockpit was not enough to remove the tension in every muscle of his body. As he had done many times before, Gourgen concentrated on the flying task. The risk to others simply could not be allowed to affect his flying.

"Two meters, still no swing."

The signal guide commanded even slower lateral movement as well as some downward adjustment.

"They want us down a little," repeated the loadmaster. "About one meter."

Gourgen just thought about lowering the collective to reduce their height.

"That's good. Hold here."

Karapetyan scanned all his cues several times to monitor the movement of the helicopter. His concentration on the task of minute control inputs intended to hold all the needles in exactly the same position, kept the big machine in position while the ground crew did their job. Below them, a platoon of men worked at near frantic speed to fasten the principal securing bolts to hold the section in place.

"They have it. You can release the hook," the loadmaster announced over the intercom for the pilots, a significant moment for external load operations.

Gourgen depressed the red button on his cyclic control stick. The event was imperceptible in the cockpit since the weight of the load had already been transferred to the bridge structure beneath them.

"We are free."

With that announcement, Gourgen gently pushed the stick forward and raised the collective along with an adjustment of his pedal position to counteract the increased torque on the main rotor.

"You want the controls?" Gourgen asked his copilot and best friend, Anatoly Demjanovich Grishchenko, one of the principal helicopter test pilots with the Gromov Flight Research Center in Zhukovsky, Russia.

"Sure."

Gourgen released the controls and held up his hands to signal the cockpit crew he no longer was flying the aircraft. "Let's land in the field. We will wait until we are released. Peter," he called to his loadmaster.

"Yes, Gourgen."

"When we are on the ground, would you be so kind to go out and check with the supervisor to make sure we are finished here. We can still make home this afternoon, if we leave soon and get some fuel in Kiev."

"No problem."

Tolya maneuvered the big machine to land in the large, open field they used for staging during this job. Once the aircraft stopped moving and the collective was full down, the forward entry door advisory light illuminated signaling the departure of their loadmaster.

Gourgen watched out the left side window as his loadmaster jogged away from the helicopter through the tall field grass until he was clear of the main rotor disk. Although the eight, whirling, main rotor blades were eight plus meters above the ground, the habit of moving quickly past the reach of the blade tips had become instinctive to everyone working around helicopters.

They watched as the two men conferred. The construction supervisor checked with several members of his crew, and they monitored the progress of the work. Gourgen checked the fuel totalizer, and then looked over his shoulder at his flight engineer. He pointed to the fuel quantity indicator. The flight engineer scanned several of his instruments, then held up his left hand with his thumb and index finger close together. They did not have much time left before they would need to shutdown the big engines to save fuel for the short flight to Kiev.

"They need to make a decision soon," said Gourgen to put words to what all of them were thinking.

"We have been down here for a week and a half," Tolya added.

"You would think they would be glad to get rid of us."

"They always like to be safe," said the flight engineer. "They will probably make sure every nut and bolt is in place, just in case something really weird happens."

Gourgen waited another five minutes. Even at flat pitch, what the pilots called flight idle; the huge Soloviev engines were burning a lot of fuel.

"That's it. Let's shutdown," commanded Gourgen.

The flight engineer pulled both throttle levers back to the ground idle position to let the engines cool for a few minutes. He stepped through the various switches and procedures to prepare for a complete shutdown of the engines. Before the final shutdown steps could be completed, the loadmaster headed back to the aircraft.

"Let's hold here," Gourgen said.

They waited for the loadmaster to enter the aircraft. He ascended the stairs into the spacious cockpit and plugged his headset into a spare panel. They all turned to look at him.

"Sorry it took so long, Gourgen," he began. Gourgen waved his hand to acknowledge the courtesy, but let it pass. "He wanted to make sure they had everything in place."

"There you go," interjected the flight engineer.

"Yes, well, they have the main bolts done, and he has released us."

"Let's get this beast spun up and everything secure for the transit."

The loadmaster left the cockpit as the crew returned the aircraft to its normal flight configuration. They waited for a few seconds until the loadmaster reported his readiness for flight, meaning all the doors and ramp along with any remaining loose equipment were secure.

Gourgen motioned with his right hand as if signaling his cavalry troop to move out in the prescribed direction. Anatoly gradually raised the collective until the helicopter was in a stable hover. They all checked their instruments to confirm readiness of the machine, and then he pushed the stick forward and added more collective as they transitioned to forward flight.

Anatoly banked the big helicopter to pick up a heading toward Kiev airport to their north. They waved to the ground crew on the bridge as they passed over them. The flight took a quarter hour.

Arriving at Kiev International Airport, Anatoly landed the helicopter on the runway to minimize any potential damage due to the hurricane force winds of the main rotor downwash. He taxied into the assigned parking space and called for the shutdown. As the flight engineer worked through his procedures, Anatoly stayed with the controls until the main rotor stopped. Gourgen unbuckled his seat harness and took off his headset.

The flight engineer and navigator completed their tasks. Gourgen was the first to stand behind his left seat. He arched his back to stretch his tight muscles. His medium height and build along with his loose clothing masked his strength. His curly, salt and pepper, close cut hair, fine-featured face and swarthy skin marked his Armenian heritage. The contrast came into focus when the nearly a head taller Grishchenko stood next to him. Anatoly's thinning, light brown hair and roundish face gave him an older appearance although the two men were less than a year apart and right at 50 years of age.

They met midway through their university education. They both started flying at the same time and remained close friends through the years of enormous change in aviation and in their country. While they worked for different segments of the industry, Gourgen at Mil and Tolya at Gromov, they were the closest of friends, personally and professionally.

"That was interesting," said Tolya.

"You will be ready for these precision external load operations in short order," Gourgen answered.

"I do not get much of this type of work at Gromov. All research stuff . . . strange things the engineers want to look at. I need more of this. It looks like fun."

Gourgen chuckled. "Fun, yes, but hard work as well . . . too many people depending upon your control inputs."

"Isn't that the way it always is?"

"I guess. Let's go find something to drink. I worked up a thirst." Gourgen turned to his crew chief, "Let's get the machine refueled so we can get home this evening."

"As you command, my captain," he answered causing all of them of laugh.

As the crew gathered outside the massive helicopter's forward hatch entry on the left side, a man in coveralls came up to them. "Comrade Karapetyan?" he called.

Gourgen held up his hand. The man passed a folded piece of paper. Gourgen read it.

"Appears we may have another mission before we return to Moscow. I need to call a telephone number, but the message says there is a heavy lift at some nuclear power plant just north of Kiev."

"Chernobyl?" asked Tolya.

"Yes, probably, I guess."

"That plant is near where I grew up as a boy. Several childhood friends work at that plant. They want us today?"

"I will have to call."

The one call indicated on the note turned into a half dozen calls. As the aircraft commander, he made the decision to take the assignment although it probably meant staying another one or two nights. The crew of five other men would probably not mind the extra stay since it was only Thursday. Gourgen knew they all enjoyed unique work, and the proposed job qualified as unique.

"Well, what is it?" asked Tolya.

"We are to proceed to the engineering village that supports the nuclear power plant . . . the name is Pripyat, I think."

"Pripyat River runs past the Chernobyl plant. That is the one . . . about 70 kilometers almost due north of Kiev."

"Once there, we land for a meeting with the engineering team at the village party headquarters."

"What is the lift?" asked the loadmaster.

"They want us to lift a six ton electric motor for some pump and drop it through a hole in the roof."

"Six tons, that is some motor."

"One of their main feed water pumps, they said.  They are trying to make final preparations for some big test in a few weeks, and this motor replaces one that has been causing them some problems."

They all nodded their heads although they had not been asked a question. Gourgen smiled. He knew he had judged the situation correctly.

The flight across Kiev to the plant took only 20 minutes. From their altitude of 500 meters, the plant had been clearly visible on the bright spring day.  The large red and white striped exhaust stack on top of the massive, white buildings was a beacon for them to navigate toward on the horizon.  Other large buildings came into view.  According to the telephone information, they had four working nuclear reactors, and they were in construction on the fifth and sixth units.  The pristine, white apartment buildings among the trees about one kilometer south of the main plant identified the support village of Pripyat.  They circled the plant and village twice to make sure they had a good visual image of the facility layout.  A large, grass field among the trees was just as they described. Anatoly landed the big helicopter in the middle of the clearing.

Several men walked from the nearby buildings to greet them.  A medium build, medium height professional looking man with dark, close cut hair lead the group.

"I am Anatoly Sitnikov, Deputy Chief Operational Engineer, of this plant," the man said as he extended his hand to Gourgen.

"I am Gourgen Karapetyan, the aircraft commander."

"May I introduce Mister Bryukhanov," he said motioning toward a medium build, plain looking man.  "He is the station manager of the Chernobyl Nuclear Power Plant.  This is Chief Engineer Fomin," he added referring to a blockish man with a reddish, over pressurized face. Sitnikov then moved his hand to a tall, strong looking man dressed in the uniform of a firefighter. "This is Major Telyatnikov, the commander of the Pripyat Fire Company."

Gourgen introduced Anatoly and the rest of the crew. The flight crew followed the four local men toward several small buildings. The shrubbery around the closest building was the best manicured of the whole village from what Gourgen could see. It had to be the village headquarters of the Communist Party; their buildings were always the best looking and cared for in any village.

After a short orientation briefing on the purpose of the power plant, they jumped directly into the discussion of the task at hand. The lift item was indeed a six metric ton, electric motor for a coolant circulation water pump, one of eight massive pumps for each unit that moved cooling water to the reactor core for steam production. Using drawings, they described a small platform erected inside the plant underneath one of the large, reinforced, concrete, roof panels that the helicopter would need to lift off first. The task was to lower the motor through the hole in the roof onto the platform. Once bolted onto a base plate to secure the motor, they would release it. From that point on, the interior crane would move the motor to its proper place for attachment to the pump impeller assembly in the primary coolant feed system. The helicopter lift would save them considerable time, weeks or several months, over the conventional ground handling process.

Lifting the roof panel would be relatively easy for the huge helicopter. Each panel weighed about one metric ton, plus it already had lifting eyes cast into it since a construction crane lifted them when the building was assembled. The tar used to seal the seams between panels and cover the panels themselves had already been removed in anticipation of the lift. The plant managers had quite a bit of confidence in using a helicopter for this task.

The hole in the roof that needed to be opened up was located near an interior corner close to the tall exhaust stack they had seen on the flight into Pripyat. They worked with the engineers to calculate the clearances they would have.

The main rotor blade tips would be sweeping a circular arc just 7.5 meters from the trellis structure supporting the stack. The main rotor would also overlap the adjacent Turbine Hall roof. The fuselage would be parallel to the roofline about 5 meters from the building.    In addition to the task of threading a heavy load through a small hole, they would have to watch their clearances very closely. They needed light winds for such a close quarters, precision task.

"Any other questions?" asked Bryukhanov.

"Since we are here, we would like to see more of the plant, especially the reactor," said Tolya. "None of us has seen a nuclear reactor, nor been this close to one."

Several of the locals chuckled. "It is a common question from visitors. Since time is of the essence, would you mind if we waited until after the motor is inside the Pump Room?"

Anatoly looked to Gourgen, who shook his head. "No problem."

"Any other questions?"

Anatoly held up his hand like a schoolboy. "Yes. I believe a childhood friend works here. Would it be possible to see him?"

"Who is it?"

"Lelechenko, Aleksandr Grigoryevich Lelechenko."

"Ah, yes, our deputy chief of the electrical shop," answered Fomin. "We shall check on his duty status." He nodded his head toward Sitnikov to check on the man's work schedule and location. The answer did not take long.

"Aleksandr Grigoryevich is currently working the second shift," announced Sitnikov. "He will not get off duty until after midnight. He is also scheduled to assist with the pump motor placement assuming the motor is inside the hall tomorrow morning."

"He is one of our very best electrical engineers," said Fomin. "He is usually involved in any major project at this plant. He has been here from the beginning, 10 years ago."

"We grew up together in a little village 45 kilometers northwest of here," Anatoly said, "on the Ukrainian border with Byelorussia."

"Let us do this," interjected Bryukhanov. "I would assume there is insufficient daylight remaining today, and you would probably like to make this lift early in the morning when the winds will be the lightest."

"Yes," answered Gourgen.

"Then, if you will agree, we shall let Comrade Lelechenko have a good rest while you lift the motor. When you have placed the motor inside the Pump Room, we shall call him to meet you here. He is certainly capable of leading your tour, that way you can do two things at the same time."

"That should be just fine."

"We have made arrangements for you and your crew to stay at our little visitor's quarters for the night. It is quite comfortable. They will serve your meals as well, and take care of any special needs."

"Excellent."

"Anything else?" asked Bryukhanov.

"We shall need to borrow your drawings for our planning," said Gourgen. Fomin pushed them across the table to the pilots. "I think we have what we need. There is more planning we must do this evening to be prepared for a lift of this nature in the morning."

"Very well, then, we are adjourned."

The Mi-26 crew excused themselves and returned to the helicopter. The five-member crew huddled over the drawings in the lighted, cavernous, cargo bay of the aircraft. They carefully remeasured clearances to all significant objects in the vicinity of the roof opening. They also crudely defined angles to checkpoint features that would help the pilots properly position the big machine. The fine detail movements would be handled by the loadmaster lying on his belly looking through an open panel down the attachment cable holding the large motor. For this task, they all felt better controlling the placement. As such, the helicopter's crewchief would position himself on the roof near the hole, so he could look inside the building, receive guidance instructions from the plant crew on the platform, and quickly translate them into hand signal commands to the loadmaster looking down at him. Neither of the pilots would be able to see the hole, the load, nor the crew chief.

When they made their final calculations, they realized the platform was perfectly placed for them to use their longest lift line

— a 30-meter, twisted strand, steel cable. They normally carried three lengths — 10, 20 and 30 meters.

All were confident in the situation. The power plant crew had done this before. The lift task, although a bit peculiar, was well within their capabilities, and the capacity of the Mi-26 helicopter.

The professional flight crew made an early night of it after they ate a light meal. They would rise at 05:00 to make the final preparations for the helicopter, so that they could lift the pump motor at about 08:00. The last few logistical coordination elements were completed with the plant crew prior to retiring.

# 3

*07:10, Friday, 11.April.1986*
*Chernobyl Nuclear Power Station*
*Pripyat, Ukraine, USSR*

The sun was just beginning to peek over the trees. The cool skin of the helicopter had condensed the moisture in the air to shroud the large machine in a sparkling coat. They all helped complete the preflight mechanical inspection to make sure the aircraft was ready for the day's work. One last time, they went over each step of the lift sequence including the signals for the fine movement of the load once it began to descend into the Pump Room of the Central Hall building. They were ready.

Gourgen had more experience with this aircraft type and this class of lift, however these jobs did not come along every day. Anatoly wanted the opportunity. They agreed to let Anatoly fly the mission. Gourgen would act as his copilot and spotter.

A young man came running out from the Party headquarters building. "Sitnikov wanted me to tell you everything is ready in the Central Hall."

"Thank you," answered Gourgen. "Let's get that chunk of steel in place."

They took their positions. Anatoly repositioned the helicopter. Several men including their crew chief were on the roof of Unit No. 4 Central Hall. They installed a four-cable harness to the panel, then attached a short, insulated lifting rod. The insulation would protect the crew chief from the high voltage charge built up in the helicopter and the instantaneous grounding that would occur when the lifting eye neared the hook. He had performed the hook-up task many times and was prepared for the loud report of vaporized air when the high energy, electric arc closed the distance between the hook and the cable eye.

The helicopter lifted the roof panel to the ground, not far from the pump motor still covered in a protective shroud, then Anatoly landed next to the new motor. Their loadmaster disembarked to hook up the load and ensure everything was ready for the lift. Their crew chief and now roof spotter waved from high above them on Unit No. 4 Central Hall.

"Everything set?" asked Anatoly as doors closed.

"Everything is ready, Anatoly Demjanovich. You are cleared to lift. I will be on the headset over the hook."

"Here we go."

Anatoly raised the collective, the lever in his left hand that increased the trust of the main rotor. The helicopter responded precisely to commands. He carefully positioned the aircraft over the load lifting the 30-meter cable until it was taut. He adjusted his position based on commands from the loadmaster to ensure the pump would not have any swing when it was lifted off the shipping pallet. The load came off cleanly. Anatoly directed the helicopter straight up until the load was above the roof of the Central Hall. The hole in the roof – their target – was clearly discernible, along with their crew chief standing back from the opening. As Anatoly gradually moved the helicopter and its suspended load toward their target, the roof spotter knelt down to brace himself against the high winds of the rotor downwash. As Anatoly tried to retrim the control forces, so he would not have to fight against the resistance forces in the stick, a couple of inadvertent control bumps jerked the aircraft slightly, but enough to cause the load to move beneath the aircraft.

"You have too much swing," called out the loadmaster.

Their crew chief stood up moving away from the roof opening, not wanting to be near the swinging motor.

"I need to put it down," Anatoly announced. He started to move the helicopter away from the building.

"Wait," said Gourgen. "Try partially lowering it onto the roof to stop the swing. If you don't let all the weight down, it looks like it will hold."

"It is six tons, Gourgen," called out the loadmaster. "It has momentum."

"Aaah, you are right."

"I am going to the ground."

By the time Anatoly moved away from the building and lowered the motor toward the ground, it was swinging several meters in an odd, figure eight pattern. As the heavy motor touched the ground, it dug a trench in the grass and started to tip over on its side.

Patiently, listening to instructions from the loadmaster looking through the hole in the belly down the cable to the motor, now at a precarious angle, Anatoly made minute corrections to steady the motor in an upright position. He took a few deep breaths to relax himself, and then started over again.

The motor came up steady as a rock. As they approached the roof opening with the suspended load, the crew chief lay on his belly with his head over the edge. He checked the interior to ensure they were ready to receive the motor. He then rolled over on his back. He stayed that way until the pump entered the hole.

Anatoly concentrated on his checkpoints on the exhaust tower and the adjacent building. Gourgen scanned the entire area to watch their position. The loadmaster's commands came over their headsets as he watched the cable for any telltale signs of trouble and their crew chief on his belly staring alternately down the opening in the roof and back to the helicopter above him. The hand and arm signals from the roof were translated into words by the loadmaster. Anatoly moved the aircraft precisely and smoothly.

"The load is inside the roof," announced the loadmaster.

The announcement was of vital significance. From this point until they released the load, many lives would, once again, be directly dependent of the actions of the pilot. His total maneuvering room was a rectangular space, two meters by four meters, and his final target spot was just 1.5 meters square. If either of the engines even coughed, he would have to use whatever energy he could pull up and try to yank the load clear. The normal option of pickling the load – just releasing it – was no longer available. Dropping the six-ton, electric motor, now inside the building, would undoubtedly collapse the receiving platform, sending several workers to their death, and substantially damaging important machinery and piping inside the building. Even more sobering, most of the pipes contained highly radioactive water under pressure as the reactor was still operating at full power.

Anatoly showed no signs of the added pressure. He focused on his checkpoints and made each control input smooth and deliberate. The aircraft remained rock steady.

"He is indicating we are close," said the loadmaster. "Slowly. Slowly. Hold it," he barked.

Anatoly responded to the command arresting the last of his descent rate. "How does everything look?" he asked as he kept his attention on his station keeping.

"Engines and systems are perfect," the flight engineer responded.

"Your position is good from my angle," said Gourgen.

"It appears they are securing the motor on the platform. Once they have it bolted down, they will release the cable."

They waited in their position for nearly 10 minutes as the workers anchored the motor. For those minutes, the big helicopter was essentially secured to the building. If an engine failed or any other serious problem developed, they would release the hook and cable to allow the aircraft to move away from the building. In that event, another option, landing on the roof, would not be a good idea. The massive, 35 metric ton, helicopter would crash through the roof like a stone through tissue paper.

"We are free."

"Remember to lift the cable straight up until we are clear," Gourgen reminded Anatoly.

"Thanks. I probably would have forgotten."

Anatoly manipulated the controls perfectly as the helicopter rose straight up until it passed the top of the exhaust stack, then he transitioned to forward flight. By prior arrangement, their crew chief would remain at the plant and make his way from the roof to meet them in the control room for their tour of the plant. Once clear of all the obstacles and stabilized in forward flight, Anatoly let go of the controls for the first time to move his joints.

"That's hard work," Anatoly said.

"Yes. It is. You can't blink, and you can't move. After a while, it starts to hurt."

"I think I was at that point. I guess we should land back at the village square."

"Sure. We asked for a plant tour, plus didn't you say you wanted to see your school friend?"

"Aleksandr Grigoryevich, sure. What time is it?"

"Nearly ten."

"It took us better than two hours for that lift."

"It was a bit unique with all that stuff around," said Gourgen.

They landed at the same spot they departed earlier. The shutdown was normal. The big machine had done its job. They worked together to inspect various important locations on the aircraft to make sure there was nothing abnormal beyond what the cockpit instruments could tell them.

A large automobile stopped abruptly, screeching its tires, in front of the Party headquarters building. The plant manager, Bryukhanov, jumped out of the car and nearly ran toward the aircraft. His face and eyes displayed the smile.

"Perfect," he shouted. "Absolutely perfect. You saved us many weeks."

"Glad we could help," answered Gourgen.

"The motor is secure on the platform. It will be installed later today. We have a very important test coming up in a few weeks. The new motor will return us to full pump capacity. You have saved us weeks," he repeated.

"Has Aleksandr Lelechenko been notified I am here?" asked Anatoly.

"Yes, yes. He should be here shortly. Is there anything we can do for you?"

"Just the tour and maybe some lunch, then we will be off,"

Gourgen answered. "We all want to get home. We have been away for two weeks."

"Lelechenko will take good care of you."

"Thank you."

"No, thank you. You have saved us much valuable time. Safe journey," Bryukhanov said, then turned and walked smartly to his waiting automobile.

They waited as if at attention until the door to his car closed behind him. The sun was an hour or so short of its zenith. The warmth transformed to hot. They entered the cargo bay, pulled out a couple of removable windows on the opposite side to allow the breeze to cool the interior. The pull-down, canvas, bench seats offered sufficient temptation for a short nap.

"Perhaps we should call your friend," said Gourgen.

"You are right. I shall go."

Anatoly was halfway to the Party headquarters building when a balding, confident man emerged from the woods. A smile grew on the man's face. Gourgen could imagine the smile returned from Anatoly. The two men embraced as brothers touching each cheek in the European style. They talked for several minutes before Anatoly motioned toward the helicopter. Gourgen stepped outside.

"Gourgen," Anatoly said as they approached. "This is my childhood friend, Aleksandr Grigoryevich Lelechenko. Aleksandr Grigoryevich, this is the world's best pilot, Gourgen Karapetyan."

"Hero of the Soviet Union," said Lelechenko as he shook Gourgen's hand.

"How did you know?"

"Your compatriot," he answered motioning to Anatoly, "is very proud of you. I feel like I know you."

"A pleasure to meet you."

Lelechenko nodded his head in recognition. "Are you ready for your tour?"

Anatoly introduced the remainder of the crew. They walked to the Party headquarters building. The flight crew waited outside while Lelechenko disappeared inside. As he returned, a small bus drove out from behind the building.

The scale of the plant struck all of them as they left the last trees behind the bus. The massive buildings looked much bigger on the ground than in the air. They seemed to go on forever – four fully operational reactor units, plus two more under construction. The buildings seemed almost too large. What could possibly be that big?

The bus stopped in front of a three-story portion of the complex that jutted out from the larger buildings. Two rows of windows marked the upper floors. They entered through a small side door, ascended two flights of stairs, and entered a door marked, CONTROL ROOM, UNIT NO. 4.

The enormous console stretched the length of the large, long, rectangular room. The overwhelming array of dials, instruments, lights and switches seemed to be endless. Men dressed in white laboratory coats with white, brimless caps stood or sat along the console. The wall in front of them contained a host of displays – the center was filled by a matrix of colored lights that looked like some gigantic game board. An almost anti-climactic set of tables and chairs were barely noticeable at the back of the room. The light green paint between the displays and covering the console support made the room appear more like a surgical suite than the control room of an electrical power plant.

Lelechenko led the small group to the back of the room. In a subdued voice, he began, "This is where it all happens. From this room, the operators can control every aspect of the plant's operation."

"There does not seem to be much actually happening," observed Anatoly.

"It may not seem like it, but we are running at full, normal rated, power . . . about 1,000 megawatts of electrical power while the reactor is running at 3,000 megawatts of thermal power."

"Is that good?"

"It is the best in the Soviet Union."

"So, how does this thing work?" asked Gourgen.

"Well, let me see if I can explain it. The array of lights in the middle represents the reactor itself. Each light is a control rod, the means by which the operators control the nuclear reaction in the pile and thus the heat output. The blue streams are the primary cooling loops. The ones on top are actually carrying the steam produced inside the reactor. The steam and water in those pipes is very hot and highly radioactive."

"Then, how do you replace the pump?"

"First, we are not replacing the pump, only the motor that drives the pump. The water line remains intact. If we had to replace a pump for some reason, we would have to shutdown the entire unit. There are no isolation valves as such, only a check valve to keep pressurized water from back-flowing when a pump is not in operation."

"What are those big round displays?"

"At the other end, you can see symbols for the drum separators. They separate any remaining water droplets from the steam that goes to turn the turbines that produce the electricity for the grid."

"I have heard that before," said Gourgen. "What is the grid?"

"In simple terms, the grid is a network of stations that interconnect all the generation plants, so that particular power plants can be taken off-line for maintenance. In fact, that is why the primary pump motor that you lifted in this morning is so important. Normally, we run with five or six primary pumps running for full power operations. We have a very special test to do in a few weeks that the engineers say all eight pumps are needed, just in case."

"Special test?"

"We have never done one of these before, so everyone is eager to see what happens. Our fuel stacks are nearly spent, so we need to shutdown anyway to replace the nuclear fuel. The test is rather important. The operators will reduce power first, then we shutoff electrical power to or from the grid to simulate a major electrical failure. The plan calls for us to use the momentum of a turbine wheel as it spins down to generate enough electrical power to keep a bank of the primary coolant pumps – four – on-line as well as power for the control room. The intent is to keep critical systems running until the emergency diesel generators can be brought up to full capacity . . . that takes about 50 seconds."

"Sounds important."

"That it is. There are several tricky parts, but it seems pretty straight forward."

"Can we see some of the plant?" asked Anatoly.

"Sure," Lelechenko said, then waved to one of the men who seemed to be in charge.

The plant's deputy electrician led the flight crew through a set of interior doors into a long wide corridor that extended both directions for probably a kilometer in total length. It was well lit in contrast to many hallways throughout the country and was most likely the main pathway inside the plant connecting all the units of the power plant. Lelechenko turned right leading the group down the shorter end of the long hallway. A hundred meters down the hall on the left side, a wide, metal, stairway rose through the ceiling to several platform levels. They ascended the stairs to the first level and entered the door.

They walked out onto a balcony overlooking a large hall. Machinery of various types lined all the walls. The center of the room was occupied by what appeared to be an enormous metal plate with criss-crossed deep ribs for reinforcement and blocks of black material in between the ribs. There were also four large lifting eyes. A heavy, overhead crane provided the lift capacity.

"What is the big plate?" asked Anatoly.

Lelechenko chuckled. "We call it, the five kopeck piece." They all laughed. The *pyatachok*, the Soviet five-kopeck coin, was the largest of their monetary coins. "It is more properly called, the biological cover. Beneath that plate is the reactor itself, well, actually 20 meters below the cover. We call it, the pile, since it has many blocks of carbon along with the fuel stacks themselves and the array of control rods needed to moderate the nuclear reaction. Once we shutdown the reactor and let it cool, that cover will be removed so the fuel can be replaced."

"How long have you been running on this fuel?"

"This batch . . . about five years. The fuel is supposed to last five to ten years, but we have been running at high power virtually the entire time. That is why we only got five years."

"Five years," laughed Gourgen. "If we had fuel to last five years, they would keep us flying for the entire time." Gourgen's entire crew laughed and added their quips.

"Where is our pump motor?" asked Anatoly using the possessive to identify the unit they lifted in this morning.

"In the left pump room," answered Lelechenko. He walked along the balcony to the left. They descended a half set of steps and entered through a small empty room with double doors opening out on both sides. It had to be a buffer room for fires or other emergencies that required isolation of one side or another.

When they entered the pump room, the metallic smell of steam and ozone from the electric motors along with a tinge of lubricating oil enveloped them. The loud whine of more than one pump assaulted their hearing. This was a place where machine work was done.

The most dominant feature was the tower of hefty scaffolding holding the new motor on a platform halfway to the ceiling. Another overhead crane was positioned over the motor and its lifting hook attached but not holding the motor's weight.

The other three primary coolant pumps were arrayed in a zigzag pattern. The massive pumps occupied the entire room. The large diameter pipes stretched from the reactor room through the array of pumps to what looked like an enormous boiler. A white shroud completely covered the space where the number three pump was and where the new motor would be installed.

Lelechenko shouted. "This is the left pump room. The right pump room is beyond the far wall. These pumps move the coolant water from the turbine condensers to the reactor." He swallowed hard to soothe his throat from the shouting. "Each pump moves 7,500 cubic meters of water per hour. When the reactor is running at full power, as it is now, six pumps are running — usually three in each pump room."

"That's a lot of water," responded Anatoly.

"Yes, it is."

"Those are the boilers?" Gourgen asked pointing toward two large drums mounted on the left wall.

"Those are the drum separators, I told you about in the control room, where any remaining water is removed to produce dry steam for the turbines. Even a small water droplet in the steam could be catastrophic to the high-speed turbine blades. The turbine could literally explode."

"Is steam produced in there like a boiler?"

"No. Steam is produced in the reactor and collected in those drums."

"What is the shroud for?" asked Anatoly pointing to the white covering in the middle of the room.

"It is to protect the workers from any radioactive water that might leak from that pump while the new motor is being installed. The old motor has already been removed and completely sealed."

"Doesn't this radioactivity worry you?"

"No, not really. We know how to protect ourselves," he answered. "Let us move through. It is too loud in here." Lelechenko led them again along the balcony walkway through another buffer room.

The largest of the rooms they visited was occupied by eight large turbine casings four on each side with a complex of pipes, valves, pumps and other equipment. A heavy hum filled the room. It was loud, but not as loud as the pump room.

"This is the Turbine Hall for Units Three and Four. Steam from the pump room powers these 250 megawatt electric generators," explained Lelechenko. "All eight turbines for both units are currently running at full capacity. These four," he said pointing to the set closest to them, "are part of Unit Number Four." He paused to let his audience absorb the scene. "We can also cross-connect them. Steam generated in Unit Four can be routed to any group of the turbines in this hall should the need arise."

"You can feel the power," Anatoly said.

"Yes, it is impressive. I have worked here since the beginning, and I am still amazed by the power of this place."

"How do you stand the noise?" asked Gourgen.

Lelechenko smiled. "I am practically deaf. Let's go outside." He led the way for the group. Back in the long hallway with the doors closed behind them, the noise levels were substantially lower. "It is very loud in there with all that machinery. I suppose you get used to it."

"Like the turbine engines on our helicopter," Gourgen added.

"And, the rotor noise."

"So, there is noise everywhere, but I do enjoy working here. It is a constant challenge keeping all this machinery running."

"Maybe you will get a short rest after your test while they are refueling your reactor."

"Yes, perhaps, but we could get real busy depending on how this test goes," answered Lelechenko.

"Everything will be perfect," added Anatoly.

"While we have had a few problems and a couple of minor accidents in the ten years I have worked here, we have never had any significant problems. Motors and switches fail, but they are quickly replaced. We always get the best stuff."

"Like a helicopter," Gourgen said.

"Yes, like your helicopter. The number three pump motor failed just last week. The new motor was here three days ago, and we requested a helicopter to lift it the next day. You received the tasking, and there you have it."

"That is pretty good."

"Like I said, we generally get the best equipment and support . . . one of the reasons it is so nice working here."

"And, close to home," Anatoly added.

Lelechenko smiled. "Yes, Tolya. I am close to our home. I live here in Pripyat now . . . it is much more convenient . . . and, I do go back occasionally, but not so much anymore now that my parents have died."

"It has probably been 15 years for me, so I am sure you have been back more than I have."

"Yes, but not by much."

Anatoly explained for his friends. "We hunted in this area and fished the Pripyat River. We never went hungry, did we Aleksandr?"

"No, we did not. This has always been bountiful country even in the hardest of times."

Gourgen knew he had to be referring to the trauma of the world war and the German occupation although none of them could remember that time. It was hard since many crops were burned to prevent them from falling into German hands, but the game and fish could still be found.

"We should be going, if we expect to make it back to Zhukovsky this afternoon," interjected Gourgen.

"Indeed, Gourgen. I think Galya is planning to have our usual Friday night event," said Anatoly. Gourgen nodded his head.

They walked back through the control room to ask a few last questions before they departed by the same path they had arrived. The crew went directly to the aircraft to prepare it for flight.

Gourgen spoke first. "Thank you for taking the time to show us the plant."

"You are most welcome."

"It was great to see you again, Aleksandr Grigoryevich. We need to do better keeping in touch with each other."

"Yes, we must. It is not often I get to see one of my schoolmates, and especially one who has been so successful."

"Nonsense. Look at this," he said sweeping his arm across the scene. "You live in this beautiful place and work on such important equipment. You are most fortunate."

Lelechenko nodded his head in recognition. "Come back and stay longer, Tolya."

The flight back to Zhukovsky, the Government's flight test center and locus of aviation research, took nearly five hours. They arrived late in the afternoon with the sun just barely above the horizon. They agreed to land at the main airfield instead of the Mil flight test facility north of the city. It was good to be home, and the extra 20-minute drive from the Mil test facility to Zhukovsky did not have much appeal.

# 4

*20:35, Friday, 11.April.1986*
*Building R4, Apartment 44*
*Zhukovsky, Russia, USSR*

"Milla, I'm home."

The usual inviting smells from the kitchen were missing. Normally, Ludmilla would have prepared their evening meal. The rich, earthy aroma of bread baking along with other spices she commonly used would offer a comforting welcome.

"In here, Gourgen," she answered from the bedroom.

Gourgen entered their bedroom to find his wife packing the last few items she needed into a small leather case. She turned from her task to embrace her husband. They touched each cheek then kissed in the simple, familiar manner of a couple that had been together for nearly 30 years.

Gourgen sat on the edge of the bed. "We have Friday night at the Grishchenko's."

"Not tonight. Dimitri wants to go to the *dacha*. He tells me Viktor Sergeiyevich Korolyov will be visiting his mother. They want to talk rockets and space."

"Where is Dimitri?"

"Outside probably pacing back and forth waiting for me."

"I did not see him."

She looked at him. "He is packed and ready. Are you going with us?"

"We left the aircraft here, so we could get home at some reasonable hour. I must move the machine north. They need to work on it tomorrow and Sunday. Plus, I told Tolya we would be there tonight."

"I cannot, Gourgen. I promised Dimitri. I was not sure if you would return today or not. I made arrangements. We will go out with Sergei and Natasha."

"Then, I will join you tomorrow at perhaps mid-day, after I move the aircraft."

Ludmilla finished the last of her packing, closed the top and latched both fasteners. Without words, she walked out of the bedroom leaving Gourgen to follow her.

In the kitchen, she removed a small container of sliced, cured meat from the small refrigerator. She began slicing several thick slabs of black bread from a half loaf. Gourgen was surprised to see a relatively fresh looking tomato so early in the year. He wondered where it came from, but did not ask. She prepared two sandwiches for him.

"How was your trip?"

"Interesting."

"You have done these before, Gourgen," she said as she placed the plate on the small kitchen table and sat across from him. "What was so interesting?"

Gourgen took two quick bites followed by some tea. "Last week and early this week we lifted a number of very large bridge sections into place. That was fairly routine." He took another bite of his sandwich, but this time he finished chewing and swallowing before he responded. "Wednesday, when we stopped at Kiev for fuel, I received a message. We were needed at a place called, Chernobyl, or actually Pripyat, north of Kiev and Chernobyl."

"Isn't that near where Tolya was born?"

"Yes, we met a childhood friend of his."

Ludmilla watched her husband eat and waited patiently for him to continue. It was dark, and she glanced out the window as if to check the lighting.

Gourgen swallowed, and then said, "We had to lift a very big motor for a water pump at the nuclear power plant." Her attention peaked. "We had to lift this thing, thread it through a small hole in the roof and place it on a raised platform inside the building."

"Nuclear power?"

"Yes."

"Isn't that radiation? Isn't that dangerous?"

Gourgen placed the last of his first sandwich on his plate and held up his hand. He swallowed his bite. "No, Milla. It is a power station. They produce electricity . . . quite a lot of electricity I might add."

Ludmilla stood and walked to the sink feigning attention to a few dishes already rinsed. "Yes, but they use nuclear engines to generate that power," she mumbled.

Gourgen considered whether to correct her terminology and more importantly whether to continue this particular line of discussion. He took a few more bites as he weighed his options. "Did Dimitri talk to Viktor Sergeiyevich?"

"Don't change the subject on me."

"Milla, I just wanted to know if Dimitri talked to Viktor."

"Yes, he talked to Viktor," she snapped with some irritation.

"What is Viktor Sergeiyevich doing now?"

"Gourgen," she protested.

"Milla, please."

"What his father did!" She returned to her task. When it became obvious there was nothing substantive left for her to do at the sink, she skulked out of the kitchen.

Gourgen finished his sandwich and cup of tea. He stared out the window at the falling veil of dusk diminishing the details of the other buildings beyond the window. He considered the thorns bothering Ludmilla. He had flown many missions of all types, some dangerous, some not so dangerous. Why was the mission at Chernobyl bothering her more than all the other higher risk missions he had flown?

Ludmilla was fussing with the clothes in her case, moving one item from one place to the next, than back again. Gourgen stood in the doorway for several cycles. Neither chose to acknowledge the other for several minutes.

"Milla, what's wrong? What's bothering you?"

She did not alter her pointless task. He had not seen her like this in many years, certainly not since he had flown that last series of structural limit demonstration flights on the new Mi-28 attack helicopter. The most recent mission was minor in comparison to other experimental flights. What was it she felt, she saw, she sensed, that made her so worried?

"Milla?"

She stopped, stood very still with her head down. He could not tell whether she was actually looking at anything in particular. He noticed the small contractions in her chest. A tear descended her cheek.

"Milla, what is bothering you?"

His wife turned defiantly toward him. Her cheeks were wet with tears. "You fly around the country, and you are perfectly happy. You are doing what you love to do. And, you have no idea what it does to me."

"Why is this different? We have been through this thousands of times. So, what is so different?"

"I heard from Galya that you two were at this radiation place. I did not understand it at first, not until you told me what they did there. It scares me, Gourgen."

"Tolya's school days friend has been working there for ten years and nothing has happened to him. They know how to run the plant. They have been doing it safely for years."

"It scares me," she said as she stomped her foot.

Gourgen waited for a few seconds to let the heat pass. "We only lifted a pump motor through the roof. It is done. We do not have to go back."

Ludmilla nodded her head, and then returned to fidgeting with her clothes. The knock at the door broke the moment. "That must be Natasha," she said, then closed the top and latched it. "You will join us tomorrow?"

"Yes, about mid-day, I expect."

"Say hello to Galya and Tolya, and the others. Enjoy your little Friday night party." Ludmilla kissed her husband.

Gourgen wrapped his arms around her and pulled her tightly to him. He kissed her more passionately, to leave her with a clear image of his feelings.

Ludmilla nodded her head in silent recognition, then left.

Gourgen took his flight overalls off, then the rest of his clothes. He drew a hot bath. Easing himself into the hot water, he soaked, letting the warmth relax every muscle and joint. Ludmilla's fear stuck with him like a massive spider web tangled all around him. He still wondered why this mission bothered her so much, why this task more than all the others? She was a very good, devoted woman, who had stood by him over the many years of difficult times, distractions and mistakes. She had long since accepted his avocation. There was something else, but what?

The water cooled. He washed quickly before the water became cold, to remove the last residue of sweat, oil and kerosene fuel from the day's mission.

He dressed in a slow, meandering manner still troubled by Ludmilla's apprehension, or was it something more? The clock on the wall told him he was nearly an hour late for the Grishchenko's. Everyone would be there, and they would most likely give him a hard time for being late. The walk in the early evening air felt good. The Grishchenko's lived in a first level apartment, three buildings south of them. Kids played under the lights. This was a happy place, but he longed for the pine scent of their *dacha*. Tomorrow.

# 5

"Good evening to you, Galya," Gourgen said as Anatoly's wife, Galina, opened the door to their apartment in Zhukovsky.

"And, good evening to you, Gourgen. Where is Milla?" she asked.

"She needed to get away. She promised to take Dimitri to the *dacha*. Viktor Sergeiyevich Korolyov is apparently at his parent's place. They left with Sergei and Natasha. I will join them tomorrow afternoon. Are the others here?"

"Not yet. Everyone is late tonight."

"Good, then there shall be no grief for me."

"So, since you have nothing else to do, you came to the party," she chuckled.

"Yes, yes. You caught me," answered Gourgen as he kissed each cheek, and then mustered up a serious expression. "Galya, what did you tell Milla?"

"What do you mean?"

"When I told her where Tolya and I had been, she started to cry. She was very upset about something."

Galina looked into his eyes several seconds before she answered. "I know what goes on there."

"What?"

"Nuclear stuff."

"Yes, but it is safe."

"So they say."

"Now, she is very worried. I have never seen her like this."

She searched his eyes again. "I will make it right with her when you return Sunday night."

"I would appreciate it. It is over and done. No need to worry."

"As you say then."

Gourgen turned his head as if to look for his friend through the wall. "Where is Tolya?"

"In the living room with Boris and Nicholas." Gourgen started to leave, but Galina touched his shoulder to stop him. "Gourgen," she said softly, "let me tell you why Milla is so upset." She paused for a nod of his head and assured attention. "Just last week, more stories of very sick people and even fatalities among nuclear workers have circulated among the wives. We are all thankful that our husbands are not in that industry. One of the wives has a brother who is suffering miserably as he dies, and the Government will not even acknowledge his injury."

"What happened?" interrupted Gourgen.

"He was exposed to that nuclear material somehow. I think she said some sort of accidental spill of something or other."

"An accident, Galya. There was no accident at Chernobyl."

"As you say, but that does not lessen the worries all of us have when we hear about this nuclear stuff . . . things we cannot see, or touch, or smell. Things that will kill you."

"This place was clean and modern. The workers were all very healthy. That power plant was a well run electricity generation facility."

"Just try to understand what is on Milla's mind. Comfort her."

"Good advice, I should think."

"Yes, now go find Tolya and the boys."

Gourgen walked down the short hallway past the kitchen and made an even shorter right turn past two small bedrooms. The two boys sat in chairs listening to their father. They all looked up.

"Uncle Gourgen," shouted Nicholas as he jumped up, and then embraced the man they always thought of as their uncle although they were not related.

"Good to see you, Nicholas Anatolyevich. How is school?"

"Tolerable," the teenager said causing a flurry of laughter. He looked around quickly wondering why everyone was laughing, and then joined them. "I do what I must to get to flight school."

"Good for you. And, how are you, Boris?"

The older brother was nearly as tall as his father and in his last year of his university education. He would soon graduate and enter the Air Force as a communications officer.

"Quite well, Uncle Gourgen. Thank you."

"Good."

The knock at the door and Galina's greetings announced the new arrivals. Anatoly Kovatchur, their friend, neighbor and fellow test pilot, entered the room effervescent as ever, along with several other pilots and a couple of the wives. Anatoly had been a successful fighter pilot in the Air Force, fought in Afghanistan, watched friends return home in coffins, and then became a test pilot for Mikoyan-Gurevich. He was five years younger than Gourgen and Anatoly Demjanovich, and still had not found the right woman to marry.

"Now, we are one big happy family," bellowed Anatoly. The strong, medium built man shook everyone's hand in the Western style.

Galina and the other women brought platters of small sandwiches. As was usually the case with the pilots, there were also glasses of orange juice and bottled water, no vodka or other alcoholic beverages, since most of them had to fly the next day. They ate sandwiches with laughter, and talk of children and school with aircraft and flying liberally mixed in the topics. The group always enjoyed the camaraderie of true friends.

"So, Tolya," said Anatoly in his strong voice, "Gourgen tells me you are now a heavy lift expert."

"Gourgen exaggerates."

"Now, now, no need to be modest."

"It was just a rather large electric motor for one of their coolant pumps."

"Six metric tons," bellowed Kovatchur. "I should say, large. So, tell us about your experience."

"This story is not as good as your night missions in the mountains of Afghanistan," said Grishchenko.

"Nonsense. Being strapped to a building with no place to go is not exactly a cakewalk now is it. So, get on with the story. We are all waiting to hear about it."

"Come on, father," said Nicholas, "we do want to hear about this."

"All right." He took a drink of water. "After we completed the bridge repair task south of Kiev, we were asked to lift this heavy motor at the Chernobyl Nuclear Power Plant. The electric plant is quite close to my childhood home . . . before I went to the university. They wanted us to lift this motor and drop it through a hole in the roof. Because of the nature of the lift, we used a 30-meter cable to hook it to the helicopter. The actual flying had to be very precise."

"The rotor blade tips were within about 7 meters of the building," interjected Gourgen. "It does not take much error for the blades to impact the steel. If that had happened, it would have been a real mess."

"How big was the hole?" Boris asked.

"About two meters by four meters," answered Anatoly.

"So, let me see, now," Kovatchur said. "You have this six ton, pump motor dangling 30 meters beneath the aircraft, and you must place it into a two by four meter hole."

"Yes."

"Incredible."

"It was not just me. It takes a team. The Mil Two Six has an engineer watching the engines and systems, a navigator who handles communications, of course, Gourgen and me. He let me fly this one." Everyone laughed. "He takes this bridge section in the wide open spaces, and gives me this thing."

"You said you wanted to gain more experience with long line lifts, so there you have it."

"It was like threading a needle, holding the thread several centimeters away, and . . .," he paused for the laughter, "and, you must do it blind with someone else giving you directions."

"Impressive."

"Who was giving directions?"

"We had our crew chief on the roof of the building looking down into the hole and back up to us. The loadmaster was lying on his belly in the cargo compartment looking down through a hole near the hook. He could see the motor plus see the hand signals from our roof spotter."

"As you know," added Gourgen, "the Mil Two Six is a rather large aircraft. In the cockpit, we sit about ten meters in front of the hook. There is no way for us to see the load."

"And, you dropped this motor into the building?"

"They built a platform about halfway to the interior ceiling. We had to place the motor on the platform."

"Inside the building?" Kovatchur asked with incredulity.

"How big was this platform?" asked one of the other pilots.

"One point five meters square," answered Gourgen.

"So, now, let me see," Kovatchur paused moving his hands to emphasize the relationships, "you have to place this six-ton motor on a one point five meter square platform inside a building with a two by four meter hole in the roof using a thirty meter cable ten meters behind you, and all of this you cannot see."

"Yes," Tolya responded. "Even at that, our wheels were within a few meters of the roof when we finally reached the platform."

"Why the platform? Why not just drop it in place?"

"I guess they wanted to use their overhead crane for the fine placement installation."

"Plus, we would have needed a 60 or 70 meter cable which would have made the threading the needle task substantially more difficult," Gourgen added.

"What about the radiation from the reactor?" asked Galina with some apprehension.

"Radiation is scary stuff."

"Well," said Tolya pausing to consider his words, "my childhood schoolmate, Aleksandr Lelechenko, has worked at that plant for ten years, and he is healthy as can be. We were only there for a day. He said it was perfectly safe."

"Did you get to see it?" asked Nicholas. Anatoly nodded his

head. "What did it look like?"

"Like a big, steel and concrete building with a massive steel plate in the middle of the floor."

"You could see the reactor . . . glowing perhaps?"

"No. We could only see a lot of machinery, pumps, motors, valves, pipes and turbines."

"The entire plant is huge," Gourgen said. "There are four, fully functioning, reactors at the plant."

"I have never understood how they make electricity from a nuclear bomb contained in some building," Galina said.

"First, it is not a bomb. It cannot explode," began Tolya. "The way Aleksandr Grigoryevich explained it to us, the nuclear fuel heats up and boils the water circulated through it to form steam. The steam is bled off to turn the big turbines that produce electricity in kind of the reverse process of a motor."

"What if something goes wrong?" asked Galina.

"Aleksandr Grigoryevich said they have many safety systems. He said they have safety systems for the safety systems."

Everyone laughed. The pilots were satisfied, but the women were not.

"If it is so safe, why do they need all the safety systems?"

The room fell silent. The women looked at Anatoly Demjanovich. The men looked at their feet except for Anatoly who held his wife's eyes. Everyone now recognized the seriousness of Galina's question. She was worried about her husband. All this science and technology did not make her happy. She had never been comfortable about things she did not understand. Galina worried about her husband every day he had to fly. She tolerated aircraft, but she had never accepted them as objects of safety.

"Galya, the plant is a complex of machinery. The operators cannot see into the reactor. They need instruments to know what is happening, much like we must have instruments to tell us what is happening inside our engines."

"We do not need instruments to see if the fire is right for cooking. We do not need instruments to know if we are hot or cold. Why do we need these things that we cannot see or feel? Why do we need to make life so complicated?"

"Electricity, Galya. You grew up in the same conditions I did. We did not have running water or any electricity. My parents never accepted electricity."

"Perhaps, they were right."

"Galina, we are all better off with electricity, running water, aircraft, automobiles, and yes, even nuclear-powered, electricity plants."

"Maybe, but why do we need nuclear power? I can boil water to make steam. I don't need all this atomic stuff we cannot see, and we cannot control without more fancy systems that no one understands."

Gourgen recognized the tone. Galina and Ludmilla had shared their concerns. He would let Anatoly handle this one, and he wanted to hear the outcome. Perhaps, it would prepare him better for further discussion with his wife in the country tomorrow.

"All we did was lift a motor," Anatoly said finally in frustration.

The men chuckled without looking the women in the eyes. Galina was the first to get up. The other wives followed her. All the men including Boris and Nicholas stared at the hallway through which the women had disappeared. They looked at one another.

"Well," said Kovatchur, "I guess Galya is not a lover of complex things."

"It worries her as I am sure it does the other wives. They worry about us. They see the cemetery between us and the airfield continuing to fill up with lost comrades. So, yes, she does not like the things we do."

"Don't you worry about something going wrong?"

"No, Nicholas. None of us do. If we worried about what might go wrong, we would probably never fly or get out of bed in the morning."

"Life has risks," added Gourgen. "Life would not be much worth living without risks. We work hard to understand those risks and control the conditions that affect them."

"Mother still worries," Nicholas said. "We listen to her sobbing sometimes in the night when you are on some particularly dangerous mission. We worry about you."

"Thank you, son. All of us know life is not easy. Flying adds a certain, seductive spice to life. It is just something we love to do. Each of us," Tolya said waving his arm at the assembled pilots, "is good at what we do. There is no one better in the world. We are proud of what we do for our country, and yes, there are risks."

"So, why couldn't they get the motor in by themselves?" asked Kovatchur.

The group laughed hard, ate the remaining sandwiches and refreshed their drinks.

"Ah, they worry a lot," Anatoly said.

"No. I want to hear the answer to my question."

"As you say then, so they told us, it would have taken them several weeks to manhandle the motor into place. We did it in two hours. They have some big test coming up toward the end of the month, and they needed the motor replaced, installed and qualified in order to accomplish their test."

"Why did you want to do this assignment, Tolya?"

"There are some flight tests coming up that I felt I would be more prepared for if I had some operational experience of a similar nature."

"Sounds reasonable."

"What are you working on?" asked Gourgen of Anatoly Kovatchur.

"We are doing some performance enhancements to the MiG-29. The Sukhoi boys have managed to successfully test vectored-thrust nozzles for the Su-27, and the Air Force is pushing Mikoyan-Gurevich for more maneuverability."

"Sounds like fun."

"Hard work."

"Oh sure, you come back from those flights with a smile on your face. It cannot be that bad."

"Sure, and my flight suit is soaking wet."

"From wetting yourself."

The group laughed hard, again. They loved to poke fun at one another.

"From sweat, you idiot. Like I said, I work hard up there."

"You ought to try something like that Chernobyl task," said Grishchenko.

Anatoly chuckled. "You are right, Tolya. I really should try it. You have not invited me to fly with you for quite some time."

"We will have to find an appropriate mission for our good friend," said Gourgen. "Won't we, Tolya."

"Most definitely. He is getting too cocky with his noise maker and its big afterburners."

"I have had enough," Kovatchur said and stood up to leave. "I must fly tomorrow."

The others followed suit. They thanked Galina and Anatoly for their usual hospitality. They also gave Boris and Nicholas a slap on the back and a vote of confidence.

Gourgen was the last to leave and gave Galina a big hug. He whispered to her, "Your husband is an exceptional pilot, Galya. He will always do the best he can. No need to worry."

Galina pulled back from him. "Thank you, Gourgen. You are a good friend, but I still worry."

# 6

*12:45, Saturday, 12.April.1986*
*40 kilometers west of Moscow, Russia, USSR*

The sunny, warm spring day and the sun's zenith made traffic scarce. Everyone going to the country had already arrived. The last 30 minutes of the journey made Gourgen's open windows an actual pleasure. The dominant scent of pine trees carried the rich earthy aromas along with short bursts of other forest fragrances. A brown, light wool jacket was the only addition to his cotton, summer, slacks and shirt he wore. Gourgen could feel the coolness of the wind on his ears and cheeks, but he still felt warm. The spots of sunlight gave him small eruptions of radiant heat.

The repositioning flight of the big Mi-26 from the main airfield at Zhukovsky to the Mil Flight Test Facility to the north had been routine. A short test flight on the Mi-28 had gone equally as well. All the test objectives had been met, and the flight was completed ahead of schedule. It was not the day's flights that occupied his thoughts most of the way to their cottage. It was last night's argument with Ludmilla.

The shadows of the overhanging branches offered minute cool blasts that amplified the smells. The presence of the forest kept Ludmilla's worries at an appropriate distance, but never too far from his consciousness.

The high, black, wrought iron fence along the right side of the road with its ornate gate marked the estate of Mikhail Sergeiyevich Gorbachev. As he always did when he passed this stretch of road, he looked through the fence and openings between the trees, across the broad meadow to the far treeline, hoping the catch a glimpse of how the high and mighty lived. This attempt ended, as all the others did — nothing. The thicket of trees indicated the end of Gorbachev's property.

Gourgen entered a dense portion of the forest, a little over one kilometer, where the narrow, two lane roadway tunneled through the mass of green. The darkness at mid-day brought an urge to turn on his headlights. On the other side of the forest tunnel, a large meadow along the banks of the Moscow River on the right side of the road opened up to illuminate the row of cottages on the opposite side. The mixture of modest picket fences, manicured shrubbery and a rainbow of blossoms identified the small, informal community where Gourgen's family along with many others spent the weekends and holidays.

Turning off the asphalt onto a one lane, dirt road, Gourgen worked his way through the three rows of square plots and tiny homes to a meandering tire path like some well-disciplined column of cows wearing the grass thin in perfect parallel lines. The two-story *dacha* that his family called home appeared in a thinning of the trees. He pulled off the path into a little cubbyhole cut and worn into the vegetation just for his automobile.

As he passed the thigh high, narrow, white picket fence into the yard, Ludmilla came out carrying a large pan of water that she spread into the flower garden.

"You made it," she said looking away from him.

"Yes. It was a very pleasant drive."

"Good."

Gourgen looked around to take a quick inventory of those present. "Where is Dimitri?"

"With Viktor Sergeiyevich," she answered as she passed him back into the house without a kiss or even connecting with his eyes.

Ludmilla's mood broadcast a preview. He could expect perhaps a greater dose if his mother was here. Sasha Petrovna identified more closely with Ludmilla than she did with her own son. On sunny spring days, she usually took long walks through the forest ignoring the pleas of her eldest son to recognize her 75 years. Maybe Ludmilla had not had time to pump her up. The short steps and light footfalls coming toward the front door told him he was not so lucky. Gourgen sat down at the large, heavy wood table in the middle of the yard.

"Sonny," she said as she advanced toward him, "why are you doing this to Milla?"

He looked up at her while her eyes remained down as she watched each step as if she needed to avoid placing her foot on something. "What, Momma?"

"You know what! Do not play ignorant with me."

He knew precisely what the topic was. "Momma, it was a simple mission. We lifted a motor into a building. I have done flights like that hundreds of times."

"Not the flying, Sonny. I do not mind so much as Milla does. What of these invisible rays, or some such?"

"Milla worries too much," he said dismissing her question. Gourgen stood and walked toward the house. "I am going to take a nap. It has been a hard week."

"You do not walk away from your mother."

Gourgen stopped halfway to the small alcove of a porch serving as their entryway to the front door. He hesitated wondering whether he should really get into this. He could never win an argument with his mother. Resistance faltered. "Yes," he said turning around to face her.

"See, Milla is right. How often do you take a nap? Rarely, I tell you. Something is wrong. Those rays did something to you."

"Momma, please. Ludmilla is not correct. There was no danger. We were there for an afternoon and a morning. There are people who have worked there and lived there for ten years or more. There are children playing in the streets. They are not in danger."

"Milla is still worried, so I am worried."

"There is no need to worry, Momma. I am fine. I just want to take a short rest to relax."

"Maybe so, Gourgen. Maybe so. But, I think you need to reassure Milla. Maybe you need to make love to your wife."

"Mother, please!" he protested although the suggestion was quite appealing to him.

"Just trying to help."

"Thank you. Now, may I go take a nap?"

Sasha Petrovna waved her hand, palm down, as if she was shooing a fly from the butter.

Gourgen walked into the house. The smell of freshly baked bread warmed the darkened interior. He found Ludmilla kneading another clump of bread dough. He wrapped his arms around her, pressed himself against her backside, and cupped her soft, full, left breast in his right hand. She did not respond to his embrace and continued with her task. Gourgen kissed her on the cheek. Through her thin smock and apron, he could feel her nipple rise to his touch, but she made no effort to recognize his attention. Gourgen kissed her again and whispered in her ear. "I am going to take a nap."

Ludmilla nodded her head to acknowledge his announcement, but nothing else.

He climbed the narrow L-shaped stairway to the second floor. Four bedrooms, twice as many as their apartment in Zhukovsky, filled the second floor. On one end was his parent's room that now only his mother used. On the opposite end was a slightly smaller room that barely allowed a double bed for Ludmilla and him. The two bedrooms in the middle served as a small dormitory for children or guests. When all the children came, even the living room filled with sleeping family. The construction of a large, sitting room would add some more sleeping room, but that would take most of the summer to complete.

Gourgen did not bother undressing nor getting under the covers. He lay spread-eagled on the bed and instantly passed into sleep.

Voices and laughter from the yard woke him. He checked his watch. He had slept for three hours. He crossed his legs and placed his hands behind his head as he listened to the chatter outside. He could easily recognize Dimitri and Viktor Sergeiyevich Korolyov, and two small children who had to be Andrei and Ivan, which meant at least Sergei, the eldest of their four children, and Ivana, his wife of four years, were here. A few admonishments to the two small boys re-established his mother's presence. He smiled as he listened. He could not tell whether either of their two daughters, Natasha or Galina, made it to the family *dacha* for the weekend. He would know soon enough. At the moment, he was perfectly content to absorb the family from the blissful comfort of his bed.

Gourgen rose from the bed, poured some water in the washbasin, and rubbed his wet hands on his face several times. After drying his hands and face, he joined the family. Everyone was as he had heard them. To his surprise, Galina, their youngest daughter, sat quietly beside her mother. Natasha was the only one missing.

"There is Grandpa," shouted Andrei.

The two grandsons ran to Gourgen. He scooped them both up, one in each arm, and kissed them both on the cheeks. The boys reciprocated as they nearly choked him.

"Did you have a good nap, Father?" asked Dimitri.

"Yes, I did, and I needed it too."

"Tough week?" asked Sergei.

Gourgen glanced at Ludmilla, who simply stared back at him. This appeared like it was one of her more defiant moods. He left her piercing eyes for the inquisitive expression of his eldest son. "Not really . . . just long."

"So he says," muttered Ludmilla.

Sergei glanced over his shoulder to see his mother's eyes. She met his eyes, and then returned to Gourgen.

"Why is Mother so worried?"

"Anatoly Demjanovich and I flew a heavy lift mission at the Chernobyl Nuclear Power Plant, north of Kiev. It was a huge motor for one of their coolant water pumps. We had to lower it through a hole in the roof."

"That doesn't sound bad," Sergei said glancing at his mother again.

"Your mother worries about the radiation. The wives have been talking about nuclear accidents and the injuries."

"Was there any?"

"No. It was perfectly safe."

Sergei turned to Ludmilla. "If he was exposed to radiation, he would be very sick right now. So, father is probably correct."

"Maybe it wasn't enough to make him sick. Suppose it was enough to make him sick later."

"Milla, there are hundreds of people who have worked there for ten years, and they are not sick."

"There you have it," Sergei said. "Now, let us talk about something else."

Ludmilla shook her head, stood and stared at Gourgen, then Sergei, and walked into the house. Natasha followed her mother. Ivana looked around at the males, and then rose to join the other women.

"So, Viktor, how do you like the Space Institute?" asked Sergei.

"It is fantastic. I now understand why my father liked rocketry so much."

"How is your mother?"

"She is just fine and feisty as ever."

"Excellent. Is she out here this weekend?"

"She and grandmother live out here, now." The ability to live in the country was a true sign of the rewards the Government heaped upon the family of Sergei Korolyov, considered the father of the Soviet space program. "These days, they only use the apartment in the city when they need to be in Moscow."

"Viktor says I should go to the Institute as well," announced Dimitri.

"Perhaps you should," Sergei answered. "What does father say?"

Dimitri looked at this father, who returned a neutral expression.

"We have not talked about it, yet. But, I know he will support it."

Ludmilla, Natasha and Ivana began bringing food out from the kitchen. The boys rose to help. In just a few minutes, the table was full. They had pickled herring, boiled eggs, two types of bread, sliced tomatoes, boiled potatoes, and a large pitcher of orange juice and several bottles of water.

Viktor Sergeiyevich said, "I shall be going."

"Please stay, Viktor," answered Ludmilla.

"Yes, please do," added Dimitri.

"No. My mother is probably expecting me. I shall see you later."

"Oh, Viktor. We can tell her you are staying."

"No. I really should be going."

As Viktor disappeared into the shrubbery and the family said good-bye to him, they sat down. Gourgen, as the patriarch of the family after his father's passing several years earlier, sat at the head of the table. Ludmilla sat to his right, and Sasha to his left. Alexei and Ivan sat between Sergei and Ivana.

They talked about school, about current events at work, about the beautiful weather and about a swim in the still cold Moscow River. They laughed as they talked and ate. Even Ludmilla began to laugh. Gourgen felt better when he saw her laugh, and the sparkle returned to her eyes. The family made life worth living.

They enjoyed the spring afternoon and the sharing common to their family. Each of them found pleasure in the lives of the generations — parents, siblings and children.

As the women cleared the dishes, Dimitri decided he wanted to do something else. "Father, come with me to the Korolyov's. Viktor Sergeiyevich said he has photographs of the work they are doing on the new *Energia* booster for the *Buran* re-entry vehicle."

"I have seen pictures, Dimitri."

"But, he is working on the rocket motors just like his father. I want to do what he does. I want you to see them."

Gourgen sensed more in his youngest son's request. "All right."

Dimitri led his father along the narrow path and through the fence that once sealed the *dacha* of the famous leader of the Soviet space program. The Korolyov family lived next to the Karapetyan family since World War II. When Sergei Korolyov was alive, the security around him made informal, casual visits virtually impossible.

Gourgen had known Korolyov was someone very important, but for nearly two decades, he knew nothing of what the renowned man did to become so important. Any reference to him was simply,

The Chief Designer, which to Gourgen meant he was an engineer and leader of some design bureau, and yet despite many private but risky inquiries, he never did find out what the short round man did for the State. It was not until the year prior to his death in 1966 that Gourgen learned he was the founder of the Soviet space program, the designer and builder of the most powerful rockets in the world at the time, and a man so important to the State that he was forced to live in anonymity. The security continued until his two boys went off to the university to begin their careers and families. His oldest son, Nikolai, had been killed in an airline crash several years after his father's death. Viktor carried on his father's work. Once the security surrounding Sergei Korolyov faded, the two families developed a closer relationship.

The Korolyov *dacha* was roughly twice the size of the Karapetyan cottage complete with indoor plumbing, and a gas line for heating and cooking. Dimitri walked confidently up the half dozen steps, across the porch, to the front door, and knocked. Viktor answered the door.

"Is this a bad time?" asked Gourgen, two steps behind his son.

"No. We just finished. Come in," he said standing back and opening the door wider.

"I want my father to see your photographs," Dimitri said.

"Sure."

Viktor was 15 years older than Dimitri, but did not seem to mind indulging the teenager's curiosity about rocketry, space and the future. Gourgen paid their respects to the matriarch before they went to the study. The rich woods of the floor, the walls, the desk and chairs marked the room of a powerful man. The walls were completely covered with shelves of books or photographs that could serve as a chronicle of the Soviet space program. Gourgen always marveled at the accomplishments when he entered The Chief Designer's study. The good thing in all of this success was Viktor did not appear to be intimidated by his father's fame.

The three men poured over the impressive photographs of Soviet space launch vehicles, large rocket engines, the Soviet version of a space shuttle and other significant engineering work. Gourgen was as much impressed by the depictions of vital national systems, as he was the existence of such detailed photographs outside some secure building or complex.

Dimitri's incessant questions and Viktor's patient answers convinced Gourgen of his son's avocation. They talked of the university. Viktor offered, without a request, to help get Dimitri an interview for entry into the Space Institute, the country's and the program's internal university and engineering complex. He would have to stand on his own merits and potential.

After an hour of discussion and bidding their good-byes, father and son made their way back to their *dacha*.

At the fence, Dimitri stopped and turned to face his father. "Do you see why I want to join the space program?" he asked.

"Yes, son. Your desire is clearly apparent. You must prepare yourself for this interview. You must also recognize that you may not have what they want. Just because you know Viktor Korolyov does not guarantee you anything."

"Yes, but my father is famous too . . . a decorated Hero of the Soviet Union."

"In aviation."

"It does not matter."

"Perhaps."

"Will you help me, too, father?"

"Of course, Dimitri. I will do whatever I can to help you achieve your dream."

"Excellent. Then, I shall have no problems."

Dimitri turned and continued along the narrow path as Gourgen started to offer more words of caution and reserve, but did not want to say them to his son's back. Their youngest son was plainly effervescent for the remainder of the weekend. His excitement made everyone feel better, including Ludmilla. Gourgen was thankful for his son's excitement and the relief from Ludmilla's dire mood. They returned to Zhukovsky Sunday evening.

# 7

*14:15, Friday, 25.April.1986*
*Mil Flight Test Facility*
*30 kilometers north of Zhukovsky, Russia, USSR*

The day had gone exceptionally well for Gourgen. The team managed two very productive development flights on the Mi-28. Even the engineers from the Moscow design office had been pleased. The past hour spanned an energetic and enthusiastic discussion about the next series of flights to be flown on the prototype advanced attack helicopter. The mechanical and aerodynamic elements of the machine were maturing well. It was the fancy new electronics the Government wanted that had been giving them fits. This day was different. Everything worked perfectly. Gourgen told himself many times during the planning session, they only needed a good string of days like this day and they would be ready for the Government testing.

"Gourgen," called one of the flight test engineers, "telephone."

Gourgen finished his discussion about a pending test, and then walked into the next room. "Karapetyan," he said.

"Gourgen, this is Tolya."

"So, what can I help you with, my friend?"

"I completed a preparation flight this morning on that new test rig I have been telling you about. Can you come down this afternoon and fly it with me? I would like you to try it."

"Can you hang on? I will check with the engineers. I think we are complete for the day, but I need to check with them."

"Sure."

Gourgen placed the handset on the wooden desk and entered the engineer's room. He asked several of the permanent staff. The answer was the same. He returned to the telephone. "Looks like I am done for the day, well, actually for the weekend, so I can be down there in about an hour."

"That will just about be right. They are turning the aircraft now. It will probably not be ready until two or three, anyway."

"I will close up here and join you shortly."

Although he had no more flights for the day, he had planned to go to the main engineering offices in the city.. He made several calls to change his planned informal meetings with various engineers, then said good-bye to his colleagues, wishing them a good weekend. He found his aging, white, Zhiguli sedan among the line of other similar automobiles, and placed his flight equipment bag in the rear seat. Gourgen stopped at the gate to allow the guards extra time to open the security barriers, then exchanged a few kind words with the two, long-time Interior Ministry guards who manned the gate.

Traffic was unusually heavy on the main north-south highway for the mid-day hour. He waited for a break, pulled across the northbound lanes onto the median, then waited another minute or so for another break to turn left into the outside, southbound lane. The tail of a spring storm had passed an hour earlier. The sun's warmth brought a veil of steam to the asphalt highway. The moist, earthy wetness offered an aroma of freshness and renewal. The new, green array among the trees confirmed Gourgen's favorite season. He did not drive fast. In fact, most of the traffic passed him with ease. He was perfectly content to enjoy the country scenery, the smell of spring, and the pleasant, speed-induced breeze circulating through the car's interior.

The next major area of inhabitation was the aviation community of Zhukovsky and the massive Ramskoye Aerodrome – like a combination of both American flight test facilities at Edwards and Patuxent River. All the aircraft design bureaus – the big guys, Antonov, Tupolev and Ilyushin; the fighter groups, Sukoi and Mikoyan-Gurevich; and the helicopter designers, Kamov and Mil – had hangars and flight test facilities at the large government flight test center. Mil and Kamov had their main flight facility north of the city, just outside the perimeter highway, and only used Ramskoye when there were specific government evaluations to be conducted. The community also provided a home to the Gromov Flight Research Center, the Soviet counterpart to the American's National Aeronautics and Space Administration, at least the aeronautical part; and TsAGI, simply, the Central Aerohydrodynamic Institute, with its myriad of wind tunnels, computers, water tanks, and other paraphernalia of aerodynamic research. The entire aviation community was named for Academician Nikolai Egorovich Zhukovsky, who founded TsAGI in 1918 and was known as the father of Soviet aerodynamic research and many say the father of Soviet aviation.

Gourgen passed through the primary residential area on the north side of the city with its dozen or so apartment towers and the principal buildings of the flight test center to the main road intersection that was actually a 'T' juncture. To the right was the large TsAGI complex, and on the left, at the northeast corner, was the Gromov establishment. He turned left, driving down the length of the Gromov facility to find a parking spot. Gourgen retrieved his flight equipment bag from the back seat of his car, then walked the 60 meters to the closest building.

The guard at the pilot's entrance gate did not recognize him, forcing Gourgen to pull out his government identification card. He worked his way through the dark halls, past the various offices and laboratories, to the pilot's office. Greetings flew as he weaved his way to Anatoly's desk.

"So, you have a new toy?" he said as he approached.

Anatoly motioned toward the chair beside his desk. "I think you will like this thing. We have been working on the equipment and test procedures for what the West calls, tethered hover testing. In essence, they attach you to the earth by a massive cable. A special load cell, that measures tension, is placed at the bottom of the cable and electrically connected to the test equipment. They change the cable length to establish your hover height, and then you pull on that cable like you are trying to lift the earth. They record the force generated, do some calculations, and then they tell you how much power you produced. A quick precise way to determine hover performance – lift capacity. Pretty slick, huh?"

"Ever since you brought that up, I have thought about it. I suspect the equipment might have many uses, not just for testing."

"I suppose, but that is not what we are trying to do here."

"No. I understand. I have just been thinking."

"Well, it works, and I wanted you to try it before we do the certification testing."

Gourgen held the eyes of his friend as he thought about the mechanics of using the test rig. "What about alignment? If the angle is not precisely vertical and remains that way, the load values will be less due to the angular component of the lift vector."

Anatoly smiled broadly. "Precisely. So, we developed a series of potentiometers in a fixture that is attached around the hook that determines the cable angle quite accurately. The signals go to an indicator in the cockpit with a set of crosshairs for the pilot to keep centered." He waved his hands like a magician. "There you have it – precision hover position. The ground guys also watch those angles so they can back calculate any corrections to the data."

"Hey, I am impressed."

"I thought you would be. As you say, there are potentially other uses for this stuff."

"I can see a few."

"Let's go fly," Anatoly said with the excitement of a child with a new toy. He placed one telephone call, undoubtedly to the flight line, and established that the aircraft was ready. "They are waiting on us. We will use this as another test condition."

They walked through the building toward the aircraft hangar. "What aircraft?" asked Gourgen.

"For this, we are using a Mil One Seven – more power."

"That should work."

"We have just one load cell, well, just one type – we have several spares – for the moment. We plan to obtain a family of these devices for light, medium and heavy helicopters."

"I can't wait to see the one for the Mil Two Six."

Anatoly laughed. "Right. We will need a Mil One Seven just to lift the load cell."

They both laughed at the image of a load cell the size of a small automobile to withstand the forces associated with measuring the Mi-26 helicopter's maximum lift capacity of 20 metric tons – 20,000 kilograms of mass – almost four times the capacity of the Mi-17.

The two pilots stopped to talk to several of the mechanics and then the flight test engineers. They all agreed on the test conditions they would fly. There was no need for any other on-board crew, so Anatoly and Gourgen would be the only two in the aircraft. The tether cable had been adjusted to place the helicopter at 20 meters – just under one rotor diameter – and, not quite out of ground effect, but nearly so.

Anatoly pointed out each element of the test equipment from the load cell, a brass cylinder the size of a four liter can, at the end of the cable stretched out directly in front of the aircraft, to the strange cage of thin steel bars built around the conventional lifting hook. The cockpit instrumentation was far from standard. The test center added many unique instruments for one project or another. Many of the standard instruments were missing altogether or had been replaced with some instrument for a different purpose.

After they completed the cockpit orientation for Gourgen, Anatoly pulled a large card from his flight suit pocket and placed it in a small holder on the instrument panel in front of them.

"Here are the points they want us to hit," Anatoly said pointing to the card. "Our current weight is seven point two tons. For this flight, the torque meter is set for 100% at maximum power for twelve tons. We will use a baseline torque with nominal tension on cable and centered. From that point, increase torque in 5% increments to 100%, all the time keeping the crosshairs," he said pointing to the special indicator, "centered, then call each mark." Gourgen nodded his head in agreement. "The controller will acknowledge your mark, then call when they have all the data they need. You hold the point until they are complete." Again, Gourgen nodded his head. "Any questions?"

"It seems pretty straight forward."

"Yes. It is actually much easier than the old way with theodolites, or the really old way with measuring line."

They both laughed at the crude methods they used decades earlier. The new equipment promised many improvements as well as increased accuracy for flight testing.

Anatoly called the ground controller, passed some starting condition information, and then waited for the indication of readiness and the clearance to start.

"Let us get this machine running," Anatoly said when he was satisfied with the conditions.

Gourgen quickly stepped through the engine start procedures. He was quite familiar with the Mi-17 having done some, maybe even most if he went back to figure it out, of the original development and certification testing for the Mil Design Bureau.

The two friends and veteran test pilots remained attached to the earth for 90 minutes. They completed the defined test card in good order. Gourgen asked for some other test conditions to measure the load cell values when there was an angle to the cable. He intentionally displaced the helicopter's position to 3/4 of the scale, and then used similar torque values at essentially the same weight. The system proved to be sensitive enough to measure the small angle effects.

After securing the aircraft, they returned to the hangar and sat down with the test engineers and mechanics. They debriefed the flight, then entered into an expansive discussion about the uses of the equipment in a non-test environment as well as variations on the configuration to enable other tasks for both test and operational.

"This contraption around the hook," Gourgen pointing to a drawing, "could be used the help us with external lifts as well."

"My thoughts precisely."

"Perhaps, you would not have had to work so hard on the motor lift a few weeks back."

Several engineers laughed along with the two pilots. They had undoubtedly heard the stories from Anatoly.

"It is getting late," announced Anatoly. "I need to get home to help Galya."

"Yes, right," Gourgen said. "Thank you for the enlightening flight, gentlemen. You have done some very good work. This will help all of us."

Gourgen followed Anatoly to his desk, watched him secure his flight gear, push some papers around the desk, then nod toward the door. Just outside the gate, Anatoly turned right. It was only about two kilometers to the apartments, a comfortable walk in the late afternoon.

"I have my automobile. I drove down from Moscow. Remember? Do you want a ride?"

"Sure."

Anatoly was always a bit tight in Gourgen's small Zhiguli, but he never complained. Traffic was light in the aviation community even though it was a Friday evening.

"That is some good stuff."

"Yeah. A couple of the engineers worked up the equipment with the mechanics. They pulled parts from various places. The load cell comes from some rocket in the space program, so they tell me. The potentiometers were developed for the Su-27 engine exhaust nozzles."

"It works."

"Like you said, we could have used something like that for that lift at Chernobyl."

"That, plus a small video camera or two to give us a picture of what the load is doing. It is one thing to be attached to the earth; it doesn't move." They chuckled at the image. "A real load moves."

"Right you are. We will have to work on that. Perhaps, the engineers can find some other parts."

They pulled into the parking area between their two apartment buildings.

"Are you and Ludmilla coming over?"

"Sure."

"So, Milla's going to make it this time?"

"Ah, she is all right. She worries more as she gets older, but she has settled down."

"Good, then we will see you both shortly."

Gourgen waved his left hand to acknowledge his friend. He walked up the five flights of stairs to his apartment – one of four on that floor.

"I am home."

"In here," Ludmilla said from the living room. She sat with Dimitri on the modest couch with books and papers scattered across the table in front of them. "This mathematics is pressing my capabilities. You need to help your son."

"What is it this time?"

"Differential equations with complex variables."

"Whoa. How about tomorrow?"

Dimitri shot up in an instant. "Thank you, father. No problem."

Ludmilla just shook her head as their youngest child left his work on the living room table. He offered some fading farewell for the evening that was barely recognizable.

"You make it too easy for him," she said.

"He has had a long day in school, and I have had a long day in the air. We have all weekend to help him learn his mathematics."

She stood, wrapped her arms around her husband, and then kissed him. "How was your day?"

"Interesting. I just finished flying with Anatoly Demjanovich on a new test rig they have come up with for certain performance testing." He surveyed her attire. She wore a simple, button-up, print dress. "Are you ready to go to Tolya and Galya's?"

"Is it just the usual group?"

Gourgen nodded his head. "I think so."

"Then, I am ready."

He nodded his head, again, and then grasped her hand to lead her toward the front door. They stopped in the kitchen to pick up a loaf of freshly baked bread, a small block of cheese, and a liter bottle of water.

The coolness of the spring evening added an invigorating refresher. They held hands like school kids as they had always done even in the hard times. Their 30 years together had not deteriorated as many marriages did with time, pressure and stress. They always seemed to find a way to resolve any differences that might rise between them. Greetings among friends, colleagues and neighbors brought the protective comfort of a community around them.

The regular group filled the apartment of Galina and Anatoly Grishchenko. Laughter and spirited words amplified the rich aromas of various breads and cheeses, the tang of orange juice, the faint sting of vodka, and the peculiarly earthy odor of beer. Although the test pilots were quite careful with alcohol when they were flying, they were also known to celebrate at the end of a hard week's work.

"Milla and Gourgen, you are late," shouted Anatoly Kovatchur. "We started without you."

"As I can see," Gourgen responded glancing to the half full bottle of beer in his hand. "Tolya kept me late."

"Oh, do I detect our comrade in a lie?"

"Naw."

"Well, my friend, Tolya made it nearly on time."

"This is his home," came Gourgen's retort.

Ludmilla left him to join several of the women in the kitchen. The wives often retreated to the kitchen when the pilots became a little rowdy.

"Where are Boris and Nicholas?" asked Gourgen hoping to deflect the attention of their late arrival.

"At school," Anatoly answered with a curious tone as if to say, why are you asking.

"Hey, did you hear about Nicholas' little trouble?" barked Leonid.

Gourgen took on a concerned expression. "Serious?"

Anatoly was smiling, so it was not bad.

"He found him some girl trouble."

"The good kind of trouble," added Anatoly.

"Seems our host's youngest boy got caught in a compromising position by the girl's brother."

"Oh, oh."

"Yes, indeed. Our not-so-small hero gets into a fracas with her brother. No serious blows, but clothes get torn, and eventually all three of them are half naked in a pile on the floor."

"I can see this coming," said Gourgen. "Then, what happened?"

"So, the story goes, they all start laughing so hard their sides ache. The brother stands up, gathers up the sternest expression he can, and says, 'just be careful,' and then walks out leaving the two lovers to their desires."

"And?" Kovatchur said.

"No need to get sordid, here."

"Sounds like Ludmilla and me."

"Gourgen Rubenovich Karapetyan," shouted Ludmilla from the kitchen.

Everyone began laughing. Even the women in the other room could be heard.

"He is in trouble, now."

"This must be really good."

The wives streamed into the living room. They poked at Ludmilla and giggled.

"We were young and wild. . . ."

"Gourgen Rubenovich," Ludmilla growled, "don't you dare."

Everyone knew Gourgen did not like to be called by his patronymic name, which added to the laughter. Even Ludmilla could not resist the levity.

"I had just obtained her father's permission to marry the lovely Ludmilla, their eldest daughter. I was so proud of myself. We found ourselves in a secluded part of the forest near her family *dacha*."

"Oh, no," said several of the women.

"We know what happened next," gurgled a couple of the men.

"Yes, well, there we were like two wild animals," he paused

for effect causing Ludmilla to leave the room with her face several shades of blush, brighter. "Passion took any last inhibitions from us. We were rolling around in the leaves with various stages of undress. I get my hand tangled up in her *brassière*. We are laughing so loud, it must have attracted the attention of her mother who was in the forest collecting berries. In an instant, there she was standing directly over us like some commissar having just discovered a coven of traitorous conspirators." The laughter turned to tears as everyone added their variations.

Gourgen struggled to contain his own laughter. He eventually held both hands as if he was surrendering himself. "Please, please," he said trying to find at least some reduction in the cacophony of hilarity.

"So, did she snip it off right there?" asked Anatoly Kovatchur, adding to the noise.

"Please, please," Gourgen repeated, shaking his hands above his head to gain some reduction in the noise level. It took several minutes, probably due to fatigue rather than loss. "No one said a word. I started to apologize, then she held up her hand – stop – like a traffic policeman. I did not budge, did not twitch a muscle. Then, Ludmilla, who is half naked, begins to giggle, and it builds. In a few moments, her mother starts to laugh. I am looking at both of them, then I start to laugh. Ludmilla and I look at each other, wrap our arms around each other, then when we look back, her mother is gone."

"Yes, dear boy, but did you do the deed?" asked Galina which burst the laughter beyond all previous levels.

Tears of joy rolled down everyone's face. Gourgen held his side as he laughed hard. He could see that moment in time so clearly, as he always did. Among the laughs, jabs, and aching of their sides, Gourgen shouts, "Yes." That put several on the floor. Gourgen regained control faster than the others.

He left them to find Ludmilla in the kitchen. He wrapped his arms around her. She made a feeble, perfunctory attempt to hit him, then gave into his embrace. He kissed her on the cheek.

Ludmilla turned in his arms. They kissed passionately. He whispered, "I love you."

She returned, "I love you."

Someone shouted, "Now, they are going to do it in the kitchen." They started giggling as the others packed into the small kitchen. No one could move. The laughter felt good. It was a good group, a close group of friends that shared their lives and enjoyed the camaraderie of fellowship.

Gourgen and Ludmilla stayed with the others for several hours, sharing little stories about their lives. This was a night for enjoyment. They left the party and returned to their apartment. Dimitri had left a note that he was staying with a friend. They fell into each other's arms and finished what had begun hours earlier.

# 8

*23:15, Friday, 25.April.1986*
*Chernobyl Nuclear Power Station*
*Pripyat, Ukraine, USSR*

"Good evening to you, Alexsandr Fyodorovich," said Yuri Tregub, the 2nd shift operator of Chernobyl Unit No. 4. "Welcome to the delayed party, and thank you for coming early," he added in some feigned sense of humor.

Alexsandr Fyodorovich Akimov – the veteran, middle aged, 3rd shift operator – looked slowly around the control room confidently absorbing the indications of all the instruments as well as the status board. "Good evening to you, Yuri. You are not finished with the test," Akimov said with authority. He did not wait for a response. "Where are we?" he asked as if he did not already know.

"Well, the test did not go quite as planned. The sequence started, as the test plan required, at 13:00 this afternoon. Power was reduced from 3,000 megawatts thermal to 1,600 at which time the Number Seven turbogenerator was disconnected. The Emergency Core Cooling System" otherwise called the ECCS, "was disconnected an hour later."

"Disconnected?"

"Yes. If you recall Alexandr Fyodorovich, the engineers were concerned about thermal shock if the system dumped a massive amount of cool water into the hot core."

"But, that is our last line of protection should something go wrong."

"As you say, but everything will be as planned."

"I hope. What else?"

"The MPA," the maximum design-basis accident protection system, a complex network designed to enable an orderly shutdown of the unit including the reactor at a high power condition, "has been switched off to avoid triggering the ECCS. Also, both emergency diesel generators have been shunted along with the operating and start-up transformers in order to disconnect the unit from the grid."

"Is anything working?" Akimov sneered.

Yuri laughed hard. "Sure, the reactor is at 1,600 thermal, pumps one and four in the left loop and pumps five and six in the right loop are running, and the Number Eight turbine is still on-line," he looked up to the display wall, "at 80%."

"So, what happened to the test? This was supposed to be completed on the first shift. We should be preparing the reactor for refueling, now."

"Shortly after they brought the power down for the final stage of the test, somewhere around 14:00, the load dispatcher in Kiev requested that the unit not be removed from the grid."

"Why?"

"No reason given. I can only surmise there was some industrial demand that needed to be satisfied."

"And you left the ECCS disconnected?"

"Yes, Alexsandr Fyodorovich. The control valves have been closed, chained and locked as Fomin's test plan instructs."

"I was not trained for this," Akimov growled. "What if something goes wrong?"

What the two experienced operators did not know, because of the abnormal shutdown procedures being utilized for the run-down test, the conditions for an accident were already well underway.

The normal, nuclear fission, by-products of enriched uranium 238 ($^{238}U$) fuel were producing a condition called, the Iodine Well. When the actual fissionable portion of the enriched fuel – uranium 235 – is split to release its enormous heat and bevy of neutrons, it produces tellurium and iodine. The unstable iodine decays with a half-life of 6.7 hours into xenon which in turn decays with a half-life of 9.2 hours into cesium. Cesium, one of the principal hazardous waste products, has a half-life of about two million years and will eventually form a stable atom, barium. It is the xenon, however, that causes the most problems in controlling nuclear fission reactions. Xenon absorbs neutrons, the trigger elements of fission –more neutrons . . . power increases – less neutrons . . . power decreases.

In all $^{235}U$ fission reactors, the by-products were continuously produced as a direct function of the power levels or neutron flux. In this case, xenon was being produced at a rate consistent with their 3,000 MW(t) operating condition, well in excess of the reduced power when Akimov prepared to assume control. The peak xenon levels would be naturally reached about 11 hours after the start of the test – midnight.

The excess xenon was absorbing more and more neutrons, thus pushing the reactor to a sub-critical state approaching shutdown. In their effort to complete the run-down test, the operators would be driving against an enormous headwind to hold a low power level.

At this point, shortly before midnight, on Friday, 25.April.1986, the condition inside the reactor was technically still recoverable. The Iodine Well, or peak xenon level, made low power level maintenance very difficult – nearly impossible. If they had abandoned the run-down test at that time, an accident could have been avoided. With the pressure to complete the test, more extraordinary intervention would be required, although as each minute passed they raced toward the point of no return.

Yuri looked around the room to see who might be listening. Alexsandr instinctively did the same. "I was not trained for this either, but Dyatlov," he said, motioning with his head toward the deputy chief engineer under Fomin, "is here to supervise the remainder of the test."

Akimov glanced around again to find Anatoly Stepanovich Dyatlov pacing at the back of the control room with his hands clasped behind his back and watching his foot falls. "Oh, great. Won't he be a big help," Akimov said.

Yuri chuckled softly to avoid attracting attention. "You will be all right."

The two nuclear reactor operators stared at each other

wondering why they were violating their training and instincts.

"So, when did you restart?"

"I picked up operations on my shift with the reactor holding at 1,600 thermal. At ten past eleven, about 40 minutes ago, we finally received concurrence from Kiev to disconnect from the grid, so we restarted the test. I held at 1,500 thermal 20 minutes ago knowing that we had shift change coming up." He pointed to the open page in a binder. "Here is where we are in the test procedure."

"Give me a rundown, one more time, of our systems status before we resume the test."

"As you wish. I have already informed you the ECCS has been disconnected. I must remind you the valves have been chained per the test plan to avoid inadvertent opening. The MPA has been disconnected since the ECCS is blocked out. All this has, again, been in accordance with the test plan in order to ensure repeatability of the test, should you need to repeat it," Yuri Tregub said as if to vindicate what he considered to be an abnormal condition. "The Local Automatic Control system has been acting up a little. We have had some trouble maintaining the power level," due to the build-up of xenon internal to the reactor. The human operators could only see the symptoms of adverse processes already underway. "You may need to go ahead in manual mode. Both emergency diesel generators have been blocked along with the operating and start-up transformers, as I said earlier."

"Have you ever operated with so many protection systems disengaged?" asked Akimov.

"No, but it is exactly in accordance with the test plan," he answered, again a bit defensive of an abnormal condition.

"Yes, well, neither have I. What if the beast gets away from us?" Alexsandr asked in an almost pensive, rhetorical manner.

"It won't. Anything else?" Yuri pointed toward the status board. "As you can see, we have four," of eight, "coolant pumps on-line. The number three pump, the one with the new motor, has been fully tested and is operational. Other than those items, we appear to be tracking to plan."

First Alexsandr then Yuri looked at the large clock on the wall in front of them.

"It is nearly midnight, so I will take control."

"Alexsandr Fyodorovich has assumed control," announced Tregub for the benefit of all those in the control room. "Do you mind if I stay behind to watch the test?" he asked.

"Not at all."

Akimov leafed through several pages of the test plan book before he spoke. "All right, comrades. We have a test to run and a beast to put to sleep. Let us get on with our task. Begin reducing power," he commanded.

The dials on various instruments crept down gradually. Akimov walked from control panel to control panel as he scanned the instruments and monitored the status board lights on the wall in front of him. His scanned hesitated on the large wall clock as if to assimilate the time associated with test procedures with the real time on the clock.

**00:23**

"Alexandr Fyodorovich, we are getting some fluctuations" announced Leonid Toptunov, the reactor control engineer.

Akimov stood behind his controller. The reactor now acted like a common pole magnet. Each move the controller made caused the reactor to move in the opposite direction. It was not responding properly. "Switch off the Local Automatic Control."

"LAR off," the controller responded as he moved the large red levered switch to the OFF position.

"Screw her down."

"There she goes. The reactor appears to be responding, now."

"Good. Continue reducing power. When we get to 200 megawatts, we will throttle off the number eight turbogenerator and record the inertial rundown output. Are all the instruments ready?"

"Yes."

"Excellent."

The thermal energy of the reactor continued to decrease at a reasonable and steady rate. The progress looked good. Just as Akimov turned his attention to the steady printouts from the Skala-7 computer, buzzers then alarms went off. He immediately turned back to the panel.

"Power just dropped to 30 megawatts."

"All right. Let's get the power back up. We are too low."

They watched as the control rod indicators displayed the retraction of various long rods from the reactor core in their effort to increase reactivity. At first, the reactor responded, but then dropped again. The Iodine Well and poisoning of the reactor with the highly absorbent xenon led them into the trap. The fluctuations in power were an indication that the automatic system moving control rods in and out of the reactor could not keep up with the xenon poisoning, especially at such low power levels. The combination of switching to manual control and the excess xenon levels now made low power virtually impossible to control. The test drove them to attempt to stablize the power level to facilitate the run-down test.

Dyatlov charged forward. "Imbeciles," he shouted. "You have done something wrong." The deputy chief engineer stomped up and down the length of the control console, blurting obscenities at no one in particular.

"We must get the power up," commanded Akimov, "or we will sink deeper into the Iodine Well."

The Iodine Well became like a strong vortex dragging them deeper into a state of irreversible progress toward catastrophe and infamy.

"The rods are coming out, but we are not getting reactivity," announced Toptunov.

"Iodine," Akimov said more to himself using the reference to the primary decay product rather than the actual, neutron-absorbent xenon.

Dyatlov shouted, "You idiots. You have let the power get away from you. Get it back up now."

Akimov ignored him as he focused his concentration on the

indicators. He could feel his heart rate increasing. This was not good. They watched as the rods continued to withdraw from the reactor core in their attempt to increase power. Akimov glanced at the large wall clock in the middle of front wall prominently positioned among all the other displays.

**00:36**

Time became a critical commodity, and they all knew it. The core continued to decay at an increasing rate. Instead of increasing power, the reactor was now succumbing to the products of decay. Without the automatic controls, the human masters headed toward a reversal of rolls; they would soon become the slaves of their nuclear master.

"Get pumps two and seven on-line," commanded Akimov. "We need to cool the core."

The controllers did as they were commanded. Water flow through the reactor core was now much higher than the power levels warranted as they fought with the contradictions caused by the xenon poisoning.

Power levels crept slowly back up to 200 MW(t) as more rods were withdrawn from the core. They were approaching their reactivity reserve limit of 30 rods with 180 rods pulled completely out. The reactor should have been running at much higher power – actually near full power – with so many control rods pulled from the core. They were fighting against the Iodine Well and xenon poisoning. They all recognized the threat, but none of them knew why. Progress told them they were making way in the struggle to extricate themselves from the Iodine Well. The symptoms led them to a fictitious image of normalcy.

**00:52**

"Let's see if we can hold it here," Akimov said.

They waited. Dyatlov continued to curse something or someone unseen.

What they could not see was their false sense of security. The instruments told them they had stablized the reactor, but the contamination of the core picked up its deadly pace. They had no instruments to give them that most critical detailed information. Akimov looked at the clock again.

**00:58**

"Is she going to hold?" said Toptunov, more to himself than as a question.

"I don't know. The Iodine Well appears to be more extensive than we think. We need to get the reactor shutdown."

"What about the experiment?" shouted Dyatlov.

"I am tempted to abandon this damnable experiment. Here we are struggling to control a large reactor at very low power with most of our emergency protection systems disabled just for some damn fool electrical experiment," Akimov barked, then looked over his shoulder to see if Dyatlov was listening. The man was probably oblivious to the precipice of the abyss they stood so near to at that moment.

**01:03**

"Engage the number eight circulation pump," commanded Akimov as required by the test plan. They would need all eight pumps on-line when the actual run-down portion of the test began since one entire loop would be lost when the simulated failure occurred.

Water flow through the reactor core continued to climb and yet the temperatures in the core would not come down. The abnormally high flow rates caused pressure in the reactor to decrease. Instead of the normal boiling, steam production causing good mixing in the water channels, the water began to flash boil resulting in a thin boundary of steam between the hot fuel face and the passing water – a condition the engineers called, film boiling.

**01:06**

"Number three pump," commanded Akimov.

The last of the huge circulation feed pumps was activated. They were now pumping 60,000 $m^3$/hr of water through the convulsing reactor – 16 million gallons per hour, enough to fill an Olympic size swimming pool in three minutes. The normal flow rate at normal operating power levels was 45,000 $m^3$/hr. The signs were there.

The No. 4 reactor at the Chernobyl Nuclear Power Station was doomed. Although none of the humans recognized the true gravity of the situation. Without much awareness, only 18 rods now remained in the core; 12 rods beyond the prescribed reserve limit for full power operations, and the best they could manage was only 200 MW(t). On top of that, the cooling water circulation loops were now in a serious breach of operating protocol, but still in accordance with the run-down test plan.

With the circulation pumps running at such high flow rates, pumps can cavitate. A slight fluctuation in line pressure for any reason – there could be a host of possibilities at this stage – water at the pump impeller face could boil causing a precipitous drop in flow through the pipes and thus the core. Even more perilous, once a pump at high power begins to cavitate, it vibrates with rapidly increasing violence until it is shutdown or fails, often opening cracks in seals or pipes, or opening the feedline completely. Either way, the result they feared would become a reality.

### 01:06:20

The point of no return. The long, nearly 20 minute, fuse of the bomb was now lit and burning. The human controllers of the nuclear leviathan had become the slaves. The illusion of control kept them calm. They refused to recognize or acknowledge the signs all around them. They had lost control of the nuclear monster a few walls away from them in the Central Hall. Any action by the human slaves, from this point on, had only one outcome. The only question now was when.

The xenon poisoning consumed more and more of the core's reactivity, and at an increasingly rapid rate. Temperature continued to rise while pressure dropped. Inside the inferno barely contained, water began to decompose forming its constituent elements – oxygen and hydrogen gas. The constituent gases began to accumulate. The explosive mixture collected into ever expanding bubbles. The process took on a life of its own. As more hydrolysis gases were formed, thermal transfer from the overheating core dropped along with the cooling water pressure. The circulation pumps began to vibrate, imperceptibly at first, as the hydrolysis gas bubbles migrated throughout the entire circulation cooling system.

**01:22:30**

Toptunov, puzzled by the conflicting indications on the control panel before him, walked the several meters to the Skala-7 computer, continuous form, printout accumulating in the output box. He started with the most recent information line.

ORR=18, he read.

Confusion mounted rapidly. He glanced up at the wall indicators. He shook his head. "There must be a mistake," he muttered to himself.

The minimum Operational Reactivity Reserve, by regulation and practice, was 30 rods. Toptunov saw the conflict. With 193 of 211 control rods completely removed from the core, they should be generating in excess of 3,000 MW(t) and yet they were barely managing to maintain 200 MW(t). There could only be one answer, but Toptunov refused to believe it. There was no escape from the Iodine Well. At this point, the xenon poisoning of the core made the nuclear control impossible. The film boiling at the fuel elements kept the enormous heat generated from being effectively transferred to the massive volume of water coursing through the reactor. The fuel rods began melting and distorting. Still, Toptunov hesitated.

"Get on with the test," shouted Dyatlov.

Akimov looked to Toptunov who continued to leaf through the computer printouts and could only shake his head, then to Dyatlov. "There is something wrong."

"There is nothing wrong, you idiot," barked Dyatlov. "You just let the core get too hot. Shutdown the Number Eight turbogenerator, so we can get this damn test done before you mess up everything. There will be body parts on the platter if you don't get this test done."

"Perhaps," Akimov murmured, not diverting his concentration from the instruments before him.

"Perhaps, hell, you indecisive bastard. We must get the test done so we can shutdown the reactor and cool the core."

Akimov continued to scan the instruments that were now a mass of contradictions to him. What he, or anyone else in the control room of Unit No. 4, did not know was, the instruments accurately represented the destruction rapidly progressing within the massive nuclear bonfire in the Central Hall.

Akimov's mind told to him to attempt a rapid shutdown of the reactor. His perception of the best path to that objective was to complete the test since all the emergency systems he would normally utilize for such a shutdown were intentionally disabled. He placed his finger on the appropriate line of the experiment checklist and read the next few steps. Akimov reached for the communication lever to the turbine control room. "Let's proceed. Oscillograph on," he commanded the instrumentation team in a small booth built as a duty office in the Turbine Hall.

"The oscillograph is running," came the response.

"Shutdown Number Eight" he called to the Turbine Hall.

"As you command," answered Yuri Kershenbaum, the senior turbine control engineer on duty.

### 01:23:04

The steam throttle valve to the only active turbogenerator was closed. The momentum of the heavy turbine rotor began to coast down still providing electrical power for critical systems. As Akimov saw the line pressure to the No.8 turbogenerator drop, he pushed the MPA (maximum design-basis accident) button as required by the checklist.

The water in the primary cooling loop lost the last of any demand. The pressure dropped. The combination of high temperature and falling pressure along with the high speeds of the main circulation pumps, struggling to push as much water as possible, caused the water to boil throughout the system. The pumps began to cavitate. Vibrations from all eight pumps began to shake their mounts and the connecting pipes violently. The floor of the reactor control room began to shake like some high frequency earthquake.

Silence filled the control room. Blank, confused and disbelieving stares passed from one man to another. No one could find the courage to admit what each of them suspected. The consequences of the images filling their thoughts defied human comprehension.

Water flow in the coolant loops dropped rapidly since the pumps were designed to pump water, not steam. The melting core began to slump into itself. The neutron flux rose sharply as the dying reactor surged with power.

"We've lost her," shouted Toptunov over the rattle of the control room.

"What the hell," said Akimov more to himself.

"You fool. What have you done?" shouted Dyatlov over the din.

"We have a power surge. Hit the AZ button!"

**01:23:40**

Akimov leapt for and depressed the large, red, emergency power reduction system button. The drive motors on all 193 of the withdrawn control rods wound up to maximum torque trying to drive the critical control rods into the core. The control rods were their only method available to absorb the neutron flux and stop the reaction. Each rod indicator froze within seconds showing only 2 to at most 2.5 meters of insertion as they jammed up against the now distorted fuel channels. The high absorbency sections of the rods were still well above the core. The stainless steel, graphite plugged, rod tips increased reactivity even further. Power within the reactor surged, again. The remaining water in the core boiled violently, rapidly splitting into its constituent elements of hydrogen and oxygen.

Akimov saw the rods hang up and dashed for the switch to the control rod servo-drivers. He turned the power off to allow the heavy control rods to fall by gravity into the core. They did not move a millimeter. The reactor began to consume itself.

Akimov shouted, "I don't get it!"

Hydrogen gas exposed to such high temperatures began to

detonate. The 500-ton biological cover, affectionately known as the *pyatachok*, or five kopek piece, began to dance like the pressure relief valve on a kitchen steam cooker. The more than 2,000 blocks of 350 kilogram absorbent material bounced up and down like some strange crowd of excited people.

**01:23:50**

The explosive gases began detonating in the pipes, pumps, valves and other collection points. The rumblings seemed to come from the bowels of the earth. Everything shook. Shock waves in front of walls of flame spread rapidly through the primary cooling system.

The human slaves now became distant and helpless observers as the massive structure shook violently. Pipes ruptured spraying thousands of gallons of highly radioactive water across the pump room and flowing into every space water could go.

**01:23:58**

The wall of flame made its way into the enormous drum separators — large collection tanks designed to collect and dry steam for the turbines, and met a large accumulated volume of hydrogen and oxygen gas.

The explosion, with the force of many thousands of pounds of TNT, burst the tanks blowing out walls, the roof and anything in the way of the rapidly expanding fireball.

**01:24:00 (23:24 GMT), 26.April.1986**

The enormous accumulation of hydrogen gas in the core erupted. The 500-ton *pyatachok*, was tossed hundreds of meters completely through the roof of the Central Hall into the air like a coin flipped at a sports game. The uranium core now molten along with the white hot graphite moderating material and anything else in its path blasted through the opening.

Large chunks of uranium fuel and graphite blossomed like some giant flower through the remaining inadequate structure into the cool night air of the Ukraine. The fragments streaked across the night sky. To the few ex-military men within range to observe the event, it resembled the largest explosion of white phosphorus they had ever seen.

The white hot pieces ignited fires everywhere, but most seriously on the tar covered roof of the Turbine Hall. They burned through concrete slabs or steel panels. The nuclear inferno spewed fragments and cinders in the huge fireball with such force that the collection of radionuclides rose to the stratosphere well above 10,000 meters.

The humans in the control room were stunned.

"What the hell was that?" asked Dyatlov.

"What is going on?" asked the dazed and confused Akimov. "We did everything right. What happened?"

The *pyatachok* returned nearly to its original position sending a cloud of dust and debris into the air. The impact produced another shudder through the building and caused huge cracks in the reinforced concrete to spread farther or open wider. The biological cover, intended to contain high radioactive materials, now rested askew with an incredibly large opening from which the nuclear volcano ejected its invisible death into the atmosphere.

# 9

*01:24, Saturday, 26.April.1986*
*Chernobyl Nuclear Power Station*
*Pripyat, Ukraine, USSR*

The monstrous, white hot, azalea blossom where Unit No.4 once stood lit up the night sky. The spectacle alone turned every head within several kilometers and awoke many sleeping peacefully in Pripyat. The sound of the explosion accentuated the scene. A billowing, boiling cloud illuminated by a bluish-white light from below ascended to the heavens above the Northern Ukrainian countryside.

Fires erupted everywhere the nuclear fuel and burning graphite landed. Trees, small buildings, automobiles and almost any object began to burn. The flames on the roof of the Turbine Hall leapt hundreds of meters into the night sky as the roofing tar burned adding its thick black smoke. The jagged and grotesque remains of the Unit No. 4 Central Hall punctuated the horrific scene.

The Pripyat firefighters did not need alarms to trigger them to action. The sound of the explosion attracted the attention of the duty crew. Their colleagues were scrambling into their garb and running to the trucks before the last fragments fell to earth.

Alarms from the operating units began to light up the control panel at the station. An on-site assessment was not needed to issue a general alarm. All available fire fighters in the Pripyat-Chernobyl area were called. Major Leonid Petrovich Telyatnikov, the chief of the Pripyat station, was called at his *dacha* in the country even though he was technically on holiday.

As the two duty fire trucks raced toward the power station, frantic actions inside the stricken plant marked the struggle to regain control. As technicians in the Turbine Hall shook off the concussion of the explosion, then raced to figure out what happened, they tried to call the control room, but communications lines to the controllers had all been severed by the explosion. Within minutes, chunks of black material – the enriched uranium fuel and graphite moderator – burned through the reinforced concrete roof panels. Molten tar began dripping from nearly every roof panel seam. The men in the Turbine Hall did not wait for instructions. The problem was immediately obvious. They grabbed anything and everything to extinguish the fires rapidly spreading throughout the building. The fires joined faster than the men could eliminate the flames. They could not tell among the smoke that the black chunks were burning through pipes and igniting lubricating oil. The temptation to abandon the Turbine Hall grew quickly along with the spreading flames, thickening smoke and violent waves of nausea consuming their bodies.

While brave men fought fires in the Turbine Hall with little equipment and no protection from the intense ionizing radiation, the half dozen men in the control room were blinded by the nearly complete cutting of the instrumentation and communications lines. They remained dazed, speechless and motionless as eyes scanned the blank, frozen or red indications and displays. Their thoughts grappled with the enormity of what had just happened to them.

"This cannot be," said Akimov.

"What the hell have you done now?" shouted Dyatlov.

Toptunov went to his colleague. "Something has exploded, Alexandr Fyodorovich. There are fires. We need the fire fighters."

Akimov nodded his head. Toptunov pressed the fire alarm although he had no idea it accomplished nothing.

"We did everything right," Akimov mumbled more to reassure himself than to inform anyone else.

"Yes, well, something dreadful has happened."

"Get water to the reactor," commanded Dyatlov. "Cool the core down. We cannot lose control."

Akimov and Toptunov scanned their instruments. Many indicated zero. Some were frozen at their last settings. There was nothing to control.

In the Turbine Hall, chunks of concrete ranging from dust to slabs larger than a man littered the floor. The air was thick with the biting smell of ozone like some huge electrical fire. Breathing was difficult. While the flames could be extinguished, the invisible fire of the intensely radioactive objects scattered around the room could not be seen nor extinguished with the simple implements of man.

Molten tar continued to drip down through the holes in the roof adding to the fires. An enormous slab of roof concrete nearly the size of a turbine casing finally broke the last of the reinforcing rods holding it, opening the largest hole in the roof. The large block fell to the floor causing the room to quake and severed the lubricating oil feed line to the No. 8 turbogenerator.

Hot oil sprayed across the room. A steady, voluminous stream of oil pumped from the open wound. The accumulating hot oil found a piece of burning graphite and ignited. Flames shot through the roof. Thick, black, oil smoke filled the Turbine Hall. The peculiar blanketing odor of partially burnt petroleum mixed with the now ever-present ozone to produce a more ghastly assault on any remaining ability to smell.

Several men screamed as the flames ignited their clothing. Human commands shouted could barely be heard. Igor Kershenbaum's turbine machinery engineers and technicians, although reasonably trained to extinguish minor fires, were overwhelmed by the inferno enveloping them. The fires presented an immediate threat, but the far greater injury came from the invisible and imperceptible high energy particles bursting from the uranium fuel and burning graphite fragments scattered around the large room.

Without hesitation or apparent concern for their own safety, the men adjusted their actions to the changing perception of threat. Several switches were thrown to shut off the lubricating oil feed pumps. Slowly, they began to make progress.

The first of Telyatnikov's fire fighters arrived and sprang into action as they had been trained so many times. The team worked like a precision instrument. The flames surrounding the chunks of dark material on the ground were extinguished although the real fire continued to spread its invisible poison. Hoses were connected to primary supply lines. The roof of the Turbine Hall appeared to be the greatest threat since the wreckage of the Central Reactor Hall looked beyond salvation. The brilliant bluish-white light illuminating the sky above them attracted their attention, but the yellow and orange flames among the billowing black smoke on the roof of the Turbine Hall focused their professional minds. Flames were their lot in life.

Hoses snaked behind the fire fighters as they made their way to the burning roof. Recognition came quickly. They yelled for more fire fighters. As the operators in the Turbine Hall fought their battles, the fire fighters began the torturous process of extinguishing the flames on the now gooey liquid pools of burning tar. The same dark chunks littered the roof but were not of immediate concern. Large holes could be seen in the Turbine Hall roof emitting their own thick black smoke.

Kershenbaum's turbine operators and Telyatnikov's fire fighters shared many things beyond the flickering tongues of fire around them. Their eyes began to sting and water. Their throats dried to the point of pain and difficulty swallowing as their saliva disappeared. Nausea soon took a mounting presence. Each man attributed their symptoms to the heat of the fires and the extraordinary exertion demanded of them. What they did not know was their symptoms actually came from what they could not see.

The dark chunks that seemed to be everywhere and varying from pea size to a large grapefruit began to take an exacting toll. The emissions covered a broad range of radionuclides, a veritable cornucopia of particles from alpha and beta to gamma rays, and the ever-present neutrons to the mind-boggling contamination of cobalt-60, strontium-90, iodine-131, cesium-135, among many others, each emitting their own ionizing radiation. The particles easily penetrated the clothing and fire protection gear of the men. None of the men had respirators to make some attempt to filter out the inhaled particles. None of them carried dosimeters to detect the invisible hazard. The bombardment of the normally resilient human cells was instant and complete.

Living human cells can tolerate ionizing radiation to varying degrees. Bone marrow, the source of blood cells – oxygen carrying hemoglobin, disease fighting leukocytes and blood clotting platelets – represented some of the least tolerant cells. The mucous linings of the mouth, nose and throat and especially the stomach and intestinal tract were also readily susceptible. The alveoli of the lungs soon lost their pliability and permeability. The skin turned various shades of brown as the process of necrosis commenced. They called it, a nuclear tan – an industry colloquialism.

Real damage to human cells depended upon a direct relationship between the intensity of the ionizing radiation traditionally measured in roentgen, and the duration and extent of exposure. These factors combined with the normal cellular regeneration rates of various human cells defined the exposure limits. Tolerance limits vary but are generally set at fractions of up to five roentgen per 24 hour period. Survival becomes questionable above 200-300 roentgen in an entire life time.

The dark material scattered within a 500 meter radius of the remains of Unit No. 4 emitted 5,000 to 15,000 roentgen. For those few at the Chernobyl Nuclear Power Station that night who saw the eye of the nuclear volcano, they were exposed to in excess of 30,000 roentgen. Many of the heroes that night absorbed a fatal dose of radiation poisoning in very short order. The first vestiges of a most gruesome and agonizing death began to accumulate.

As the heroes fought the fires, the control room was surprisingly unaware of the enormous magnitude of the disaster.

"We did everything right," Dyatlov now muttered, adding his own incredulity to the others. "We did everything right."

"I think the reactor has exploded," said Toptunov.

"No," protested Akimov. "That simply cannot be true. We must get water to the reactor. We must cool it down."

"If it has exploded, we cannot get water to it. We need more than water now."

"Nonsense. We need the electricians here to get the pumps running again. Get Lelechenko and his crew up here right now."

Akimov turned to face a bewildered Dyatlov. "Anatoly Stepanovich, I will call the electricians, however I would suggest we contact Comrade Bryukhanov and Comrade Fomin. They must be notified that we have had an accident."

Dyatlov stared at the shift foreman. He struggled with his recollection of events searching for a mistake that he might have to answer for or worse yet be accused of high crimes against the State before a judge. "Yes. Most certainly. You are correct." The deputy chief engineer dialed the number by trained repetitiveness. "Viktor Petrovich," he said softly allowing the Plant Manager to bring himself to full alertness, "we have experienced an accident."

"What?" answered Bryukanov.

"There are a few fires. The fire fighters are hard at work."

"How serious?"

"We do not know just yet."

"I will be right there. Have you contacted Nikolai Maksimovich?"

"Not as yet. I called you first."

"Good, then call him. I shall be right there," he repeated as if the message had not been received the first time.

Dyatlov dialed the correct number for Chief Engineer Fomin. No answer. He dialed several more times with the same result. Frustrated and confused, he noticed the pungent smell of ozone. Thinking he may not have remembered the number correctly, Dyatlov looked up the number and using his finger to hold his place, dialed each number carefully – same result, no answer. He tried several other possible numbers, to no avail.

While Dyatlov tried to find the Plant Chief Engineer, the professional and impromptu firefighters waged a heroic war against the flames. They continued to make progress although for many their nausea quickly turned into vomiting. For a few, the vomiting was violent and without discharge. As the urge continued to consume them, foamy red blood came up, and yet they refused to leave the fatal task at hand. Their entire insides felt as if they were on fire. Pain grew in nearly every joint in their bodies as they moved swiftly to contain the flames.

Twenty minutes after the explosion, the first few injured men arrived at the Pripyat Medical Clinic. Doctor Valentin Belokon, the duty physician, examined two men. Their skin was dark and dry, blistered in several areas. They vomited blood. Their bodies were swollen including their tongues, mouths and throats making speech and breathing difficult. Their blood pressure was perilously high along with their heart rates. Instinctively, Doctor Belokon knew what caused this damage. To confirm his silent diagnosis, he found a 250 roentgen radiometer. As he switched it on without audio and passed it over each man, the needle shot beyond full scale.

Belokon ordered several intravenous fluid drips for each victim along with injections of morphine. He left the room to call the plant manager. No answer. He called the control room of Unit No. 4 on a dedicated medical emergency line that happened to be still working.

"Akimov."

"Comrade Akimov, this is Doctor Belokon at the Clinic. Have you seen Comrade Bryunkanov?"

"No, doctor, but I have talked to him. He was informed of our minor accident and is on his way down here."

"Minor accident!" Belokon shouted. "I have two men in my clinic who are suffering from acute radiation poisoning, the most severe cases I have ever seen beyond a textbook. Both men have been so extremely exposed they are not likely to live more than a few days. I suspect you have a major radiation disaster. How many more men have been exposed?"

Akimov's knees nearly buckled, his mind numbed by the doctor's information. How could this be? We did everything right, he told himself. What is happening here? "I am not sure, doctor. There are fire fighters here, now – perhaps a dozen, I suppose. My normal crew is 18."

"You need to get the people out of there, if it is not too late. Get protection."

"Yes, sure. I do not understand, doctor. This cannot be."

"Yes, it can, comrade. I have the proof in my treatment room," he spat and hung up.

Akimov's confusion mounted. The information around him told the engineering story although the consequences of that story were beyond the worst nightmare of any nuclear engineer. He wanted so much for the story to not be true . . . to be something much less than his worst nightmare. If he wished it hard enough and long enough, perhaps it would not be true.

Viktor Petrovich Bryukhanov, the Chernobyl Nuclear Power Station Manager, entered the Unit No. 4 control room. Akimov glanced at the clock.

### 02:30

Bryukhanov looked pale as he scanned the room probing each set of eyes as they turned to him. He locked onto the humble stare of Dyatlov.

"What have you done to my plant?" Bryukhanov demanded.

Dyatlov wrung his hands in front of him as though water might squeeze out of some invisible rag. "We did everything right, Viktor Petrovich, just as the test instructions told us. Isn't that correct, Akimov?" The shift foreman nodded his head, not wanting to say anything. "We are still attempting to determine the damage and what caused it. I suspect hydrogen gas accumulation in the drum separators."

"Is the reactor intact?"

"Yes. We think so."

"Think so," shouted Bryukanov. "You do not think with the nuclear reactor. You either know or you do not, and you will find out. You must cool the core."

"We are having some electrical problems getting the coolant pumps restarted."

"You must get water to the reactor. Get water to that thing, and get someone into the Central Hall to confirm the reactor is safe."

Dyatlov nodded to Akimov, who in turn directed Toptunov,

the reactor control engineer who did not have a reactor to control, to perform the task.

Leonid Toptunov left the control room calmly, then jogged down the long corridor toward the Central Hall and his doom. He wove his way around debris. Doors were blocked. On his fourth route attempt, he unfortunately reached his objective. He stepped onto a work balcony 15 meters above the floor.

The intense heat, the overwhelming sting of ozone, the bright bluish-white light and the burning fire within his entire body pushed him back, but he fought those sensations placing an arm over this face as if that might help. What he saw defied anyone's imagination. He scanned the room as quickly as he could. The image imprinted permanently in his mind and would stay with him for the few remaining days of his life.

Toptunov tried to run back to the control room, but found he had no strength. Each movement of his joints became difficult. The nausea welling up from deep within him added to the sense of profound fatigue he felt.

"Well," demanded Bryukanov as Toptunov returned to the control room.

"What happened to you?" asked Akimov before Toptunov could answer. His skin had turned brown, his eyes were red like the after effects of the worst possible alcohol binge and his face and body were swollen. The reactor control engineer could only shake his head.

"Well," repeated Bryukanov. "Speak up, man. Tell us the reactor is safe, and all this is some dreadful over-exaggeration."

Toptunov shook his head in disagreement as his nausea continued to mount. "The reactor is destroyed," he said softly fighting for strength.

"Nonsense," answered Bryukanov. "You must have it wrong." The plant manager turned to his deputy chief engineer to discuss something of no importance.

Akimov leaned toward his friend and colleague. "Are you all right, Lenya?"

"The reactor is destroyed, Alexandr . . . utterly destroyed." Toptunov struggled with several attempts for a deep breath. "The *pyatachok* is two thirds off its place," he whispered. "The core is completely open and burning," he said, fighting for air. "The Central Hall is completely destroyed. There is barely anything recognizable." His knees nearly gave way. Akimov held his colleague adding significantly to his own exposure. "The Hall is completely open to the sky."

Blood drained from Akimov's head. He felt faint. This simply cannot be, he told himself. We did everything exactly as instructed, Akimov replayed the thoughts again. The consequences were just beyond imagination.

Vorobyov, the Civil Defense chief for the plant and Pripyat, joined them holding a 250 roentgen radiometer in front of him as if it was too hot. "We have a major disaster," he announced. The others turned toward him. "There is very intense radiation everywhere."

"That is crazy," responded Bryukanov.

"This is a 250 roentgen radiometer, and my readings are off the scale everywhere."

"Your instrument must be faulty."

"I do not think so. We must evacuate the plant and the city."

"All this incompetent thinking. Go away and find a proper functioning instrument. Do not come back until you have accurate information."

Vorobyov stared back with abject incredulity. He had more important things to do than waste his time trying to convince a reluctant manager.

The evidence mounted quickly in Akimov's mind. Everything except his wishful thinking told him the reactor was destroyed, and they faced a disaster of unworldly proportion. He guided Toptunov toward the door. He needed to get his reactor control engineer some much need medical attention. Once that was done, he felt compelled to do his own assessment. He wanted to check on the Turbine Hall and the circulation feed pumps.

"I must call Moscow," announced Bryukanov as Akimov and Toptunov left the control room. The plant manager found the proper telephone and dialed the number from a card he extracted from his pocket. He waited for the connection and several rings. "Comrade Marin, sorry to disturb you so early in morning. This is Comrade Bryukanov at Chernobyl. We have had an accident."

"How serious?"

"We are still trying to determine the extent, but we had an explosion we believe came from one or more of the separator tanks."

"Is the reactor safe?"

"Yes."

"Any injuries?"

"We are still doing an assessment. We do not have a clear picture as yet."

"Very well. I shall be in my office in an hour. I want a complete report by then."

"As you say . . . ," said Bryukanov, his response terminated by the disconnection tone. He checked the clock.

**03:10**

They had an hour to figure things out. Bryukanov gave numerous commands, most of which had no meaning as he continued to discount reality.

The firefighters pressed their struggle against the consuming symptoms of radiation poisoning. Many of them continued to disregard the warning signs, attributing their feelings to the heat of the fires and the intensity of the battle. Still, none of them had protective clothing, respirators or other equipment. Everyone of them, to a man, failed to recognize the greatest threat by far. The intense radiation would take an exacting toll on the first group of heroes at Chernobyl.

Akimov returned to the control room. His skin several shades of brown darker, and his previously white smock covered with black soot. He looked to Bryukanov and Dyatlov. "The reactor is destroyed."

"You idiotic incompetent," shouted Bryukanov. "That is

impossible. You are confused and mistaken. Instead of wandering around this important facility, why don't you concentrate on getting the circulation pumps back on line. We need water to cool the reactor."

"There is no reactor to get water to, comrade."

"Stop arguing with me and get those feed pumps working."

Akimov stared at the senior manager. Wasn't he listening? Akimov fought his own nausea and fatigue. Then, turned to the task he had been ordered to do. He tried absent-mindedly to use the telephone to reach the pump room. The absolutely dead line reminded him of their communication situation. He dispatched one of the technicians.

The man returned with a report that the electricians had found a live terminal board, cross wired the pumps and would soon have one or two available. Akimov directed several of his maintenance crew to open key valves. They had to be opened manually since the rewiring task was too great for electrical operation. Primary attention focused on the pumps. Akimov, feeling his strength wane, sat down at the control panel for the first time since the explosion.

"We also have some wildly conflicting reports," Bryukhanov stated more for the others in the room. "Who is the best reactor physicist in the area?"

Akimov thought for a moment. "Probably, Sitnikov."

"Yes, yes, you are quite possibly correct."

Akimov twisted slightly at the indirect rebuke. Sitnikov knew more about RMBK-1000 class reactors than just about everyone else on site combined. He had been the deputy chief operational engineer for the entire plant since the start-up of Unit Two. No one questioned his knowledge or expertise.

"Get him down here. I want his assessment."

Akimov's only acknowledgment was his quick reference to the contact list of telephone numbers and dialing the appropriate one on their outside telephone. Sitnikov had been awakened by the explosion and was fully dressed finishing a very early breakfast before he headed to the plant to see if he could be of any assistance.

Lelechenko entered the control room. He looked terrible. "We have Pump Two ready, Alexsandr Fyodorovich, and we should have Pump Eight ready in another few minutes. Most of the necessary valves are open. We shall open the others shortly."

"Go ahead and start up Number Two."

Aleksandr Lelechenko left. Akimov felt compelled for some strange reason to follow him to the left loop pump room, the closest to the control room. The electrician quickly descended the metal stairway to the pump room floor. Akimov froze in shock at the sight.

The bite of high ozone concentrations assaulted his nostrils, throat and lungs. Smoke curled into what used to be the left loop pump room. A bright bluish-white light illuminated parts of the remaining structure above them. The orange flicker of flames added a surreal quality to the light.

Nearly all the roof was gone. Major chunks of the walls between the pump room and the Central Hall were piled or scattered among the pipes. Two of the pumps, Three and Four, could not be seen. They were either gone or buried. The Number One pump had major dents and debris around it probably making it unserviceable. Only the Number Two pump actually looked like a motor/pump combination.

The distinctive whir of a large electric pump in the background provided the first encouraging sound since the disaster began. "She is spinning up," Lelechenko shouted up to Akimov. "You should have coolant water, now."

Akimov returned to the control room fighting for each step against the mounting fatigue in every muscle of his body and the pain in every joint. He checked the appropriate instruments; there were no indications. He reached for the start/stop button for pump two, hesitated as he considered the wisdom of blindly pushing it, then decided to leave it.

"Number Two Coolant Pump is running," announced Akimov. "We are pumping water into the core."

None of the humans could possibly know the real situation.

There was no water left in the core, and no water would ever reach the core on the Unit No.4 reactor. All the coolant pipes as well as just about anything else in proximity to the reactor core had either been completely severed or melted. They were indeed pumping water, 7,500 cubic meters per hour, but the water was gushing from multiple breaks and flowing into the lower reaches of the plant.

"Three and Four will not make it . . . too much damage. We will work on the others."

"Good," answered Bryukhanov. "Let me know when you have more."

Valves were being opened and closed at an incredible cost to human life, but the men performed their tasks with unswerving dedication. While good men were exposed to lethal radiation to get the primary circulation system working, they did not know their efforts had absolutely no value. They were accomplishing nothing.

The No. 2 Coolant Pump, followed shortly by another of the eight original coolant pumps, was pumping highly radioactive water not back into the reactor to cool it, but instead into the spaces and channels beneath the reactor, spaces that carried vital electrical and communications lines. The human slaves had no way to know that every single water line to or from the reactor had been catastrophically severed beyond any practical repair. And yet, they persisted under the illusion of progress and benefit to pump water with the false hope of helping the situation.

The Deputy Chief Operational Engineer of the Chernobyl Plant, Anatoly Andreyevich Sitnikov, arrived at the Unit Four Control Room. "There are large chunks of what appears to be graphite and possibly core fuel scattered about within a kilometer of the plant," he announced as he entered the room.

"Nonsense," barked Bryukhanov. "I asked for you to come down early, Anatoly Andreyevich. I need your expert assessment of the reactor's condition. I also need you to be objective and factual. We have had far too much emotion tonight."

Sitnikov nodded his headed, then turned to the wall displays and control panel. He conferred quickly with Akimov, then departed on his mission.

The telephone rang. Dyatlov answered, "Unit Four." He listened. "Yes, sir." He held the telephone handset toward Bryukanov. "Moscow calling for you, Viktor Petrovich."

"Bryukanov."

"This is Marin. What is your status?"

The Plant Manager instinctively checked the clock to see whether he had missed his required call.

**03:55**

"Yes, minister. We are still collecting information. I have just dispatched our best expert to determine the extent of damage."

"Tell me what you have."

"We are making good progress with the fires. They should be under control, soon."

"Do you still think it was a collection tank explosion?"

"Yes. Excess hydrogen, I suspect."

"What else?"

"We also have coolant pumps on-line. We are pumping water to cool the reactor."

"Good. Now listen. We are forming a special commission to investigate this accident. They should arrive there later today. Until then, make sure the reactor is kept cool all the time. Do you understand?"

"Yes, sir," Bryukanov said as the telephone line went dead.

**04:30**

The Chernobyl Plant Chief Engineer, Nikolai Maksimovich Fomin, finally entered the Unit No. 4 Control Room. "What a mess," he announced.

"Yes. And now, we have a government commission coming to investigate."

"What the hell happened?"

Akimov listened for the answer while he feigned attention to the non-functional control panel.

"A hydrogen explosion in one or more of the drum separators."

"Is the reactor OK?"

"Yes. We restarted the coolant pumps."

Fomin turned to his shift foreman only to see the back of his head. "What is the state of the reactor?" he asked Akimov.

Bryukanov answered, "Shut down."

Fomin wanted to hear an answer from Akimov, but chose not to pursue it. Major Telyatnikov, dressed in his heavy, waterproof firefighter's gear, marched awkwardly into the control room. His firefighter's suit was completely wet, as was his face. More troubling was the swollen, puffy shape of his face, his bright red eyes and dark brown skin tone. The normally, very fit, vigorous man seemed to wilt when he came to a stop. All eyes in the control room were on the fire chief.

"All the fires have been extinguished including those in the Turbine Hall. The damage to the Central Hall, the main pump rooms, and portions of the Turbine Hall is severe and perhaps irreparable. The remainder of Unit Four and portions of Unit Three have sustained major damage. Several of my men had to be taken to the medical clinic. Most of my men are quite ill. The best we can determine so far is, one known fatality, a technician by the name of Khodemchuk, I believe. We have evacuated Comrade Shashenok; he is not likely to survive."

"You do not look well either, Leonid Petrovich," observed Bryukanov. "Perhaps you should be evaluated at the clinic as well."

"All of my men are ill. Doctor Belokon shall assume responsibility. I am clearing my men out. I have asked Chernobyl Station for support from Kiev to provide fire protection since I have no able-bodied men left."

"You have done heroic service, Major Telyatnikov. Thank you. Now, please let Doctor Belokon take care of you."

"I shall. I might. Doctor Belokon is suffering as well. You should seek additional medical assistance from Kiev, and possibly Moscow."

"Thank you for your concern."

Telyatnikov nodded his head and left the room with a defeated posture. Bryukhanov and Fomin looked at each other with puzzled expressions.

The foreman's telephone rang. Akimov felt too weak to answer it, but finally did. He listened, then turned to Bryukhanov. "Major General Berdov has arrived and would like both you and Comrade Fomin to join him at the Party offices in Pripyat."

"Very well. Keep water going to the reactor."

"By all means," answered Akimov feebly.

The five hours since the explosion had been very costly in human lives. Khodemchuk died instantly in the initial explosion. Shashenok died at 06:00 that morning from massive radiation exposure. Telyatnikov, Akimov, Toptunov along with all the Pripyat firefighters and Unit Four technicians would eventually succumb to horrible, agonizing deaths over the next few weeks and months as virtually every living cell in their bodies turned to mush.

# 10

*05:45, Saturday, 26.April.1986*
*Chernobyl Nuclear Power Station*
*Pripyat, Ukraine, USSR*

The office of the First Secretary of the Communist Party Committee for the town of Pripyat had become the *de facto* command center for the disaster response team. Bryukhanov and Fomin arrived at the building joining various key leaders of the Pripyat community, but military uniforms dominated the rooms. The most senior official at the moment was a tall, gray-haired, handsome man in the military dress uniform of a major general and bedecked with medals. The general poured over maps of the area spread across a large table. He ignored the Plant Manager and Chief Engineer for several minutes until he decided sufficient waiting time had passed.

"You two must be Bryukhanov and Fomin."

"Yes, we are," answered Bryukhanov, "and, who are you?"

"I am General Berdov," he answered with pride. He was actually Major General Gennady Vasilyevich Berdov, the Deputy Minister for the Ukrainian SSR, Ministry of Internal Affairs (MVD) – a unique organization similar to a combination of the FBI and the National Guard in the United States. "By 07:00 this morning, I will have more than a thousand security troops deployed around this place. By that time, we will have sealed off every road. I need to know the extent of damage."

Bryukhanov cleared his throat. "We have had an explosion."

"I know that," Berdov snapped. "What damage?"

"Initial reports indicate serious damage to the Unit Number Four Central Hall as well as the adjoining Turbine Hall. The fires resulting from the explosion have been extinguished. We have only one confirmed fatality, however we suspect we may have a few more."

"What else do I need to know?"

"We are completing the shutdown of the reactor unit, and a government commission from Moscow is due here later today."

"Anything else?" The impatience of the MVD officer filled the room.

"No."

General Berdov stared at Bryukhanov for a very long minute, then an icy glance at Fomin. "There are reports of radiation," he growled as if he caught the two leaders of the power station in a lie.

"Minor, as best we can tell," Fomin answered, not wanting to acknowledge the true severity of what might be out there.

"I hope so. My troops are not prepared for radiological work. I have already requested a chemical warfare special unit from the Ministry of Defense as well as an MVD helicopter for an aerial survey. They will have proper instruments. We shall know for certain, then."

"Probably not necessary, but an excellent precaution," said Bryukhanov.

Berdov again bore into the two managers. "I would suggest you make a clear determination of the extent of damage. Is there any possibility this was sabotage?"

The two men looked at each other, then back to the general. Bryukhanov answered, "We do not think so. The damage appears to be from a build-up of hydrogen gas inside the primary cooling loop."

"So, the reactor is intact?"

"Yes."

"The damage, even from the village, appears to be quite severe," observed Berdov.

"Yes, well, hydrogen gas is very explosive."

Berdov's stare shot through them like some extraterrestrial lie detector scan. Somehow, he knew the plant manager was not telling him everything. However, he also knew, quite predictably, the beleaguered man was going to do everything humanly possible to make the accident less than it probably was, to protect his position and possibly his skin. General Berdov returned to his maps as well as several staff officers who had waited patiently for their commander's attention. Telephones rang incessantly as the small command team tried to collect situation reports from the deployed troops.

"Who is Bryukhanov?" shouted one of the military men.

"I am."

"Telephone."

The Plant Manager took the proffered handset. "Yes."

"Viktor Petrovich, I have completed my assessment," Sitnikov said. His voice was weak and raspy.

"Yes."

"The reactor is completely destroyed."

Bryukhanov felt his legs turn to jelly. This simply could not be. Reactors do not blow up.

"Are you there?" asked Sitnikov.

"Yes," answered Bryukhanov as he searched for a chair before he fell down. Fomin found one and pushed it under him. "How do you know this?"

"The Central Hall is a complete shambles, and the entire roof is gone . . . open to the sky. It took me quite some time to finally observe the reactor itself. Viktor Petrovich, the *pyatachok*, all 500 tons of it, has been displaced at least ten meters or more. The core is completely exposed, and there does not appear to be any signs of water."

"Water! We need water. They are pumping water, as we speak."

"No. Water will not help. We need a good moderator like boron carbide or even plain sand. We must diminish the neutron flux. The core is burning and undoubtedly melting. We need a moderator quickly, or we shall have a far worse disaster. If the molten core burns through to the ground water which is only a half dozen meters below the foundation in this area, we shall have another explosion – a far more massive steam explosion – that will rupture the earth."

"Are you absolutely sure?"

"Viktor Petrovich, listen to me," said Sitnikov sternly. "I have spent several hours making sure. I am experiencing all the symptoms of acute radiation poisoning. I am certain I have received a fatal dose. You are asking if I am sure, I have probably given my life to make sure my assessment is accurate."

The last remaining color in Bryukhanov's face washed away. His skin was nearly translucent and his eyes vacant. "What do we do?"

"You must get some type of moderator into the core to stop the reaction; that must be the highest priority above all else. Next, you must evacuate the plant, Pripyat and probably Chernobyl, perhaps even more once the radiation levels have been determined. You must act quickly. Many thousands of lives, if not hundreds of thousands, are at stake here."

"Yes. I will do what I can." The telephone line went dead before Bryukhanov could tell Sitnikov to seek medical treatment promptly. He returned the handset to its cradle, then placed his face in his hands, as much to preclude anyone from seeing the fear he felt.

"Was that Sitnikov?" asked Fomin.

Bryukhanov nodded his head without changing position.

"What did he say?"

"We are finished."

"That is what he said?"

"No. He said the reactor is destroyed, completely and utterly destroyed."

"Impossible."

Bryukhanov finally gathered some strength and raised his head. "Perhaps he was delusional. I think we should let the government commission make the determination. They will have experts with them."

"Fomin," someone called out again amid the cacophony of crisis.

It was the Chief Engineer's turn. He took the telephone. It was Akimov.

"The pumps have stopped. We are completely out of feed water."

What the hell was going on here, he asked himself? Many thousands of cubic meters of radioactive water just does not evaporate or disappear, he continued to question his mind. The human slaves remained ignorant, although they should have suspected, that the coolant water was pumped into the subterranean compartments and channels beneath the burning remains of the reactor. The only thing that had been accomplished by risking the lives of the plant's technicians was actually adding to the danger. Water and the near explosive generation of steam when the molten core reached the relatively cool ground water was now many meters closer. Furthermore, the unintended flooding of the compartments shorted out any remaining electrical and communications lines inside the plant. Not a drop of water reached the burning core.

"Cross-connect the appropriate lines," said Fomin as he instinctively checked his wrist watch.

**08:55**

"You must keep water going to the reactor."

"But, Comrade Fomin, there is no water."

"I said cross-connect the lines to get secondary and reserve water in there."

"We do not think water is getting to the reactor," said Akimov.

"That is crazy."

"We have pumped the primary loop dry, and there is no evidence any of the water reached the core."

"Absurd. You have lost your touch with reality, Akimov. I would suggest you go to the clinic for treatment. Our orders from Moscow are to keep the reactor cool. Now, either you cross-connect the lines and get water to the reactor, or someone else will."

Silence.

Akimov felt the confusion characteristic of the massive bombardment of his nervous system and brain by the ionizing radiation he had been exposed to since the explosion. He knew there was a possibility he was wrong. The last vestiges of his cognitive ability told him Fomin was wrong, not him. However, the uncertainty caused by his fatal exposure eroded whatever confidence he might have had.

"As you say, then," he finally answered.

Fomin told Bryukhanov the news. The information seemed so confusing to them as they continued to struggle with reality against the consequences of what they were being told. They did not want to believe the image emerging from the confusion and denial. They knew that if the reports were true they would be held responsible for the worst nuclear disaster the world had ever known. Neither of the men wanted history to remember them as the perpetrators of an unprecedented nuclear abuse of their country and the world. They would sit there on the periphery of the makeshift command center until the government commission and its experts arrived.

The flight from Moscow to Kiev took about an hour and a half. A flight from Kiev to the small strip at Pripyat would take 30 minutes; an automobile drive would have taken another two hours over the same distance. General Berdov had been informed that the first contingent had left Moscow several hours ago and would arrive in Pripyat in an hour or less.

The MVD troops worked quickly and professionally without knowledge nor training for the invisible threat that engulfed them. Every road, trail, footpath or rail line within a 30 kilometer radius was closed and guarded by armed soldiers. Small teams went to every apartment in the Pripyat village telling the residents to stay inside with their windows shut and curtains drawn. Any information would be passed to them by the same means.

The citizens of Pripyat, composed of a broad range of skilled technicians and their families, handled the uncertainty with professional resolve. The children had not picked up the concerns of their parents. Everyone knew there had been an accident at the plant, but none of the residents knew how serious the danger was all around them. Wives feared for their husbands still on duty long after their shift change at 08:00. Every attempt to obtain some reassuring information was met with the same circumspect paucity of content. All the information they had – the sound of the explosion, the sirens of the fire trucks and ambulances, the armed soldiers, the confinement to quarters, the unusual delay in the return of their husbands – told them something very serious had happened at the nuclear power plant.

### 12:45

The special commission's technical expert team was the first group of external experts to arrive at the beautiful Ukrainian village of Pripyat. The local crew regurgitated all the known information into categories – that which had been confirmed by multiple sources; that which had first hand observers, but not confirmed by other sources; and, all other information in various forms of hearsay, rumor or unreliable sources. They also discussed areas where they definitely had holes in the picture that began to evolve. Everyone agreed the correct precautions had been implemented. Now, the most immediate priority was to determine the extent of damage. The best method was a close-in aerial survey from a helicopter.

The initial survey flight was flown by Colonel Nestrov in an MVD Mi-6 heavy helicopter. The large, six bladed, single main rotor, aircraft was a stalwart machine for the Air Force. On board, Colonel Nestrov had a minimum crew of a copilot and flight engineer; their passengers were two noted scientists, Boris Yakovlevich Prushinsky, the chief engineer of *Soyuzatomenegro*, the Department of Nuclear Energy, and Kostya Polushkin, the chief designer of the RBMK-1000 reactor. They flew toward the plant. The scintillation from an enormous heat source blurred the atmosphere above the charred Unit No. 4. Colonel Nestrov flew a closing spiral approach around the plant. The sheared, twisted and distorted structure grew in detail as they moved closer. The evidence of the many fires popped out at them everywhere. It looked like a huge bomb had gone off inside the Unit No. 4 Central Hall. The buildings and ground within 500 meters of the Unit No. 4 Central Hall were blackened and ugly.

"We need to see down inside the building, Colonel," Prushinsky said.

The veteran pilot banked the large helicopter toward the damaged unit. He chose to fly at a moderate speed of 90 kilometers per hour at about 200 meters above the ground. The enormous heat shook the helicopter violently as it passed over the reactor building. The biting smell of ozone instantly filled the aircraft, and they could all feel the heat.

"Dear God above," came the unusual exclamation from Prushinsky.

"It is worse than I thought," said Polushkin.

"We need you to hover as close as you can, Colonel."

"I will do the best I am able to do, but I do not want to stay very long . . . perhaps a minute at most."

"That should do."

Nestrov slowed the aircraft. As they neared the edge of the building, the ozone smell and heat returned. They all felt nauseous. Nestrov turned the helicopter 90°, so they approached the cavernous hole with the right side toward the building. Both scientists pressed their faces to the windows. What they saw defied any words.

Steel beams that once defined the skeleton of the building, now appeared like some children's erector set savagely attacked. A bright, bluish-white light illuminated the interior deep within the jumble of twisted beams and broken pipes. The larger, circular, stainless steel, biological cover had been flipped like a dirty dish and now lay upside-down with only about 25% of it covering the jagged hole that used to be the refueling opening. The *pyatachok* glowed red hot from the intense heat. It was difficult to see details through the wreckage and intense light.

"Can you move a little closer?" asked Polushkin.

"We do not have much time left," announced Nestrov as he nudged the great helicopter closer.

The heat was becoming unbearable. The concentrated ozone made breathing difficult. The aircraft began to shake violently as the rotor blades cut through the enormous convective currents above the reactor. Then, they saw what they feared – the white hot eye of the inferno. Prushinsky used welder's glasses to shield his eyes;

Polushkin looked away. The broken, jagged and melting cooling pipes along with elements of the absorber control rods and fuel channels could be seen inside the angry volcano created by humans. The scientist saw what he needed to see, and what they all feared most. Containment as quickly as possible was their only option, but the first step had to be stopping the nuclear fire still spewing horrendously toxic radionuclides into the atmosphere. The extent of contamination of the countryside and indeed the planet now depended directly on how quickly they could quell the nuclear fire, then find some way to entomb the radioactive debris.

With the Mi-6 on the ground in the square in front of Party headquarters, the men exited the aircraft. They could only walk several meters before they all stopped to vomit violently. Prushinsky fell to his knees, supporting his torso with nearly buckling arms. As the strong waves of nausea passed, they returned to the command center and the anticipation of their comrades. The team members were given seats at the long table while most everyone else stood. They reported precisely what they had seen. Bryukhanov and Fomin faded into obscurity as they heard their sentence. Numerous technical questions defined in more precise detail the extent of damage and the seriousness of the situation.

"So, what are our options?" asked General Berdov.

"We have only one," said Polushkin. "We need to find large quantities of some moderating material to halt the fission reaction continuing to melt the structure and contaminate the atmosphere."

"Like what?"

"We need boron carbide, but we could never get enough of it in time. The only thing I can think of that we can obtain in substantial quantities would be sand – plain ordinary sand."

"Sand?"

"Yes. Sand will work. We need to get whatever boron carbide we can find, that would be best."

"The only way to get that much sand into the building is by helicopter, and it will take many helicopters."

A rather grim Prushinsky spoke. "General, with what I saw

over the remains of the reactor, that mess is probably ejecting enormous, unmeasurable amounts of highly toxic radioactive materials. Time is of the essence. We need to determine the radiation levels, but over the reactor, we were probably exposed to 10,000, 15,000, perhaps as high as 30,000 roentgen for a few seconds at the opening. A lethal dose is something like 300 roentgen over an entire life span. We saw blocks of graphite moderator and undoubtedly the core fuel itself scattered all around the plant. This is a radiation hazard of unprecedented proportions."

Everyone stared at Prushinsky, probably hoping that he was joking. The words sank in like burrowing bullets fired from a hot gun. They all considered what they had done so far as they assessed their own exposures. The first shaking, twinges of panic shuddered most of the listeners.

"I will place a higher priority on the proper chemical warfare specialists," said Berdov. "But, we have a battle to fight. The Motherland and our citizens are depending upon us."

"Just move quickly," added Prushinsky.

Berdov issued orders to his staff. They immediately burst into action. Several squadrons of medium and heavy lift helicopters were ordered redeployed to Chernobyl, actually to a large open field about 70 kilometers to the east of the stricken facility.

# 11

*21:00, Saturday, 26.April.1986*
*Chernobyl Nuclear Power Station*
*Pripyat, Ukraine, USSR*

Against the desires of the politicians and managers, the technicians and engineers of Chernobyl began the shutdown procedures for Units 1 and 2, less than 24 hours after the explosion destroyed Unit No. 4. With signs of radioactive contamination all around them, they knew lives were more important than electrical power.

At nearly the same time, Deputy Chairman of the Council of Ministers of the USSR, Boris Yevkokimovich Shcherbina, arrived at Pripyat as the leader of the government's special commission investigating the accident. He wasted no time.

"Status?"

General Berdov spoke first. "MVD security forces have completely cordoned a 30 kilometer radius around the plant. I have requested chemical warfare specialists."

"Chemical warfare specialists?"

"My troops are not equipped for radiological work. We need special instruments and equipment. The first aerial reconnaissance discovered the completely open and destroyed reactor, and we have many reports indicating significant radioactive contamination."

"And, the chemical warfare unit handles radiological work?"

"Yes."

"As you say then. What of the power plant?"

Berdov nodded toward Prushinsky. The Chief Engineer of *Soyuzatomenegro* cleared his throat. "Polushkin and I flew in a helicopter low over Unit Number Four. In short, it is completely and absolutely destroyed as General Berdov states. The *pyatachok* has been flipped and displaced. The reactor is open and burning."

"*Pyatachok?*"

"Sorry, Minister. A slang term we use for the primary biological cover. It is a 500 ton, stainless steel, circular retainer for about two thousand, 350 kilogram blocks of absorbent material. Normally, it is the last of several seals to contain all radioactive materials in the reactor compartment."

"500 tons?"

"Yes, flipped like a coin. When we overflew the reactor, the cover was red hot having been heated by the exposed core. There is no sign of any of the absorbent blocks. The bio cover must have been violently displaced. Although we cannot see what is happening internally to the reactor, the exterior evidence tells us the core is melting. The process will continue. The American's call it, the China Syndrome, which means that without a moderator to stop the reaction, the fuel material will generate such enormous heat that it will melt through the entire structure beneath the reactor and into the ground. When it reaches the cold ground water, there will be another explosion of steam, plus even more incalculable contamination."

"What actions are recommended?" asked Shcherbina.

"We must stop the internal reaction that is generating the heat and contamination," answered Polushkin. "This must be the highest priority."

"How do you propose we do this?"

"We need a moderator like boron carbide. General Berdov has ordered the required helicopters from the Air Force."

"General Antoshkin is due around midnight," interjected Berdov.

"What about the moderator as you call it?"

"We have ordered all the boron carbide within three days transportation of Chernobyl," answered Berdov. "It is probably not sufficient. The engineers have told us ordinary sand will work as an adequate substitute. We are looking for large sources of sand."

"Can we stop the reaction?

"Yes," answered Prushinsky, and hesitated. "We have never seen this amount of damage, Minister. We do not know what is actually happening in there, and we have no way to find out. We can only use our scientific experience and knowledge to guess . . . that is the best we can do."

"How certain of this are you?" Shcherbina asked, apparently ignoring the information.

Prushinsky nodded his head toward Polushkin, the chief designer of RBMK-1000 class reactors.

"The uncertainty is, what is happening inside the core. We have no way to determine that state precisely. Therefore, we must say there is significant uncertainty. However, Boris Yakovlevich and I both agree this is the best approach. We must get the physics under control."

"Where is the plant manager?"

"Here, Minister," he answered from the back of the group.

"You must be Bryukhanov?"

"Yes."

"How did this insult happen?"

"We are still investigating the cause. However, we suspect a build-up of hydrogen in the cooling system."

"And how does that happen?"

"Several possible ways."

"All of them, not good," interjected Polushkin. "The reactor must have overheated. Hydrogen is naturally produced by a chemical reaction between steam which should not accumulate in the core and zirconium, a principal retainer material. There are also bleeder systems to extract any incidental gases. The build-up must have been so fast the system could not handle it. This could only happen from improper operation."

Bryukhanov opened his mouth to respond but stopped when Shcherbina held up his hand.

"We shall assess blame later. What other actions?"

"We determined earlier today that the evacuation of all personnel from the exclusionary zone must be carried out as soon as possible," said Berdov.

The group continued their discussions into the night.

Sandwiches were brought in along with bottled water. Several joked about needing something stronger for decontamination, but Minister Shcherbina rejected the notion. He wanted everyone's attention on the crisis.

A list of actions was established and maintained by one of Berdov's staff officers. They defined the information they needed to develop regarding the extent of contamination along with the logistics of cooling the reactor and containing the ejecta. The evacuation plan was reviewed several times before being agreed to by the commission. The principal debate revolved around the extent of the evacuation. Was a 30 kilometers evacuation zone sufficient, or would 60 kilometers or more be better? They eventually agreed upon the lessor number until a better understanding of the contamination levels could be established.

The most heated debate came with their consideration of continued operation of the nuclear power station. Unit 4 was destroyed. Unit 3 was seriously damaged but potentially repairable. To their knowledge, Units 1 and 2 were still fully functional. The scientists and engineers recommended that the entire plant be shutdown and evacuated until the radiological situation was under control. It was then that the commission learned the operators were better than halfway through the shutdown sequence for Units 1 and 2. They argued about the enormous loss of electrical power supply to the national grid. The accident at Unit 4 took out two gigawatts – two billion watts – of electric power generation and would soon remove another two gigawatts of power. The burden on the remainder of the electric power system would be substantial. In the end, the initiative of the Units 1 and 2 operators was reluctantly praised. The radiological exposure risk was simply too great.

Major General Nikolai Timofeyevich Antoshkin, Deputy Commander of the Soviet Air Force, Kiev District, arrived after midnight. The arrival of the Air Force changed the focus of the discussions. Everyone's attention narrowed down to the use of helicopters to 'bomb' the reactor with sand until the boron carbide arrived. They also reviewed the results of the second scientific reconnaissance overflight.

The *pyatachok* was now glowing yellow, much hotter than earlier in the afternoon. The news brought a graphic urgency to their work. The heating of the biological cover was one of the few visible indicators of the enormous damage being done to the near and far environment. Reports of the human cost continued to add a very personal dimension to the efforts of the commission.

"What are you asking my pilots to do?" asked General Antoshkin.

"We need them to precisely place large loads of sand into the core of the damaged reactor," stated Prushinsky.

"What are the conditions?"

"Not good, I am afraid," Prushinsky said waiting for another question. General Antoshkin just stared coldly at the senior engineer until he continued. "The best we can determine, over the reactor, they may be exposed to 15 to 20,000 roentgen per hour. The thermal convection is substantial with several hundred megawatts of thermal energy rising fast and carrying various toxic nuclides."

The two men remained locked eye-to-eye. The seasoned military officer knew this would not be like any other mission his pilots had ever flown and probably would ever fly again. He wished this whole situation was just a bad dream.

"How precise?"

"The normal opening is 16 meters in diameter. Unfortunately, the biological cover plus debris from the collapse of the roof obstructs about half of the opening. So, the pilots must place these loads of sand in about a 7 meter hole inside the wreckage of the Central Hall."

"Do we have an expert on exposure tolerance? Any medical experts?"

General Berdov answered, "We have several medical specialist teams coming here tomorrow as well as the medical technicians with General Pikalov's troops."

"How much time do my pilots have over the reactor?" asked General Antoshkin.

"Based on our preliminary readings, I would say they have perhaps 10 to 20 seconds over the reactor depending on the level of protection before reaching their limit dose. Even at that exposure level, they will experience serious effects, but they should recover."

Antoshkin did some crude calculations in his head. "Ten seconds total time over the reactor with probably two or three loads per crew, maximum." He belched a dry, irritated laugh. "You do not want much do you?"

Several members of the commission could only shrug their shoulders. They all knew what was being asked. None of them wanted to be in the small Northern Ukrainian town immersed in ionizing radiation and struggling with a disaster of global proportion.

"Is there any other way to get the sand into the damaged reactor?" asked General Antoshkin.

"It would take far too much time to build some type of scaffolding or gantry system to transfer the required materials and place them precisely," answered Prushinsky. "The exposure and cost in human life would be far beyond our ability to calculate." Silence filled the room. "Helicopters are the only way."

"So, my helicopter pilots and crews will be exposed?"

"Yes, but . . . "

"These are highly skilled, very valuable pilots – critical members of our national defense forces. It does not take an engineer or scientist to see it will take many helicopters and many more pilots to fly over this damnable reactor – perhaps hundreds."

Shcherbina decided to tone down the exchange. "Is there a means to protect the pilots?"

"They will need protective suits, proper respirators, dosimeters and as much lead that can be tolerated," said Prushinsky, eager to appease the offended general.

"The more lead in the cockpit, the less payload they can carry."

"We must find a balance."

"Easy for you to say, now isn't it," grumbled Antoshkin as he walked away to discuss the details with his few staff members plus make the final decisions necessary to execute the mission.

"What is the status of the evacuation plans?" asked Shcherbina.

A couple of the military officers pulled on the sleeve of General Berdov and whispered the repeated question. The MVD senior officer turned his attention to the leader of the government commission. "We have ordered every available bus in the region to stage outside the city later this morning. We calculated that it should take approximately 1,100 buses. I have ordered some more of my troops to the village to carry out the evacuation instructions."

"When can you start?"

"If we are lucky, perhaps mid-morning. Realistically, probably not until the afternoon."

"And, how long to complete?"

"A few days, I should think."

"What problems do you anticipate?"

Berdov chuckled a dry, uneasy laugh. "Everything can go wrong on an operation like this. The key will be staging the transportation. I do not expect to have any difficulty with the population, but we are prepared to deal with this potential."

"Difficulty?"

"Some may not want to leave. Others will try to take their belongings or pets or some such with them."

"What do you propose to do?"

"First, we will strictly enforce the evacuation orders."

Shcherbina nodded his head and motioned for the general to amplify his orders.

"They must wear minimal clothing, and must leave everything else behind."

"Everything?"

"Yes. The concern is collateral contamination outside the exclusion zone."

"And, the pets."

"Pikalov's men have told us their fur has a high absorbency, and there is no way to decontaminate them. They must be exterminated." Conversations stopped as the somber consequences sank into the many pet owners as well as those that did not have small animals. "We will accomplish this grim task after the people have departed."

Shcherbina waved his hand. "Continue."

As the arrangements for the evacuation were being finalized, the plant personnel reported they completed the total shutdown of Units 1 and 2. The report, while encouraging that an orderly shutdown of the remaining two reactor units was done, added a sobering, depressing note. Four billion watts of electric power generation had been removed from the national electric grid in just over 24 hours.

**03:00, 27.April.1986**

The evacuation of the most critically injured of the initial group of casualties began from Pripyat to Clinic No. 6 in Moscow. They would arrive in Moscow three hours later. The special medical care at Clinic No. 6 would not be able to save any of the early casualties. Their sacrifice on the 26th of April would be punctuated by an agonizing and brutal death – some within days – the longest would survive a couple of months.

Sunday morning, the first loads of sand bags were lifted by an Air Force Mi-6 heavy lift helicopters. The logistics of the process were quite cumbersome in the early stages. They learned early that the big Mi-6, while able to lift considerable mass, was not good for accurate placement. They soon switched to the Mi-8 medium lift helicopter, the general purpose workhorse of the Air Force, and its cousin, the upgraded Mi-17.

As the Air Force officers and nuclear engineers worked on the moderation process, the civil defense personnel set in motion the large scale evacuation of Pripyat and the surrounding countryside within a 30 kilometer radius of the raging inferno hidden among the wreckage of Unit 4.

As the first buses entered the city and the citizens began the traumatic process of leaving behind the lives they had known, they watched the second group of critically ill victims leave in ambulances. Major Telyatnikov and the remainder of his firefighters were in this group along with Akimov, Toptunov, Kershenbaum,

Lelechenko and most of the 3rd shift engineers and technicians of Unit 4. The men who had so valiantly fought the visible fires in the early morning hours of the 26th became the first victims of the tragedy.

# 12

*09:20, Monday, 28.April.1986*
**Gromov Flight Research Institute**
**Zhukovsky, Russia, USSR**

"Anatoly Demjanovich, you have a telephone call from Moscow," the clerk announced.

"They must want to know how to save the world," he joked with Gourgen as he walked to the desk.

Anatoly Grishchenko did not say anything other than, hello and thank you. He turned to his friend. All humor and lightheartedness were gone, along with several shades of color.

"What was it?" asked Gourgen.

"Do you remember the man we met during that assignment at the power station?"

"You mean, Lelechenko?"

"Yes. My friend from our early school days." Gourgen nodded his head. "That was a nurse at Clinic Number Six in Moscow. He has been admitted there and is very ill. She said he wanted me to know."

"That is terrible. Do they know what is wrong with him?"

"She would not say over the telephone, but whatever it is, it is very serious. She asked me to go up to Moscow as soon as possible."

"It does sound serious."

"It probably is. I am going up there."

"I will go with you."

They took Anatoly's Moskvitch automobile up the main highway toward Moscow. When they reached the beltway loop, they turned left to travel west of the city. Moscow Clinic No. 6 was situated to the northwest of the city just inside the beltway.

"Do you think the injuries to Aleksandr Grigoryevich have anything to do with the fire they reported yesterday in *Pravda*?" asked Anatoly keeping his eyes on the cars around him.

"Hard to say. The article simply said there was an accident and fire, and the fires have been extinguished."

"But, it is a nuclear power plant."

"They did not say anything about the reactor."

They took the proper exit off the beltway. The large, seven story building stood out among the forest of pine trees surrounding it. As he often did when he needed access to controlled areas, Gourgen pinned the bright red ribbon with the solid gold, five-point, star hanging beneath it, to the lapel of his jacket. As a Hero of the Soviet Union, he was entitled to special treatment. The guards at the gate stiffened instantly when they saw the medal on Gourgen's chest, then saluted the two pilots crisply and waved them through the gate.

After asking several nurses and doctors through the corridors of the clinic, both men worked their way to the designated ward. Before they entered, the ward nurse insisted they don white hospital smocks, white caps and surgical masks covering their mouths and noses. The nurse told them about the concern for infection. Her attempt to prepare them for what they would see was not adequate.

"I think you were the nurse that called me," Anatoly said as he looked at her name badge.

"Yes. I am."

"Thank you for your effort."

Without the slightest sliver of a smile or even a flicker of brightness in her eyes, she said gravely, "It is probably the best I can do for these men." Both pilots stared back at her in disbelief. "They do not deserve what they received." Anatoly nodded his head in recognition.

As they entered the large ward segmented by drawn currents, the pungent odor of burned and decaying flesh smacked them like a bat to the forehead. Groans of pain and unintelligible mumbling from many voices and every direction compounded the surreal hell in which they found themselves. The nurse motioned for the two veteran test pilots to follow her. They passed three areas protecting three men in mortal pain.

"Here is Lelechenko," she said softly as she pulled back the curtain.

Anatoly entered the small area first. The nurse left them.

There was no way to recognize the body covered in bandages and lying on an incline — not a bed — but a cushioned board at a 15° angle. Anatoly looked at the chart clipboard hanging at the foot of the bed. It was indeed his friend, the deputy chief electrician at Chernobyl, Aleksandr Grigoryevich Lelechenko. Gourgen could feel the man's pain although no words had been said. Both pilots had seen friends severely burned in aircraft accidents. Several intravenous drips went into each arm. They looked at the bottles and bags hung above him, but could not tell what they were specifically.

"Aleksandr Grigoryevich, what has happened to you?"

His eyes smiled – an odd expression for a man in such a state. He then shook his head side-to-side slowly.

"They got me this time," he said softly through his bandages.

"What do you mean?"

"I shall die within the week."

"Nonsense," barked Anatoly trying to reject the facts before him. "What the hell happened?"

"There was an explosion at the plant day before yesterday. Fires, many fires. We think the reactor exploded."

"Exploded?" questioned Anatoly. "You told us reactors are not supposed to explode."

"So they say, but nonetheless, extreme radiation all around."

"Radiation?"

"Yes, Tolya. That is what has done this damage to all of us."

"How many?"

"I do not know for sure, but perhaps 20 . . . maybe 30 . . . mostly firemen and the operators that night."

"Did it really explode?" asked Gourgen.

The senior electrician shifted his eyes to Karapetyan.

"You may not remember my good friend, Gourgen."

Lelechenko's eyes moved slowly from Gourgen's face to the

gold star on his chest. "Now, I remember – our Hero of the Soviet Union. Good to see you again, sir."

"I wish our meeting was under better circumstances."

Lelechenko nodded his agreement. They looked at each other in silence as though they all were trying to remember where the conversation left off. The dying man looked back to his childhood friend searching for, perhaps, permission. Anatoly nodded his head that it was all right. The electrician's eyes returned to Gourgen.

"Most of us feel certain that it exploded although they tell us it did not. The radiation damage is turning our internal organs into soup. We have all vomited until only blood comes up. We cannot eat or drink. They give us morphine, but not enough to dent the pain. The engineers among us say our symptoms are classic severe radiation poisoning. So, to answer your question, yes, I think the reactor exploded."

"What are they doing about it?" asked Gourgen.

Lelechenko's eyes closed and his body shook as though an electric current was passing through his body. He must have expended enormous energy to stifle his screams of pain. They waited several minutes. Anatoly looked to Gourgen as if to ask whether they should leave.

"I hope . . . ," he growled against the pain, "I hope they bury that monster."

His eyes reopened, now filled with the redness of blood. The man's body was coming apart before their eyes and yet he resisted the urge to cry out with his agony.

"We must go and leave you in peace."

"I shall only know peace when I have taken my last breath."

"Fight, Aleksandr Grigoryevich. Do not let this beat you."

"It already has. I wanted them to end this, now, but they refuse. There is nothing they can do for me now."

"Do not give up."

"There is nothing left to give up. I shall die in the next few days. Two of us have already died. Several others are worse than me."

"Do your best."

He tried to laugh, only to cause more waves of excruciating pain. "We put out the fires. We did all we could. Now, someone else must bury the monster before it does more damage."

"Wasn't there any protective equipment?" Gourgen asked.

"There is no protective equipment for that type of radiation." Another bolt of pain shook his body. He held up his shaking hand, not wanting them to leave. "There was no time. There were fires everywhere, and we needed to get the coolant pumps running again to keep the reactor core cooled."

"If the reactor exploded, what good would the water be? Why did they do this to you?" Anatoly asked.

"Tolya, we did what was expected of us. We did not know what we know now. They needed those pumps running. The damage was enormous, but we got two pumps spun up and working – two out of the eight we had. So many lives, for two pumps, for no good."

"What can I do for you, Aleksandr Grigoryevich? How can I avenge your sacrifice?"

"No vengeance, Anatoly. No vengeance. I did what the Motherland needed me to do." Another shot of pain racked his body. They waited for the worst to pass. "What you can do is help me end this misery. I shall not survive this, and I want to end this now. You are the strongest friend I have, Tolya. Have the strength to end my pain."

His eyes searched deep. The concentration and determination were clearly evident in his eyes. They felt his pain.

"I cannot do that," Anatoly said solemnly. "You must fight this. Perhaps you can beat it."

Lelechenko just stared at Anatoly. After many long moments, he nodded his head in recognition, if not acceptance.

"We shall go, Aleksandr Grigoryevich," said Anatoly.

"I shall not see you again in this life Tolya. Take care of our Motherland."

Anatoly nodded his head, hesitated as though he wanted to

say more, then turned, pushing Gourgen out of the area. They walked out, without words, to the echoes of screams, cries and groans. The impact preserved their silence until nearly the beltway exit for Zhukovsky.

"I am sorry about Lelechenko," said Gourgen without looking at his friend.

"Do you really think it is that bad? That he is correct about the reactor?"

"Tolya, you do not do that level of damage by just a fire. You have seen pilots burned severely, and they were not this bad."

"I know that, but an exploded nuclear reactor . . . radiation poisoning . . . do you know what that means?"

"A disaster of unimaginable proportion."

They passed the Kamov and Mil flight test areas on the way south to Zhukovsky. Gourgen considering stopping to check in with the Mil flight test team, but decided it was better to stay with his friend. He would call in when they arrived in Zhukovsky.

The array of large, Tupolev and Ilyushin aircraft, vertical stabilizers on the east side of the highway marked their arrival in Zhukovsky. They watched an Su-7 takeoff and immediately circle back to pick up a chase position for an experimental Su-27 high maneuverability fighter undoubtedly on some high risk flight profile.

When they entered the reception hall of the Gromov Flight Research Institute, Gourgen called his office.

"Hello," came the simple greeting intended to protect the location and purpose of the site.

"This is Gourgen."

"Gourgen, we have been looking for you. Where have you been?"

"I went to visit a friend who is dying in the hospital."

"I am so sorry."

"What did you want me for?"

"Oh, yes. The Ministry of Defense called here. The Colonel said it was most urgent."

Gourgen wrote down the name and telephone number he was

to call. He also checked on the Mil flight schedule; no flights planned for him. He told the man to sign him out for the day. He held up the piece of paper for Anatoly to read. They went to the pilot's office for a little more privacy.

The moderate size room held 16 desks for the variety of permanent and temporary experimental test pilots assigned to Gromov. The only occupant as they walked in was one of the younger pilots who just arrived for a special test on an old Mikoyan fighter. He sat in the corner absorbed in his paperwork.

Gourgen made the telephone call. After the introductions, he listened and wrote down information with occasional glances at Anatoly and nods to the paper for him to read. The call took several minutes. Several attempts at questions were not satisfied.

"Well, my friend," he started after he hung up. "It looks like I will get my turn."

"So, it is Chernobyl."

"Yes."

"I was born and grew up about 45 kilometers from there. This cannot be happening."

"Apparently, it is, Tolya. As you can see, they want me to prepare for a 25 ton lift."

"A Mil Two Six."

"It is the only way, and even then, this lift is over the maximum external lift capacity. We will need some special test work. They want me to make a reconnaissance flight tomorrow, so I can know what I am to prepare for. I am supposed to go down there to meet with the Air Force and engineers."

"Did they say anything about the reactor or the radiation?"

"No. You heard me, I asked, but they would not answer."

"When are you leaving?"

"Tomorrow morning. They want me to fly one of our birds down there for a survey of the site. Apparently, the facilities are crude."

"Everything down there is crude."

"They want me to use our test Mil Two Four for the survey,

since it is environmentally sealed."

"Contamination."

"That would be my guess. They will probably decontaminate the aircraft when I am done."

"I want to go with you."

"Tolya, there is no reason for both of us to be at risk."

"That is the region of my birth village, Gourgen. I am going with you."

"As you say, then. I will plan for a 8 o'clock takeoff, that should put us down there at about mid-day. I will have the internal ferry tank installed tonight, so we do not have to stop for fuel."

"Do you need me to do anything?"

"No. I will have the aircraft prepared tonight. We should be at the Mil test site about seven in the morning. I will make sure there is a gate pass for you to get through security."

"Agreed."

"It should be an interesting day tomorrow, my friend. Let's get a good night's rest."

# 13

*18:37, Monday, 28.April.1986*
*Building R4, Apartment 44*
*Zhukovsky, Russia, USSR*

Anatoly dropped Gourgen off at the lobby entrance to his apartment building. Gourgen stood there facing the building, staring, but not seeing anything. He knew Ludmilla would know something had happened at the Chernobyl Nuclear Power Plant. Her fears, her concerns, her worries had come to fruition. Gourgen did not know how long he stood there.

As passing colleagues broke his trance, Gourgen headed up the stairs. He hesitated at the door trying to think of what he was going to say; how he was going to answer her questions; or what he might be able to do to assuage her worries.

"I am home, Milla," he said. There was no answer. The smell of baking fish gave him a clue. Ludmilla was in the kitchen.

She did not look up as she checked the small oven. "I know you have heard the news," she said. "It has been in the newspapers, on the radio and television, but they keep saying it is not serious."

"Yes, I have heard the news."

"Galya says you and Tolya went up to Moscow to see one of Anatoly's schoolmates."

"Is there anything you two do not talk about?"

"Not much."

"It is serious, isn't it?"

"Yes. I think so." He wanted to tell her how serious, but knew it would not help her, especially with the mission he had to fly tomorrow. "How long until supper?"

"About 30 minutes."

"Can I take a bath?"

"Sure. You should have time."

Gourgen turned on the faucet, felt the water for a few seconds until he had the desired temperature, verging on hot, then took his clothes off, adding them to the pile already in the basket. He eased himself into the steamy water. The rush of heat gave him a headache. He closed his eyes to relax, let his body adjust, and the headache passed. The thought of flying into an area of a major radiation accident did not appeal to him in the least, but the prospect of telling Ludmilla about his mission tomorrow was even less attractive.

"Supper," came her call from the kitchen. The cooling water burst upon him.

Time passed too quickly. He dried and dressed without hesitation. He joined Ludmilla at the small kitchen table. They ate silently for several minutes. Gourgen knew there was no way Anatoly could have told Galina, and no way Galina could have told Ludmilla; so, she could not know about tomorrow. Maybe he should just fly the mission, then tell her what happened.

"What do you know?" she asked finally.

"There was a fire, fairly serious from what I understand."

"That much has been in the news."

He knew he could not tell her what he had learned at Clinic No. 6. His silence undoubtedly did not give her any confidence, and perhaps even encouraged some inner suspicions.

She stopped eating, then her head dropped. "You are going down there, aren't you?"

Now, it was his turn to stop eating. He pushed his food around the plate as he fought to find the correct words. He would not lie to her, but he had to find a way to answer the inevitable questions in the least troubling way.

Ludmilla started to cry. "Oh, Gourgen. Why you?"

"They need my skills."

"There are hundreds of pilots, Gourgen, maybe even thousands of pilots that could do whatever it is they want you to do."

"Milla, I appreciate your confidence in my flying skills."

She stamped her foot hard on the floor. "You know what I mean!"

"Yes," he said with a smile, "yes, I do." Her eyes bore into his skull. "They would not tell me anything over the telephone."

"When do you leave?"

"Anatoly and I will meet at Mil tomorrow morning at seven and take off at eight."

Her head nearly hit her plate. "When will you be back?" she whispered.

"It depends on what happens down there. We are to do a special reconnaissance flight. I might be back tomorrow night, or it could be a few days. I will try to let you know, but I have no way to predict what we might find."

"Oh, Gourgen."

"Don't cry, Milla. I will be all right."

"How do you know?"

Gourgen shook his head. "I just have to believe, like I do for every flight. I study my task. I do whatever I need to do to prepare, then I simply do the best I can do to fly the mission. It is the same I do for every flight."

"But . . . radiation . . . what about the radiation?"

Gourgen swallowed hard. After seeing Anatoly's friend, Lelechenko, he worried about what they might face at Chernobyl. Radiation was invisible. You needed special equipment just to detect it, and yet it did enormous damage to any living thing. He was not particularly eager to fly into a radiation zone. "I don't know." He waited for some response other than her sobs. "I am not particularly excited about this job, but the country needs me."

"I need you," she hissed. "Dimitri needs you."

"I will be back, Milla. This is just another flight."

"It is not just another flight," she responded with heavy emphasis on the negative.

Ludmilla wiped the tears from her cheeks, then rose from the table. She cleared away the dishes even though Gourgen had not finished eating. He did not object. She quickly rinsed the dishes, then left the room.

He sat there, alone, with only his thoughts. How did things

get so crazy, he asked himself several times. Tomorrow's flights would be just the beginning. Ludmilla was precisely correct, there were thousands of pilots who could fly a reconnaissance flight or some other type of evaluation flight. The difference rested upon some very specific reason why the Government decided it needed the unique skills of a Mil experimental test pilot.

When she did not return, he checked the living room, then their bedroom. She stood at the window looking out onto the courtyard with its trees, grass, walkways and benches. Gourgen moved a few things on the chest of drawers, just to make sure she heard a few sounds of his presence. She did not move.

Gourgen moved behind her, wrapped her in his arms and kissed her neck. Her head shifted toward him in response.

"I am worried," she said softly.

"I know, Milla. I know."

"I had bad feelings about that place from the very first. Somehow, I sensed that was an evil spot."

"Evil?"

"You know what I mean. When Galya told me, you stopped there to do a priority job, I just knew it was not right. Now, you are going back down there. Not only that, but we know there has been some major accident – a fire or some such. For all we know, the reactor exploded, and there is nothing left but that radiation stuff."

Gourgen swallowed hard, trying to control his emotions, and show no reactions whatsoever. He knew she would pick up the slightest break in his voice, or hesitation in his response. He squeezed her a little more tightly and began to sway as if rocking her to sleep.

"I must go. You know that."

"Yes. The Motherland needs you."

"I do not think they would have called me if it was not of vital importance."

"You have served the Motherland, well, Gourgen. You have given your sacrifices for the Motherland. That is why they gave you that gold star and red ribbon. You have given plenty."

"I suppose so, but the Motherland needs me one more time."

"Will you be able to contact me and tell me what it is like?"

"I suspect not. If this is serious enough to need my skills, then I doubt they will want much outside contact. Also, one other thing, this is probably just an evaluation flight to make the proper preparations for the real task, whatever that may be."

"So, I won't hear from you or talk to you until you return . . . if you return."

"I will return. We are taking the Center's Mil Two Four. It is fast and environmentally sealed for operations like this."

"So, there is radiation."

"Milla, there are indications . . . ."

"What kind of indications," she interrupted.

"Anatoly's friend."

"What about him?"

"He is very ill. He will probably die within a week."

"Die?"

"Yes."

"From the radiation?"

"He thinks so, although no one has confirmed that."

"Oh, Gourgen."

Gourgen could feel the convulsions of her sobbing, then felt her tears hit his forearm. He held her tightly, kissing her neck several times, then lowering his head to her shoulder.

"Are you going to tell Dimitri and the other children?"

"I don't see how that will help anything other than to worry more people."

"What if you do not come back?"

"Then, how would this be any different from any other flight where something catastrophic might happen?"

"You know you are flying into danger . . . you know."

"The other kids are grown. Dimitri is in his last year before he goes off to a university. I have done my job as a father."

"You never stop being a father."

Gourgen felt his frustration level rising. "I know, Milla. You know what I mean."

Ludmilla extricated herself from his embrace and went to the bathroom. He could hear water running in the sink. She was probably splashing her face. Her return brought a different expression.

"I want you to make love to me," she announced.

He searched her eyes, her expression, her body. She was serious. "Are you sure?"

"Of course, I am sure. I want you to give me another baby."

"Milla," he protested.

"If I am to be alone, I want another child to preserve your blood and be with me."

"We have five children with our blood running through their veins."

"I want a child with me until I am an old woman, and the children must take care of me."

"We are 50 years old."

"I know how old we are."

"Are you sure?"

"You already asked me that."

Ludmilla shut their bedroom door behind her, then moved past him to draw the curtains. He stood still as she kissed him and began to undress him. He waited several minutes before he reciprocated. They were completely naked when she spoke again.

"Make love to me like you have never made love to me before."

Gourgen chuckled. "I am not as young as I once was."

"That has not stopped you before," she giggled.

"I will do the best for you," he said as he lifted her in his arms. He walked slowly to the side of the bed and gently lowered her to the sheets. He stepped across her and lay down beside her.

They touched and enjoyed the texture of the other's flesh. Soft words between lovers added to the sounds of their flesh growing in readiness. Gourgen made every movement in a slow, deliberate manner to heighten the sensations of their touching.

Several respites allowed sufficient recovery to perpetuate their evening of pleasure together. They mixed giving and receiving with those moments of hot mutual passion until exhaustion caught up with both of them.

"I love you," he whispered in her ear as their intertwined, wet bodies cooled.

Ludmilla rolled slightly toward him and touched his cheeks in a gentle caress. "Thank you for giving this to me."

Gourgen smiled.

# 14

*07:30, Tuesday, 29.April.1986*
*Mil Flight Test Facility*
*30 kilometers north of Zhukovsky, Russia, USSR*

Gourgen's crew chief and his assistant continued to scurry around the menacing form of the Mi-24 attack helicopter as the two experimental test pilots walked toward their sophisticated transport. This particular aircraft, assigned to the Mil Design Bureau Flight Test Center, was painted in the camouflage colors of the Soviet Air Force Frontal Aviation units except for the missing, large, red, designation numbers. Hemispheric ice and dust deflectors covered the inlets to the two, 2,200 horsepower, Isotov TV3-117, turboshaft engines. The large, 6.4 meter, anhedral wing carried no wing stores this day. Both bubble, tandem cockpits remained closed — normal procedure for the environment system. The small passenger or cargo compartment underneath the main rotor was also closed, filled for all practical purposes, by a hefty, kiloliter, auxiliary, fuel tank that would nearly double their range.

Karapetyan and Grishchenko listened calmly to the crew chief's report on the aircraft status. All systems were tested and fully functional including the weapons systems, except there were no weapons, and the twin, 30mm cannons were replaced with a closed ballast weight. The environmental system was fully serviced with the new, nuclear, biological and chemical filters installed. The system would give them protection against any airborne particles. Even the navigation system had a new map sheet inserted in the automatic location plotting system.

This was the fourth morning since the destruction of the Unit No. 4 power plant. Everyone seemed to know why these two highly respected test pilots were flying south to Kiev. No one talked about it, but there was a respect verging on reverence for them, and the mission they were about to fly.

"Ready?" asked Gourgen.

"Let's do it," answered Anatoly.

As Anatoly moved through the contortions necessary to enter the left side hatch and situate himself in the front seat compartment, Gourgen leaned into the right side hatch for the rear compartment – the pilot's station. The small passage way behind the seat connecting the pilot's compartment with the passenger compartment was sealed, as it should be. Everything was in its proper place. He went through his own contortions to settle into the comfortable, semi-formed seat.

This time, Gourgen used the checklist to go through his pre-start procedures. Neither of the two experimental pilots were accustomed to using all the systems on the aircraft. On this mission, they would need them, and they did not want to miss an important step.

The auxiliary power unit started. Once electrical power was available, Gourgen began the initialization of the navigation system, then switched on the environmental system. The active filters that would clean the air entering the cockpit took nearly a minute to heat up to the proper temperature. With the filters active, they needed the coolers working to keep them comfortable inside the sealed cockpit. When they felt the cool air coming out of the various vents, they closed and locked the cockpit hatches. The engines were started and the rotor engaged once all the systems were fully operational.

They waited several minutes for their clearance window to open through the Moscow Area Defense Network. They waved good-bye to their ground crew as well as several friends standing outside the flight test building watching their departure. The aircraft was heavy with the full auxiliary fuel tank. Pulling up on the collective, Gourgen waited until the aircraft was light on the wheels then applied forward cyclic as he continued to add power. The rear wheels broke ground, and the aircraft rotated on the nose wheel and began to pick up speed. At about 65 kilometers per hour, the nose wheel lifted off; they were airborne. Gourgen immediately retracted the landing gear. He continued to accelerate as the aircraft climbed to their prescribed 500 meter cruise altitude. They would use the maximum speed potential of the Mi-24 at 320 kilometers per hour. At that speed, the journey would take them a little over 2.5 hours.

Only required checkpoint radio calls and an occasional navigation progress confirmation provided words from either of them. Other radio traffic seemed unusually high but routine. They tracked directly to the makeshift staging field 70 kilometers east of Chernobyl. Their on-board sensors indicated only slight radiation detectable, and no known chemical or biological agents. They arrived on time. An Air Force ground controller directed them to their designated spot among the small but growing armada of helicopters in the large field. A stocky, Air Force colonel in his flight suit drove up in a small field vehicle. He waited for them to shutdown the aircraft and extricate themselves.

"I am Colonel Nestrov," the officer announced.

"I am Gourgen Karapetyan from the Mil Bureau, and this is Anatoly Grishchenko from the Gromov Flight Research Institute." They shook hands.

"We have been expecting you. Good to have you with us. Do you need fuel?"

"Not yet."

The colonel nodded his head. "If you will come with me, I will take you to our operations tent for your briefing."

Several large field tents were located in a sizable stand of mature pine trees 500 meters from their aircraft. This was definitely a military site although several civilians could be seen among the array of officers and enlisted personnel. Colonel Nestrov led them to the center tent among the half dozen grouped together. Several large maps occupied one entire side of the tent. One of the maps of the area north of Kiev and just prior to the Ukrainian border with Russia had a red circle of about 30 kilometers radius drawn around the power plant site. A green circle of about 60 kilometers nearly reached their present location. Several shaded regions blossomed to the northwest of the power plant. Gourgen immediately recognized the map as a plot of contamination zones.

They were introduced to the various officers in the tent, but Colonel Nestrov maintained the command presence.

"I trust you know why you are here?" asked Nestrov.

"Basically," answered Gourgen.

"Let me bring you up to date, then." He moved within arm's length of the contamination map. "Four days ago, a very serious explosion at the Chernobyl Nuclear Power Station produced radioactive contamination as indicated on the map. We are located here, 70 kilometers from the plant, at a safe distance. Further, the worst contamination is to the northwest."

"I grew up in Ivankov," interjected Anatoly as the colonel waved his hand past the small village of his youth. "It is a little farming village with simple people who are just trying to live their lives. They grow potatoes and wheat, and raise chickens."

"I am sorry. The village has been evacuated. It is in the hot zone."

"How could this happen?"

Colonel Nestrov turned slightly to face the two experimental test pilots. "There is a government commission investigating the cause of this disaster. Our task is containment."

"Sorry."

Nestrov nodded his head, then turned back to the map and pointed to the site of the power plant just west of the Pripyat River. "The power plant is here. Unit Number Four is the eastern most portion of the facility, other than the construction of units five and six."

"We have been there," Gourgen said.

"You have?"

"Yes. About a month ago, we lifted a six ton pump motor into Unit Number Four."

"Interesting," Nestrov said, nodding his head. "We have

managed to take a series of photographs that I will show you shortly. Air Force pilots began lifting huge quantities of sand – 2,500 tons so for – and, we just started dropping boron carbide into the reactor cavity."

"Why?" asked Gourgen.

"There is no coolant. The core was burning and melting. The sand and boron will stop the reaction and absorb the heat. The plan is to bury this mess in a concrete containment building."

"That is where we come in."

"Yes. The engineers want some means to allow for possible access to the interior should the need ever arise in the future. They also want some type of very heavy relief plate should something explosive happen inside the containment building."

"Explosive?"

Nestrov smiled as if he thought, damn civilians. "Do not worry. We are not talking about a nuclear explosion. It was steam that did all this damage. There have been several minor events as the weight of the sand collapsed certain weaker structures inside."

"As you say, then. This plate you want us to lift is 25 tons, we were told."

"The engineers are still working on the design of the building and also the cover. Here are a few sketches of what they are considering for the enclosure. Your information was correct a few days ago. The last I heard this morning, they are up to 35 tons."

"35 tons!"

"I imagine there is some variability to that number," he continued ignoring Gourgen's protest. "The plate will go right here," he pointed to the top of the sarcophagus, "in a recess that will be part of the roof construction."

"They need to be careful here if they want this plate to be lifted by a helicopter."

"What about several helicopters?" interjected Anatoly.

Nestrov laughed, probably thinking the suggestion was beyond reality.

"A possibility," answered Gourgen stopping the colonel's fun.

"However, I surmise this cover will need to be precisely placed."

"Yes."

"Then, a multiple bird lift would be too hard to coordinate."

"There is also substantial thermal turbulence over the reactor. It is not an easy or comfortable place to fly. Even with all that sand, there is still considerable radioactivity and turbulence."

"This is way beyond anything we have lifted before."

"We know," answered Nestrov. "Our weight limit is 20 tons with the Mil Two Six."

"We will need to experiment, soon, before they finish the design. We may not be able to lift 35 tons."

"The work is progressing fast. The government wants this mess sealed up quickly. Radiation contamination is serious."

"This is some of the most productive grain farming soil in the country," barked Anatoly.

"We know . . . which is why we are moving so fast."

"Why?" shouted Anatoly.

No one answered. The tent fell silent of words. Only the shuffling of paper and the clatter of a lone military teletype machine could be heard. Colonel Nestrov shuffled his feet as if he was looking for something among the small clumps of dirt. Anatoly waved his hand to go on. Nestrov stepped toward a table and retrieved a stack of several dozen, moderate size, black and white photographs.

"These are the photos of the reactor building."

Anatoly and Gourgen studied each picture. The jagged, teeth like, 'mouth' of the building made it look as though some god-like giant reached down and just ripped the roof from the structure. A bright, white hot glow could be seen in some of the photos and illuminated many of the other twisted and tortured remains in an odd manner. Debris was scattered in every direction. Smoke could still be seen rising from the wreckage even in the most recent photographs. A few shots were taken of a medium lift, Mi-8 helicopter dropping a load of sand bags into the reactor hole. Other than the edges of the adjacent buildings, the frames where windows used to be and the broad, horizontally striped, externally reinforced, exhaust stack towering above the remains of Unit No. 4, the scenes appeared surreal like some movie image of a future war. The damage was almost beyond comprehension.

"Because of the stack," Nestrov began, "the only approaches are perpendicular to the building line, and the wind has been generally out of the south-southeast. Our pilots have found the downwind approach the best so far to stay out of the plume and turbulence as long as possible."

Gourgen nodded his head. "Again, we are quite familiar with the red and white stack." Anatoly just stared at the senior Air Force officer.

"Does your aircraft have the combat filters and seals installed?"

"Yes. They were checked yesterday and this morning."

"Good. You will need them." Nestrov waited for some reaction from the civilian pilots, but received none. "You will return here and land in the northeast corner of the field. A decontamination area has been established. You will remain turning while the chemical troops wash the aircraft. With the filters, you should not have any particulate contamination. Any questions, so far?"

Both test pilots shook their heads.

"You will need to plan your reconnaissance carefully. Do not spend more than twenty seconds directly over the building. You will receive a large dose of ionizing radiation. Our pilots have been experiencing nausea, some vomiting, muscle aches and fatigue, as well as headaches. We have plenty of sealable, vomit bags. You should take several each. When you return and after the aircraft has completed decontamination, you will reposition to your current place, shutdown and exit. The medical team will give you a thorough examination."

"It is getting late," said Gourgen. "I think we will need to spend the night here. Do you have a place for us to sleep?"

"Yes. We have plenty of room. After your medical assessment, we will need to debrief your flight. The engineers should be here by then, and we will need to establish a plan and timeline tonight or tomorrow. We will refuel your aircraft, so you can leave early tomorrow morning, if you desire."

"As you say, then."

"Are there any further questions?"

"When can we take off?"

"They will stop the sand drops at 18:00. It will be about a ten minute flight for you, so you could take off any time after that."

"If you have nothing else for us, we will go prepare for this flight. May we take a few of these photographs?"

"Yes, as long as you return them before you leave."

They shook hands with the colonel and left the tent. They walked toward their aircraft. The menacing Mi-24 looked ready among the many, Air Force, Mi-6, Mi-8 and Mi-26, transport helicopters staging for their turn over Chernobyl. Gourgen was thankful they had the benefit of an environmentally sealed aircraft for this mission. As in most cases, he believed the biological effects were probably being understated, but at least they were being told about the danger.

They sat in the grass leaning against the left main wheel of the attack helicopter. They discussed various issues as well as their objective for the flight. Neither of them was particularly eager to do this mission, but they both instinctively knew they had to fly it. There was no one in the country nor the world for that matter who knew more about the capabilities of the Mi-26. They had both done incredible things with the world's largest helicopter, but this job would soon define a new and probably unique boundary to what the machine could handle.

Anatoly and Gourgen methodically checked their aircraft to make sure everything was in proper order. The indicators on the biological filters where both green. The helicopter was ready.

As their takeoff time approached, they climbed into their respective compartments, started the APU to get the air flowing and the navigation system warming up, then shut and locked their canopy doors. The engines started normally. Everything was fully operational and ready.

Gourgen waited until his watch said 18:00 straight up before he lifted the collective to begin their reconnaissance flight. They headed west toward the Chernobyl Nuclear Power Plant. The sun was setting on the Western horizon.

As they crossed a small ridgeline and the sun fell behind some low clouds in the distance, a feature in the dusk sky bloomed to prominence. A strange, huge, bluish-white beam pointed straight up as far as the eye could see. The light did not move or flicker. It was not a searchlight of any kind they were familiar with. The beam emanated from the ground directly ahead of them.

"What is that?" asked Gourgen finally.

"Maybe they have set up some lighting for us."

"Have you ever seen any lights like that?"

"No."

"Neither have I, Tolya. This looks like some serious crap, and the colonel said they have already dropped 2,500 tons of sand on this thing, and it still glows like that."

"I hope they know what they are doing."

"Me, too. Your village is to the west."

"Yes, on the other side," Anatoly said as if Gourgen did not know his directions.

As they flew closer, the beam grew in size and brightness. Flying a reconnaissance flight in twilight was not the greatest idea, but the Air Force did not want them to interfere with the nuclear moderation efforts. The last few trees passed beneath them. The large lake and the Pripyat River reflected the remaining natural light as well as the unnatural illumination from the plant.

The details of the power plant came out of the growing darkness. Only a few lights lit up Units One and Two. The city of Pripyat was completely devoid of lights. Even the streetlights had been extinguished. It looked like a ghost town. The power plant appeared to be nearly devoid of electric power. The few lights were so dim, they could have been lanterns of some sort. Only the eerie bluish-white light from the ugly Unit No. 4 presented an image of power.

Gourgen reduced their speed to half as they passed between the plant and the city. The photographs had been accurate except for that glow coming from the interior of the jagged wreckage. They could see the sand glowing, shimmering and smoldering hardly dampening the intensity of the light from the reactor.

"This is bad," said Anatoly.

Gourgen circled the building a couple of times as he slowed the helicopter further. Other than the glow, the exhaust stack with its broad, red and white, horizontal stripes, and trellis support structure occupied some prominence. The thin veil of smoke still rising from the interior wreckage of the damaged reactor floated off to the northwest. He set up for their first pass over the reactor with his approach from the south.

"Are you ready for this?"

"The sooner we get this over with, the sooner we can get out of here."

"Then, let's do it."

Gourgen pulled back some more on the stick to raise the nose and slow the helicopter to a crawling 20 kilometers per hour. The beam now lit up the interior of their aircraft. Gourgen adjusted his altitude to about 100 meters above the damaged Central Hall and slightly offset so they could look down out the left side of the cockpit. As they approached the jagged edge of the building, the aircraft began to shake with increasing violence. Heat overwhelmed the air conditioning system now on full cold. The acrid smell of ozone made it through the environmental filters. Both pilots coughed hard as the ozone assaulted the lining of their throats and nasal passages. The instrument panel blurred with violent shaking. They struggled to assess the scene below them.

The sand accumulating in the bottom of the building took on a strange translucent, yellowish hue. The glowing details of the biological cover could be seen beside the bright, open mouth of the reactor. The sand appeared to do little to dampen the nuclear fire within the rubble. The enormity of the problem facing the engineers made other considerations pale.

As the helicopter approached the north side of the building, Gourgen pushed the stick forward and pulled up on the collective to accelerate out of the inferno. He climbed to about 500 meters and set up a wide orbit around the destroyed powerplant.

"I am not particularly interested in doing that again," said Gourgen.

"How on earth are they going to cover that thing?"

"I do not know."

"A 35 ton flat plate," Anatoly said as though he was thinking out loud about the enormous problem of trying to precisely position a large object in such horrible conditions.

"I know. What are these guys thinking? What could have caused such damage?"

"It looks like some huge bomb went off in there."

Gourgen felt the rolling waves of nausea building within his gut. He also noticed the stabbing ache in many of his joints. "Are you feeling sick?" he asked.

"Yes. It must be the radiation."

Gourgen could barely reach the bags provided by the Air Force personnel. He wretched violently. The nausea continued to build. The usual relief did not come. The sickening feeling spread like a wildfire consuming his entire body. The accomplished experimental test pilot fought to fly the aircraft between the horrific expulsions from deep within his torso.

"How are you doing?" asked Gourgen once the worst seemed to be past. Not a sound came back over the intercom. The seat arrangement made it impossible for Gourgen to see what Anatoly's condition was in the front seat. "Anatoly Demjanovich, answer me."

The sound of vomiting filled his headset. "Are . . . you . . . satis . . . fied?"

"Sorry my friend. I was doing the same thing. I was just worried about you."

"Wait."

Gourgen continued to circle the glowing plant. The dusk light in the West was fading. They did not have much time left. Gourgen knew they needed to make one more evaluation pass although this time at a slightly lower altitude and directly over the reactor as if they were actually lifting the plate into place.

"Are you feeling any better?"

"Yes, a little."

"I think we need to make a practice pass directly over the spot to establish checkpoints."

"You are kidding, right?"

"If we do not do it now, it will be more difficult later in the big bird."

Anatoly thought about the situation. "All right. Let's get this done, so we can get out of this hideous place."

The cooler air felt good. There was no doubt the terrible conditions near the reactor told them no human being belonged there, but they also told them the place had to be buried. They needed to complete their evaluation.

Gourgen slowed the helicopter and descended as he turned toward the beam of light shooting skyward. He quickly judged the potential checkpoints and adjusted his altitude to about 80 meters above the remains of the Unit No. 4 Central Hall. He was now lined up to pass directly over the reactor. As they approached the building, Gourgen slowed the aircraft gradually as though they had a long-line external load beneath them.

The physiological symptoms of radiation poisoning returned more rapidly this time. Gourgen fought the mounting nausea as they passed over the edge to the building. The violent shaking of the helicopter added substantially to the headache pounding in his head. This is really stupid, Gourgen said to himself.

The veteran test pilot and Hero of the Soviet Union gently and expertly brought the attack helicopter to a stop directly over the hole of the nuclear volcano. The rising waves of heat made holding his position nearly impossible. The collective was nearly full down, and yet the five metric tons of metal still tended to rise. Gourgen used a variety of learned techniques trying to simulate precisely placing the imaginary load beneath them. The vomiting convulsions began to wrench his body although nothing came up. His head felt like someone was driving a wedge directly down the middle of his skull, and his heart pounded heavily in his chest causing his whole body to pulse with the rapidly mounting blood pressure. He instinctively glanced down at the shaking instrument panel. The numbers on the engine dials were unreadable, but the little red limit lights told him the superheated air entering the engine inlets was running the turbine temperature beyond acceptable limits. He gave up any further attempt to complete his assessment.

Gourgen pushed the stick forward. The nose dropped. They should have descended. Instead, the aircraft just accelerated. As they moved away from the building, the helicopter sank rapidly, no longer buoyed by the thermal currents from the partially buried reactor. Engine temperatures dropped quickly. Gourgen pulled up sharply on the collective to keep from descending too low and to continue their acceleration from the hell behind them.

His eyes burned and watered partly from the irritation of the ozone but more predominately from the insult of ionizing radiation. He wiped away the induced tears to set a rough course back to the staging area.

The rusty taste of his own blood took the place of his empty vomiting. His reaction was like nothing he had ever experienced nor heard of in his life. How the hell do they expect us to do this job in such conditions, Gourgen admonished himself.

Gourgen's symptoms slowly ebbed as the lights of the Air Force staging area came into detailed view. He made a wide arc to check for potential traffic. There was none. He found the area where Colonel Nestrov told them to land for decontamination at the northeast corner of the field. He had not heard from Anatoly but knew the best thing to do was get him on the ground where he could get proper medical assistance.

He found the wind direction although it was light and not a real concern. He turned into the wind for his landing approach. A half dozen men in what looked like plastic space suits waddled out to the aircraft with hoses. They directed him to position the helicopter in a slight pit lined with some heavy plastic material. They had to capture all the wash liquids.

Once he had the collective full down, he signaled the lead person with a thumbs up. They immediately began spraying what looked in the flood lights like a reddish liquid. The biological filters kept most of the smell out of the cockpit although a very faint decaying odor filled the small space. Gourgen could not tell whether the smell was coming from the exterior or interior. He checked his body. Waves of nausea still gripped him. The taste of blood filled his mouth; some had trickled out. He tried to wipe it up. His flight overalls were soaking wet. Some of his vomit stained his thighs.

The decontamination crew completed two full washes of the aircraft before they signaled Gourgen to reposition the aircraft to his parking area. Once the short transition was complete, he promptly shutdown the two engines and stopped the rotor. Gourgen scrambled out of his cockpit ignoring the pain in his joints and underestimated muscle fatigue. He opened the front cockpit door on the left side. Anatoly glanced weakly toward his friend. A red, frothy coating covered his mouth and chin.

"Medical," shouted Gourgen.

Four men in white overalls who had been walking toward them broke into a run to cover the last 20 meters as quickly as possible. Gourgen started to unstrap his friend.

"Can you move?" Gourgen asked.

Anatoly moved his shoulders in a feeble attempt but could not muster the strength.

"Medical," Gourgen now screamed.

As he fought his own fatigue to pull Anatoly from the cockpit, several hands grasped his hips and pulled him back. The medical team moved expertly as though they had done this many times. They extricated Anatoly, strapped him to a stretcher, then moved him quickly into an ambulance that had just pulled up. One of the medical technicians shone a small light at Gourgen's face to check his pupils, then pulled his upper and lower eye lids away from this eye.

"This one needs to go as well," the man announced.

Two of the medical personnel returned to help Gourgen into the ambulance. The small truck sped away jostling the occupants, but covering whatever distance it was to the field hospital. The medical people worked quickly on both of them. They inserted two intravenous drips, one in each arm; one bottle had a clear liquid and the other was a light yellowish color. They gave him a thorough triage examination. The doctor directed several additional actions.

"You are going to recover quickly," the doctor stated.

"Is he going to be all right?" asked Gourgen as his treatment diminished in intensity.

"I will check on his condition for you."

The man left. A moderately attractive young nurse began to clean him up. Gourgen began to feel better. He was not quite sure whether it was the treatment or the vision tending to him, but the result was good. The doctor returned.

"Your friend is in a little worse shape than you, but he should recover as well."

"Good."

"Now, we need you to rest."

"We are supposed to debrief the flight."

"Tomorrow. Tonight, you must rest. So, just relax. The nurses will take good care of you."

Gourgen felt safe. The warm blanket of his fatigue pulled him into sleep.

# 15

*10:18, Wednesday, 30.April.1986*
*Military Response Team Camp*
*70 kilometers east of Chernobyl, Ukraine, USSR*

"Where am I?" Gourgen Karapetyan asked the attending nurse, a young, healthy woman in the white garb of a military nurse.

"You are in a field hospital in Northern Ukraine."

"What day is it?"

"It is Wednesday, the thirtieth of April."

Time seemed oddly beyond his grasp. The disorientation and confusion brought modest but distinct waves of nausea. Gourgen knew something was wrong. He had tubes plugged into both arms, and he was in a crude but neat field hospital. "What year?"

"What year?"

"Yes."

"1986."

Some of the misty confusion began to clear. He was not as lost as he worried. "I came here yesterday?"

"Yes, you did. You flew over the reactor. You received a large dose of radiation and became very sick. We have been treating you."

Gourgen considered the information, then remembered his friend. "How is Anatoly Grishchenko?"

"He is being treated as well."

"But, will he be all right?"

"The doctors say, yes."

"What do you say?"

"It is not my place."

"However . . ."

"He was in worse shape than you. He was quite ill, but he

seems to be responding to treatment."

"Good."

"Now, you should rest," she said touching him on the shoulder. She smiled, then left the small compartment.

Colonel Nestrov walked in as the nurse disappeared. His grave expression turned into a feeble smile, then he removed his smooth, stiff, peaked, service hat and placed in under his left arm. "How are you feeling, Karapetyan?"

"Not particularly well, if you want to know the truth."

"You spent too much time over the reactor."

"Too much time. You said twenty seconds. I think we were only over the reactor for perhaps ten or fifteen seconds . . . not long."

"It does not take much time."

"No, it certainly does not."

Nestrov stared at Gourgen as if he was considering some admonishment for insubordination. Whatever his thoughts, he decided to change the subject. "What did you determine."

"That whoever did this to the Motherland should be shot."

"Yes, well, you are not alone there."

"In my humble opinion, any attempt to precisely place a heavy load will be nearly impossible . . . only luck will do it. Those are the worst flying conditions I have experienced. In addition, you are asking us to exceed the qualified, external load, lift capacity of the aircraft by 75%. No aircraft can take that."

"I need to get the engineers in here to talk to you. If their idea is not going to work, you need to tell them what you can do, so they can modify their plans."

"Bring them in, then. We did a slow fly-by to survey the site, then we did a simulated approach as though we were carrying a heavy, long-line, external load. The heat still rising from that place is incredible. Trying to precisely control the positioning of the load is beyond our capability. Something must be done to reduce the heat and radiation if we are to have any chance of success."

"The current plan is for the Air Force to continue dropping

sand and boron into the reactor cavity. The scientists tell us another few days worth of sand should have significant results."

"We will need it."

"Certainly." Nestrov looked beyond Gourgen as he thought of other things. His eyes returned to the prone test pilot. "Let me see when the doctors can release you and Grishchenko. I need you to talk to the engineers before you leave."

Gourgen nodded his head. The colonel nodded in return, then departed. Gourgen allowed himself to give in to the fatigue. He tried to eliminate all his thoughts and let sleep claim his consciousness.

He could not tell how long he had been asleep when the nurse unintentionally woke him to take his vital signs. Actually, he did not really care. She wrote down her findings.

"Your blood pressure is back within the normal range. The doctor said we can release you now. However, the doctors require that you report to Moscow Clinic Number Six for full evaluation. They are the experts, up there. We are only a field hospital. They have all the proper equipment. So, they require you to be evaluated by the experts before returning to duty. Can you get to Clinic Number Six tomorrow?"

Gourgen nodded in recognition and acknowledgment. The nurse set down her clipboard, then carefully removed the intravenous needles from his arms. Once she was satisfied with her work, she helped him sit up. Gourgen felt slightly dizzy as though he had just donated a half liter of blood. He waited for the sensation to pass, then slowly stood. His body began to compensate properly. He shed his hospital garb for his still damp flight suit.

"Where is Grishchenko?"

"Follow me," she answered without looking back to see if he was having any problems.

The nurse led him to another tent with fewer but larger compartments. More medical equipment filled the added space. She motioned to one compartment, then pulled back the flap.

Anatoly Grishchenko lay in a bed similar to Gourgen's with

what appeared to be the same tubes in his arms. He was awake.

"How are you feeling, my friend?"

"I have felt worse."

Gourgen chuckled. "That is not something I care to do again, frankly."

"At least you got a good tan."

"I did not notice," he answered looking for a mirror that did not exist. "You did as well."

"Damn radiation. Scary stuff."

"Yes. Did they tell you when they are going to release you?"

"They said later today."

Gourgen considered their options. "I will go talk to Colonel Nestrov and the engineers, so we can finish up here. If it is not too late today, perhaps we can make it back to Zhukovsky tonight."

"It will be nice to sleep in my own bed."

Gourgen laughed, again, with his friend then left the tent. He asked for directions to the operations tent where he thought he could find Nestrov. Several military personnel, too busy to take the time to assist, pointed him in a general direction that added time to his search. Eventually, he recognized a small grouping of tents. Luckily, he found Colonel Nestrov inside the same tent they started from yesterday.

Gourgen waited just inside the entrance until Nestrov noticed him and managed to separate himself from the conversation.

"They released you."

Gourgen nodded.

"Excellent. How are you feeling?"

"Not the best, to be honest, but I think I will survive."

"Yes. None of us wanted this little exercise."

"Right. The medical folks expect to release Anatoly this afternoon. We would like to return north."

"Your aircraft has been fully serviced and checked for contamination. You are as clean as it gets."

"Does that mean we are safe?"

"Yes. You are safe to leave the area . . . one of the nice features of the Mil Two Four."

Gourgen did not want to pursue this line of exchange. "I would like to talk to the engineers who are working on this giant plate."

"I will get the chief engineer down here. It will take about an hour."

"That should work. I would like to get this done, so Anatoly and I can depart as soon as he is released. We have a two and a half hour flight back."

"I will get some men on it right away," Nestrov said, nodded his head and turned to issue a set of orders to his men.

Gourgen decided a long, slow walk in the warm spring sun would make him feel better. He decided to take a counterclockwise direction around the perimeter of the field that had become a makeshift aerodrome. The assortment of aircraft parked in the field was impressive. Half were Mi-8 medium lift helicopters, the workhorse of the military. The remainder were an even mix of Mi-6's, the venerable heavy lift machine, and Mi-26's, the replacement for the Mi-6 and often referred to in the West as the C-130 of helicopters. His Mi-24 attack helicopter was the only one of its kind parked at the field.

As Gourgen walked and watched, helicopters took off headed west toward Chernobyl. New aircraft arrived, none of them using the decontamination station. They had to be really new aircraft, not just returning aircraft that had departed earlier. There was nearly a regiment's worth of rotary wing assets in this field and half again more stationed at Pripyat, probably too contaminated to be cleaned or allowed to depart the exclusion zone. None of the transport helicopters had sealed interiors like the Mi-24. Once dust and other contaminants penetrated the interior spaces and compartments, cleaning would be an impossible task. That meant most of the aircraft he saw would never leave this area, doomed to extinction.

The warm sun felt good. Watching the busy operations at the field brought pride to his heart. The accident had been just five days ago, and there was already an impressive armada of Frontal Aviation assets committed to the dangerous mission. He noticed the time as well as his mounting fatigue. Yesterday's nightmare had taken more from him than he had imagined. He made it only a third of the way around the perimeter, so he headed out into the field to shorten his return leg. He made several detours to stay a respectable distance from aircraft starting up, taking off or landing. He arrived at the operations tent 15 minutes later than expected.

Two men in casual civilian attire sat at the far end of the tent. As Gourgen entered the main portion of the tent, the two men stood. Colonel Nestrov motioned for Gourgen to come closer. Another Air Force colonel, a strikingly handsome, tall, robust man, joined them.

"Gourgen Karapetyan, this is Senior Professor Yuri Rotagov, the chief designer for the containment building, Engineer Gregori Lalingko, his assistant, and Colonel Kalasnikov, the commanding officer of the aviation regiment you see outside." They shook hands. Gourgen recognized the famous, or perhaps renown, Air Force colonel. His uncle, as he recalled, developed the famous series of Kalasnikov rifles known all over the world for their ruggedness. "Mister Karapetyan is the chief test pilot for the Mil Design Bureau and will fly the bio cover lift mission. They did their assessment flight yesterday evening."

"What did you think?" asked Rotagov.

"As I have been briefed, you want us to lift a very heavy access cover to be precisely placed in the roof of the containment building."

"Yes."

"And, it weights somewhere between 25 and 35 metric tons."

"Closer to 35 at this stage."

"Well, then, I think we have a problem."

"How so?"

"First, the maximum qualified, external load, lift capacity of our most capable helicopter is only 20 tons. You are asking us to nearly double that capacity. If it is at all possible, lifting that much weight will probably consume the useful life of the aircraft."

"We are sacrificing scores of valuable aircraft in this operation," interjected Kalasnikov.

"I understand, so wasting another aircraft would not be noticed."

The four men stared at Gourgen as if he spoke some indiscernible language.

"If that is how you wish to think of it, then so be it," answered Kalasnikov in a very calm, quiet tone.

"What do you think the maximum achievable lift weight to be?" asked Rotagov.

Gourgen stared at the senior engineers, performed some mental calculations and considered his answer. "I am certain we can do 25 tons, although we have never done that much weight before on the hook. With some work, we might squeak out 30 tons and perhaps recover the aircraft with some major refurbishment. I have no idea whether we can even reach 35 tons without building a new helicopter. Our engineers will have to complete a substantial analysis, and we would certainly have to accomplish significant modifications. If we did lift that weight, the aircraft would undoubtedly be an unusable heap of metal afterward."

"I was lead to believe the Mil Two Six set the world vertical lift record at something like 56 metric tons," Rotagov said.

"Well, your information is partially correct, Senior Professor Rotagov. The helicopter lift record was set by the Mil Two Six. However, the 56 ton weight was total mass. The empty weight of the aircraft is about 28 tons. Plus, the extra payload mass for the record flight was carefully distributed throughout the interior; it was not on the hook. There is a significant difference. Also, the aircraft used a rather lengthy rolling takeoff, and it was not a vertical lift, but a record for mass lifted by a helicopter to an altitude of 2 kilometers." He paused to get a response. None came. "As I said, the most weight we have put on the hook is 20 tons, and this will definitely be a vertical lift. So, they are not the same."

"That explains the error," Rotagov answered. Gourgen nodded his head. "Can you make 35 tons? If not, we have a very serious redesign problem."

"I would be foolish to say, yes or no. I fly these things. I do not design them. The engineers will have to determine the limits of what can be done." Gourgen considered other elements, and the group waited for his contemplation. "We surely will not be able to have much fuel on board, so we will have to get it in place on the first attempt, if we can lift it at all."

"What do you need to do for that determination, and how long will it take?"

"Under normal circumstances, I would say six months."

"We do not have that long," came the chorus response from Nestrov and Rotagov.

"With the proper resources and commitment, I suppose we could do 25 tons in a few days, 30 tons in a few weeks or so, and 35 tons, I do not know, maybe several months."

"This needs to be done as soon as possible," said Rotagov. "Every day, every minute, that thing remains open to the atmosphere allows substantial contamination of our air and our sacred Motherland. We must seal this thing soon."

Gourgen stared at the chief engineer again. No one spoke. Who ever did this should be shot, Gourgen reiterated to himself, again. All of this is absolutely crazy. The sad part is, they are certainly correct. The country, if not the world, is depending upon them to get this done soon.

"I will make a few telephone calls, if I may, while I await Anatoly's release. We will get started right away."

"Anatoly?" asked Rotagov.

"My friend and fellow pilot. He is still being treated for the radiation poisoning we received yesterday."

"I am sorry."

"So are we, but then again, we are not alone, are we?"

"No," answered the two colonels in unison.

"Can you show me some drawings or sketches of what you are thinking about for this containment building and the cover?"

The assistant engineer retrieved a roll of drawings from the table at the far end of the tent. They moved to a map table. Lalingko unrolled the drawings.

"Here are some preliminary sketches completed just yesterday. As you can see, the plan calls for reinforced, buttressed, concrete walls to be built completely around the Unit Four building. A series of interior shelves will be added to form what will become the roof. The next to last roof element will hold the heavy biological cover. A lighter weight, larger diameter, final close-out cover, of perhaps 10 tons will complete the building."

"The distance between these top two levels."

"Two point five meters."

"So, we must thread the heavy plate through the top hole and precisely place it over the second hole."

"Yes."

Gourgen laughed hard. These men are crazy, he said to himself. "We have one meter of margin to get this through. Do you have any idea how hard that is regardless of all the other detrimental conditions?"

"Yes," answered Kalasnikov.

"Well, we shall see. Is there any way to install some guides to assist the placement?"

Rotagov opened his mouth to speak, but hesitated as he considered Gourgen's suggestion. "We had not thought of that. It is not clear how we might do it, but it is worth a try. All the construction will be done by remote control using a set of gantry cranes, mechanical manipulators and concrete pumps."

"Cranes?"

"We cannot get one or several to do this kind of lift. We need the helicopter. It is the only way."

Gourgen shook his head. "Any assistance might make the difference."

"We will give it the best effort we can."

"Who could ask for more."

"Anything else?" asked Nestrov.

"I am certain there shall be other questions as we try to expand the envelope."

"Please stay in touch as you progress. We must match our

efforts," said Rotagov.

"Agreed."

"Then, we are adjourned," Nestrov announced.

"If I may use a telephone, I can make some arrangements from here," said Gourgen. "I shall set up a design meeting tomorrow morning as well as give them something to think about overnight."

Nestrov's expression turned from confidence to puzzlement. "Didn't the doctors tell you to report to Clinic Number Six for evaluation prior to returning to duty?"

"Yes, they did."

"Well, then, I would suggest you do exactly what they have told you to do."

"I thought this was a national emergency priority. The doctors can wait."

"No, they can't," Nestrov said sternly. "We need everyone as healthy as we can keep them. Losing a day to ensure your health will not be the deciding factor here."

"Very well. Then, I shall set up the meetings for day after tomorrow. Now, can I use a telephone?"

"You can use the telephone in the communications tent, next to this one," answered Nestrov. "I must caution you to keep your calls for technical purposes only, and no discussion about what has happened here, what you have seen or experienced, or why we are doing this."

"People know. It has been on the news. My wife knows."

"They know there has been an accident, but they do not know the extent of damage; and, we certainly do not want to cause a panic among the people."

Gourgen chuckled in the most sarcastic manner he could. "Right," he sneered as he turned to leave the tent.

He found the communications tent, told the chief what he was there to do, and waited patiently as the man checked on his authorization. Satisfied, the man showed Gourgen to one of many tables at one end of the tent with several telephones on each table. He briefed Gourgen on how to place a call and repeated the information constraints provided by Colonel Nestrov.

Gourgen first called the Mil main engineering offices on Sokolnichesky Street in Moscow. In case anyone was listening in, he talked to the General Designer, Marat Tishchenko, as much to inform him of the tasks they were soon to embark upon as to seek his support. The next call went to Mark Vineberg, one of the deputy general designers under Tishchenko. Gourgen gave Vineberg a more thorough briefing on the task. After some discussion, they agreed to a set of meetings as soon as Gourgen could return to Moscow, complete his medical evaluation at Clinic No. 6 and meet with the leadership team. They set the meeting time for Friday morning. He called the Flight Test Center to tell them his return plans and the need for special military tools to change certain elements on the aircraft. Lastly, he looked around to see who might be paying attention, then placed a call to Ludmilla.

"Hello," she said.

"Milla, it is me."

"I have been so worried, Gourgen. Are you all right?"

"We flew yesterday evening. Both Anatoly and I were sick, but I feel much better now. As soon as they release Anatoly, we will fly home."

"He is in the hospital?"

"Yes, more like a precaution. They say we will both recover fully."

"Oh Gourgen. I want you home."

"We should be able to make it by supper time."

"I shall look for you."

They traded, I love you's, before he hung up the handset. He returned to the command tent, briefed Nestrov and Kalasnikov on the meetings set up for Friday. They traded telephone numbers and communications procedures to be used until this job was done.

Gourgen shook hands with everyone, then left to check on Anatoly. He was feeling a little better when he was released at mid-afternoon. They took off for the return flight an hour later. This was going to be yet another unique and difficult assignment.

# 16

*22:00, Wednesday, 30.April.1986*
*Linstornborg Weather Station*
*Linstornborg, Sweden*

Evar Erickson filled his cup with strong, black coffee and returned to the Sunday newspaper from Stockholm. He had completed his hourly weather observation as required by his duty procedures. A moderate breeze blew from the east-southeast adding some chill to the early spring night. There were no weather systems in the area, so he did not have to increase the frequency of his observations. It would be a quiet night. He looked forward to reading every word in the Sunday edition including all the advertisements. It had become an odd measure of success.

Evar liked the night shift from 20:00 to 04:00. It was the most peaceful time of the day even for a remote weather and environmental observation station. It was also the only shift where he could be alone. His solitary duty enabled him to read – a true passion. Evar read everything he could get his hands on – newspapers, magazines, books, anything. He liked fiction the most — thrillers. He was usually the first to buy books by the English authors, John le Carre and Fredrick Forsythe, and the American authors, Michael Crichton and Tom Clancy. In truth, there were no favorites. Evar also appreciated a non-fiction book, now and then, if the subject attracted his attention.

The observer had finished the news section as well as the sports and business sections. It was the Arts section that caused him to stop. An article about perennial meteorite showers reminded him of the wondrous beauty the brief streaks provided across the night sky. Clouds precluded any observation of the Lyrids shower, the fragmentary remnants of the Comet Thatcher, on the 22nd of April. The Eta Aquarids shower from the Comet Halley would enter the sky above on the 5th of May, one of his duty nights. Evar could not resist the temptation.

Erickson turned off all the exterior lights and shuttered the windows to keep as much light as possible inside the small building on the medium size hill some 100 kilometers north of the big city of Stockholm. The lights of the city would be a faint glow on the southern horizon.

Outside, he stood several meters from the building and closed his eyes. The cool breeze with the ever-present scent of pine made the moment idyllic. After several minutes of letting his eyes adjust to the darkness, Evar tilted his head back and opened his eyes. The vast array of stars blanketed the sky from horizon to horizon. He picked out the marker stars, Polaris, Vega, Regulus, and Arcturus. With just his eyes, the stars were magnificent. What he really needed was a telescope, so he could explore the heavens in between observations or other duties.

Evar held his arms out with his palms up as if he was holding up the heavens. "This is why I love this job," he said aloud adding an intimacy between him and his God. "Thank you, Lord."

He scanned the dome of stars several times before he returned to the painful brightness of the interior lights. With his eyes closed, he switched on the exterior lights just in case someone might come to visit. It had only happened once in the last year, but you just never knew when some manager from the Ministry would arrive to check up on him.

As he blinked to allow his eyes to adjust to the light, he turned to face the console just beyond the wide shelf that served as his table and workbench, and now held the Sunday newspaper still spread across the top. A blinking red light caught his attention.

Erickson walked over to the left segment of the panel to read the label beneath the blinking red light. RADIATION. Something must be wrong, he told himself. The needle of the dial above it fluctuated between one and two on the ten digit dial face. It was the first time Evar had seen that warning light illuminate since his initial training course six years earlier.

Evar pulled out the manual, checked the index and found the correct page. The light was triggered when one roentgen of ionizing radiation was detected. He tapped the display several times, thinking that it might be faulty. After all, instrument failures and erroneous alarms were not particularly uncommon. He sat down, rolling his chair across the vinyl covered floor to be directly in front of the left panel.

The red light continued to blink. He stared at the dial face. The needle bounced. He thought it might pass. He tried to see a trend. If he averaged the fluctuations over the span of, say, ten minutes, then perhaps he could tell whether it was some aberration, anomaly or some strange moment intended to disturb his peace and tranquillity. Evar stared at the dial in an almost trance like state until the needle happened to remain above three for the necessary three samplings taken one second apart. The 'bong-bong-bong' of the alarm broke his concentration.

Erickson turned the page of his manual. The instructions told him to call the hazard desk in the Ministry of Interior Affairs. He dialed the number dutifully.

"Hazard desk," announced the man on the other end of the telephone line.

"This is Evar Erickson at the Linstornborg Weather Station. I have a radiation alarm on my environmental panel."

"Just a moment." the man said.

Evar could picture the duty officer checking his procedures manual, other pieces of information and perhaps other sites. Whatever he was doing took longer than he thought it should. Erickson considered hanging up the telephone and redailing to force the person to re-answer the bell.

"We have no other indications at the moment, nor do we have any reports of leaks at any of the nuclear power stations. I think you might have a faulty system."

"As I suspected. I have never seen one of these go off before."

"Recheck the system. If it still persists, you might want to take a hand-held measurement. That should tell us whether the instrument is working properly or not."

"I will do that. Thank you."

The man on the other end hung up before Evar could say goodbye. He rolled back over to the left panel. He pushed the silence button to stop the alarm. It was becoming irritating anyway. Evar looked at the needle. It was now moving in larger fluctuations between two and four.

Evar turned to the troubleshooting portion of the manual. He found the section that dealt with the radiation detection system. He read the procedures to himself, memorized the circuit number, then went to the main electrical power panel, found the correct circuit breaker, and cycled it off, then back on. He returned to the control panel, rolled to the center, paged through his computer screens until he found the correct one. Using the manual, he entered the specific instructions required to reset the system. When he reached the final step, he placed his finger on the ENTER key, turned his head to the radiation detector, and pushed the key.

In less than a second, the needle shot up to four, then five. The red light illuminated immediately, and three seconds later the alarm sounded again.

"This is not good," he said aloud, then silenced the audio alarm, again.

Evar found his master key and went to the storage room. He retrieved the hand-held, conventional, Geiger counter. He checked the setting on the lowest, most sensitive scale, left the audio on, did the required self-test, then switched it on. The peculiar clicking he had heard at the movies came to him. It showed one to two inside the building.

"This is really not good."

Evar Erickson held the small, gray, clicking, box in front of him as if it was too hot to allow near his body. He opened the door. The clicking immediately got louder. The needle jumped up to five.

"Dear God Almighty. This is real."

He rushed back into the building and dialed the Ministry.

"Hazard desk."

"This is Erickson at Linstornborg, again. This is real. I have done everything including the hand-held measurement. There is something out here."

"Stand-by."

Evar waited. The man returned more quickly this time. "We have one other site giving similar indications. I need to call the nuclear power facilities. I will call you back." The man hung up.

Erickson closed the door and switched off the hand device. He sat there staring at the blinking red light wondering what could possibly be causing radiation. Then, he remembered his Navy days. Once in a great while, one of the engineering types mistakenly pumped the bilges while they were in port and occasionally they pumped residual oil into the harbor. The event was a simple mistake and caused everyone to scramble so the contamination did not spread and foul the water. Maybe, this was like that. Some engineer at one of the nuclear power stations mistakenly 'pumped their bilges,' if there was such a thing.

Evar returned to his newspaper, wanting to think of something else. Then, a lightning bolt hit him. He jumped out of his chair and sprang to the large wall map behind the control panel. He found the four red dots that marked the locations of the nuclear power stations in Central Sweden. They were located to the west and southwest. He looked at the large dials that displayed the wind – 120° at 5 knots – east-southeast. There was only five kilometers between the hill that Linstornborg Station sat on and the Baltic Sea. There were no nuclear power stations in that direction.

Evar's mind raced. Maybe, it was a nuclear powered ship or submarine. That would mean a serious accident and lives would be at stake. He started to dial the same telephone number, then he froze. The Soviets had nuclear power stations. He had read several articles about them. They were very proud of their accomplishments in the electrification of the country, especially the rural areas, and all because of the abundant supply of electricity from the many nuclear power stations. He dialed the number.

"Hazard desk," came a new voice. The tension in those two words told him more.

"This is Erickson at Linstornborg. I am the one who first reported the radiation alarm."

"Yes, yes. what is it?"

"I am sorry. I know you must be busy."

"Yes, we are, so please get to your point quickly."

"The prevailing wind is from the east-southeast up here."

"Yes . . . so?"

"There are no nuclear power plants in that direction except in the Soviet Union."

A pause or hesitation punctuated the terse exchange. "That's it, by God. Peter," he shouted to someone else, "it's the Soviet Union." Evar heard many voices in the background. "Thank you, Mister Erickson. We must go."

"Wait!"

"Yes."

"What is going on?"

"We have radiation indications from virtually every observation station in Central Sweden, now. Some readings are higher than yours. We suspect there has been a major accident of some kind. The Minister has been informed. We are currently checking other countries, and you have given us a valuable piece of information. So, thank you for your extra work. Now, I really must be going."

"Thank you," Evar said, before the connection was broken.

Radiation scared him. He had read enough books that had something to do with radiation whether it was science fiction or the story of the bombing of Hiroshima and Nagasaki. This was something to worry about. He tried to remember the several books he read about survival after a nuclear holocaust. He found a workman's filter mask and put it on over his nose and mouth. The lungs and blood system were very susceptible to radioactive particles. Something was out there. He did not want to become a casualty.

Evar looked at the dial. It was now averaging over five. What could possibly have happened. Maybe the United States and the Soviet Union had begun an exchange of nuclear tipped missiles. Maybe this was there first indication of World War III – another cataclysm in just this century.

Erickson clasped his hands together and bowed his head. "Dear God above," he said aloud although muffled by his mask, "please protect us from whatever is out there, and please Lord, do not let this be as bad as it seems. I trust in you, Lord God. Do not let harm come to us."

# 17

*09:30, Friday, 2.May.1986*
*Mil Design Bureau*
*2 Sokolnichesky Street*
*Moscow, Russia, USSR*

As Gourgen Karapetyan had arranged, the design meeting took place at the four story, conventional, office building in Moscow. The small but distinguished group gathered in the General Designer's conference room, a dark wood panel room festooned with historic photographs of successes and notable events for the organization since its founding by Mikhail Leontyevich Mil. The floor space was fully occupied by a large conference table and perhaps two dozen chairs.

At the meeting, as Gourgen had requested, were Marat Tishchenko, General Designer of the Mil Design Bureau; Mark Vineberg, Deputy General Designer for developmental design; and Sergei Dematrov, Deputy Chief Designer for the Mi-26. Each of them possessed unique expertise and historical knowledge of the Mi-26 heavy lift helicopter.

"Good to have you back with us, Gourgen," began Tishchenko. "I understand you and Grishchenko were hospitalized after your flight." Gourgen nodded his head. "How are you feeling now?"

"Not the best I have felt, but acceptable."

"Radiation?"

"Yes. Anatoly Demjanovich is a little worse off than me. He decided to stay home."

"I hope he feels better soon."

"The doctors say he will recover."

"What about you?" asked Dematrov.

"Both of us had just about every medical test known to man,

yesterday, at Clinic Number Six. They tells us we will not have any long terms effects."

"I wonder if they are telling you the truth," Vineberg mused in muffled tones.

"There is no way to tell, I suppose, so I must accept their findings."

"Before we get too deep," said Tishchenko, "I shall ask Gourgen to give us a quick sketch of the problem."

"As you know, two days ago I flew down to Chernobyl with Anatoly Grishchenko from Gromov."

"What did the place look like?" Vineberg asked.

"Like a massive bomb went off inside the plant."

"So, there really was a nuclear explosion."

"No. They said it was steam, but the reactor is destroyed and open, spewing radioactive material into the atmosphere and across the land."

"How tragic," added Tishchenko.

"What does Gromov have to do with this?" asked Dematrov trying to change the subject.

"They are apparently doing some external load research, and Anatoly Demjanovich has been flying a few missions with me to gain experience. He will fly the tests. Plus, he grew up near the power plant."

"So, this is not their mission?"

"No. I was asked by the Ministry of Defense to fly this. I am not certain whether Anatoly will fly the actual mission with me or not. I surmise he will demand to be with me. We will cross that bridge when we get to it. Is there any objection to him flying with me?" The three senior aviation engineers shook their heads to indicate there were no objections. "We were briefed on the extent of this disastrous accident at the nuclear power plant as well as the plans for containment of the radioactive debris," he said, stretching the limits of his communications restrictions.

"So, there was an explosion," said Vineberg, again, "as the Western press has loudly speculated."

"The Press?"

"Yes. It was in the newspapers today. According to the report, the Americans detected something, apparently with their satellites, then a weather station in Sweden detected radiation a few days ago, and now Europe is aflame with condemnation."

Gourgen considered the information. He did not much care whether it was public knowledge or not, but if the radiation had been detected in Sweden, then the whole world would soon know what happened at Chernobyl. There was no point withholding facts from his countrymen when the rest of the world would have more information. "They should be angry. This insult to the Motherland, and perhaps other countries, is most tragic."

"Did they tell you exactly what happened?" asked Tishchenko.

"They said is was steam build-up, but the end of the story is the reactor is open and burning. They are trying to stop the nuclear reaction by using sand and some other substance. They want to build a sarcophagus, as they call it, to seal the wreckage and stop the contamination."

"Tell us about this plate," Vineberg requested.

"This structure will be built up around the damaged building. It will have a series of roof levels. The second to last level will have this plate."

"You said, 35 tons," Tishchenko interjected.

"Yes."

"I thought you were kidding," said Dematrov.

"I wish I was."

"That is impossible."

"Perhaps, but that is what they want us to determine."

"Why don't they use a crane?"

"They cannot erect sufficient cranes and the appropriate controls in time nor without exposing many more people. A helicopter is the only way."

"We might reach 25 tons, but 35 . . . that is crazy," said Dematrov.

"So, what do they want us to do?" asked Tishchenko.

"They want us to determine what maximum weight we can lift as soon as possible."

"We have the world record with the Mil Two Six at 56 metric tons, total weight," Vineberg said as if none of them could remember the extraordinary effort they made a few years earlier.

"Internal, not external," responded Dematrov. "The most we have carried on the hook is 20 metric tons."

"We have done overload calculations to 22 or 23 tons, I can't remember exactly," Vineberg added. "There was some margin remaining. So, perhaps we could get to 24 or 25 tons."

"Let us tell them 25 tons, then," Dematrov recommended.

"The country is in mortal danger with this nuclear reactor open and burning. The country needs us to do our absolute best," Tishchenko instructed. "I want the question – what will it take to reach 35 tons – to be answered. We must do everything humanly possible to meet this demand."

Gourgen looked at the two principal engineers as their minds considered the implications. All four of them knew what the request meant. While every aeronautical engineer has a reasonable idea of what might be accomplished, this request was far beyond reasonable. If the new one-time value could be reached, it would take an extraordinary effort in almost every area – structures, modifications, aerodynamics, propulsion and pilotage.

The Mi-26 held the world's record for mass lifted by a helicopter – 56.7 metric tons, 125,000 pounds – to an altitude of 2,000 meters using a stripped aircraft with special engines. The capacity to lift the plate was probably in the aircraft, but at what cost?

"Are you sure?" asked Dematrov.

"Yes," answered Tishchenko.

"Then, while we do the calculations, we can take some preliminary steps," Vineberg said. "We can take our test bird, strip out everything not required for a lift of this nature, and perform a series of tests to basic limits."

"What modifications do you suggest?" Dematrov asked.

"We can remove the interior hoist, remove the interior floor boards and paneling as well as the cargo handling equipment." Vineberg thought for a few moments more. "We can remove the navigator's station, all the insulation, and either the copilot's station or the flight engineer's station, or maybe both."

"That would gain us several thousand kilos, not the 15,000 we need."

Tishchenko held up his hand. "Let's start there. As the analysis goes, we may need to try many things like reinforcement of the hook or a direct strap to the transmission. Undoubtedly, we will need to work with the Soloviev Design Bureau to turn up the limits on several sets of special engines."

"As you say, then," answered Vineberg.

The meeting disbanded. The two deputy designers agreed with Gourgen on the immediate course of action. The chief experimental test pilot would proceed directly to the flight test center to begin the near term work.

The aircraft they would use already possessed the necessary instrumentation. The development work had as much to do with the pilotage required to place such a heavy load on a single cable beneath the helicopter as it did the engineering to adapt the aircraft.

Gourgen directed the specific actions over the next few days. They worked with a cable company to produce a series of special cables in 10 meter lengths from 40 to 100 meters. The longest one would give them the best chance of placing the load and minimizing their exposure to the inferno they would have to fly over. The cables were delivered in 2 days. They installed a 22 ton frangible link at the hook to ensure that if the system parted it would separate at the hook. The thought of a heavy cable releasing like a long steel whip into the fuselage was something to be concerned about.

The longest cable Gourgen had used previously was 30 meters. He would need to develop the techniques necessary to handle a load that far beneath the aircraft. Gourgen began his testing with a full crew to focus solely on the cable length techniques. They used a ten ton concrete and steel block as a representative weight. He painted a circle in the mowed grass that was one meter in diameter larger than the diagonal of the cubic weight. Lessons came quickly over four days.

"How are you feeling?" asked Gourgen when Anatoly arrived in the early morning.

"Better. I still feel a little weak, but I am ready to fly."

"Are you sure?"

"It will be the best thing for me."

"All right, then," Gourgen said as he motioned to the briefing room.

This would be the last series of flights before the aircraft underwent the prescribed modifications to take the extra hook weight. The changes would take about a week. Gourgen felt they needed at least a couple more weeks to qualify the modifications and practice with the heavier weights.

"What have you learned so far?" asked Anatoly.

"First, let me describe what we have done." Gourgen went to the black, slate, chalkboard. "Since we do not know the exact dimensions of the plate, as yet, we drew a circle on the ground with a diameter of the ten ton block's diagonal plus one meter on each side to simulate the precision needed. We have also worked up from a 30 meter cable to a 100 meter one."

"I can see this must have been fun already."

Gourgen chuckled. "How right you are. The 30 meter length was fairly consistent. Of the dozen or so attempts I have made with the 100 meter cable, I have been successful with only two. The secret appears to be in lifting the load vertically as precisely as possible, then the slowness and smoothness of the movements once the load is in the air."

"Which means we will be over that damn hell-hole longer."

"We?"

"Yes, we. I am going back with you."

"Do you . . ."

"Stop! No discussion, Gourgen. You know I have to go back. They have defiled my country, and I must see it finished."

Gourgen stared at his friend as if waiting for a flinch of some sort. He knew any continued exposure might push Anatoly's lifetime equivalent dosage beyond the point of no return. The doctors had told them Anatoly was the sickest of all the pilots so far. The experts suspected slight differences in Anatoly' genetic make-up, or perhaps one or more exposures earlier in his life, that made him more susceptible to radiation poisoning. However, he also recognized the determination in his friend. Gourgen finally nodded his head and turned to the blackboard. "If we can bring the load straight up with no initial side motion, we seem to have the best results."

"That is not easy."

"No. So, what we have done is rigged several aids. We have two video cameras looking down on the load. One looks directly down the cable with sufficient magnification. As you will see in the aircraft, we have marked the screen to give us an indication of alignment. The other camera is located along the centerline of the aircraft forward of the hook about the distance of load."

"Interesting set-up. Seems similar to the tethered hover rig we tested a few months back. How does it work?"

"I am getting better with it. The unknown will be the turbulence over the building."

"And, the radiation."

None of them wanted to hear about the dangers, but Anatoly felt compelled to acknowledge the full dimension of the problem. They would have better protection in the form special suits to avoid particulate contamination. The use of lead sheets and other protective materials covering the floor as well as other areas of the cockpit had been discussed, but ultimately rejected to maximize the lift capacity of the aircraft. They all knew the protection would not be enough, and they would just have to do the best they could.

"My biggest problem is keeping the load steady. After that, the question is the approach. Alignment and spot anticipation have been difficult. We have checkpoints here, but they will be very difficult to obtain down there."

"Are there any other tricks we can do with other cameras . . . perhaps like a bombardier preparing to drop on a target . . . known height and distance?"

"I do not know."

"Let's try it. Maybe I can think of something."

They moved out to the enormous helicopter sitting on the large concrete pad. The pre-flight inspection had been satisfactorily completed by the ground crew. Since they would only be flying around the large, grass field adjacent to the Mil and Kamov flight test centers, they would not need the navigator/communicator. The flight engineer added some safety and protection during the test phase. Eventually, the only two humans of the world's largest helicopter would be the pilot and copilot.

Everything was done in slow motion like a long distance runner setting the correct pace. Gourgen landed in the field adjacent to the hefty cube of concrete and steel. The cable had been snaked out behind the block so there were no kinks and to help the pilot see how much cable remained on the ground as he positioned the helicopter over the load and began to lift. They received a thumbs up signal from the hook man on the ground.

"Ready?" asked Gourgen.

Anatoly pointed to the two video displays mounted in the center of the instrument panel replacing the navigation and communications instruments. The image on both cameras was blurred since they were still on the ground. "This is your alignment line?" asked Anatoly.

"Yes."

"What are the circles?"

"The inside one is my target. I want to keep the load attachment in that circle. The next tells me when the load is moving too much, and the outer one tells me when to start over again. In fact, I could probably say that about the second circle. I came close to making one in the second circle, but the side motion of the load could have done damage to close in structure during the actual lift at the plant site. I have decided that I will go back, set the load down and start over again if we get movement outside the first circle."

"I see. That makes sense, but it is also a rather small circle."

"Precisely. We cannot tolerate much lateral movement on a load this heavy . . . mass times velocity, remember."

They both laughed at the school physics lesson on momentum. They also knew the reality was not a laughing matter. A mass of 30,000 kilograms, or 66,000 pounds, moving at just a meter per second could do substantial damage to just about any structure. Slow precision was the key.

"OK. Let's do it."

Gourgen lifted the collective lever in his left hand. The massive Soloviev engines responded. As the aircraft broke ground, Gourgen glanced at the video displays. The detail beneath them slowly came into focus.

"I found I do better when I use the displays," announced Gourgen. "You watch outside."

"Right."

Gourgen stopped the helicopter about ten meters above the load. He checked his instruments to be certain everything was operating correctly. He returned to the display. The load attachment moved around on the display more than on some previous flights. He looked up again to find the wind. It was off his left forward quarter and increased slightly in velocity. Gourgen slowly turned the nose of the big aircraft directly into the wind, then recentered the load beneath the helicopter and within his tracking circle. Once he was satisfied with his position stability, Gourgen continue to rise directly above the load.

"Everything is looking good," announced Anatoly.

Gourgen did not answer. He knew Anatoly did not expect a reply to a routine observation. The load continued to get smaller as the aircraft rose.

"Eighty meters," Anatoly read from the radar altimeter.

Gourgen could see the last loop of cable beginning to come off the ground. He slowed his ascent as he intently watched the display.

"Ninety meters."

Gourgen stopped the helicopter again to check his station keeping without the weight of the load on the hook. Everything continued to look perfect. He applied a slight upward pressure on the collective. The last length of cable rose from the ground. He was nearly there.

"Ninety-five meters. You are just about on the load."

Gourgen concentrated on the display. He watched the cable come completely off the ground. In another meter or so, they would feel the weight of ten metric tons tug on the great aircraft's belly. The cable snaked around with no tension other than its own weight and being jostled by the substantial rotor wash from the giant helicopter. Gourgen made control inputs to minutely change the aircraft's altitude as he watched the cable snap taut at the same time they felt a heavy tug on the helicopter.

Again, Gourgen stopped, holding tension on the cable but not trying to lift the load. He evaluated his station keeping again. All looked good.

"Everything still looks great. You are on the load," confirmed Anatoly.

Gourgen's index finger depressed the communications switch to the first detent for the interphone. "Station keeping appears to be adequate. Wind is acceptable. I am going to lift this block, and we will make a wide circle pattern to return it here."

"Sounds good. Let's do it."

As Gourgen increased the collective, they could hear and feel the engines groaning against the heavier load. Gourgen kept the load attachment centered in the inner circle. The helicopter began to feel heavy although nothing was happening other than the collective slowly continuing to rise and the engines continuing to increase power. The load broke ground and began to sway ever so slightly within the inner circle. Gourgen added more power to lift the load about five meters off the ground. He stopped once more to evaluate the situation before he would move the load.

The block swayed slightly inside the inner circle in a random, non-oscillatory manner. What movement there was, did not increase in amplitude. The load was stable. The enormous helicopter was handling perfectly.

"I am going with it," announced Gourgen.

"Ready."

Gourgen pushed forward on the cyclic. The nose dipped slightly and the grass began to move for the first time beneath the load. He released the forward stick pressure, then retrimmed the stick to hold his airspeed at about 15 kilometers per hour well below the shudder characteristic of translational lift at 55 kilometers per hour. Gourgen glanced up to his instrumental panel – everything normal. Then, he took a quick scan of the exterior and adjusted his path in a wide circle. He alternated his attention between his flight path track and the stability of the ten ton load beneath the aircraft.

As Gourgen made the minute control inputs to intercept a straight approach along the wind line toward the drop spot, a gust of wind struck the tail. The aircraft yawed causing the big machine to shake. Gourgen quickly focused his concentration on the circle display. The load swung outside the first circle touching the second circle. Carefully, Gourgen slowed the aircraft trying not to fly the load – it never worked.

"Don't fly the load," cautioned Anatoly.

"I know. I know."

The load continued to sway, occasionally passing the second circle. Gourgen gradually came to a hover. The big block moved back and forth now outside the second circle. They could feel the oscillatory reaction in the aircraft.

"Damn."

"It is not going to work," said Anatoly.

"I know, damn it."

"What are you going to do?"

Gourgen considered an attempt. Maybe, if he timed the movement of the block, he could set it down when there was no lateral velocity. He knew it was not going to work, but he still thought about trying it. A heavy load on a 100 meter cable was just too sensitive. Just the slightest disturbance caused the load to swing. There was simply too much luck involved in this work. Adding more weight to the load would only make things worse, not better.

"What are you going to do?" repeated Anatoly.

"We have no choice," Gourgen cursed. "I must put the load down and start over."

"Gourgen, easy. This is going to happen. We will deal with it."

"I know. I know."

The grass in the camera remained stationary, but the load continued to move. Gourgen gradually reduced their altitude.

"Five meters."

The block swayed.

"Four meters."

No change.

"Three meters."

Gourgen watched the load move. Fortunately, the grass remained stationary beyond the waving undulation from the rotor wash.

"Two meters."

Gourgen stopped the aircraft to watch the load. It was getting worse. Waiting would not make it better. The block was not moving in a regular pattern. He could not see an opportunity to time his final descent. In the end, he just chose the brute force path. He lowered the collective.

The helicopter shuddered as the tension in the cable released. The cable snaked violently on the display. Gourgen stabilized his hover.

"Well, that was an interesting technique."

"Do not give me any crap. It was not getting better. In fact, it was just getting worse."

"Hey, easy now. I was just kidding. You had no choice."

"This length of cable is not easy."

"Maybe we should use a shorter cable."

"Right, and put us closer to that damn inferno."

"We still have to get that plate on the spot."

"Yes, we do. Don't we."

They sat there in a hover. The flight engineer finally broke the silence. "The engines and drive train are normal."

"Thanks, chief," answered Gourgen with a chuckle. "I will get on with it."

Gourgen began the process all over again. With only a straight translation toward the intended spot, the procedures worked perfectly. He stopped over the spot. He could not believe the block sat stationary without any perceptible movement, and the block was still five meters in the air. Gourgen watched his markers and lowered the collective. Gracefully, he lowered the ten ton block precisely into the circle without the slightest lateral movement.

They repeated the process three more times with similar results. The procedures would work given some luck. The thought of doing all this over the violent thermal currents of the open reactor and the mounting poisoning of their bodies from the radiation brought a dark shadow to the mission. Gourgen pushed the thoughts out of his head. One step at a time, he told himself.

The next few steps would involve flying the twenty ton block just to confirm the maximum published external load using the 100 meter cable and the modifications of the aircraft to take the heavier external loads, assuming the design engineers could work out the details. He would also call Colonel Nestrov to give him an update on their successes. So far, so good.

# 18

*10:00, Wednesday, 7.May.1986*
*Mil Design Bureau*
*2 Sokolnichesky Street*
*Moscow, Russia, USSR*

"Good to finally see you again, Anatoly Demjanovich?" said Tishchenko, as the two veteran test pilots entered the large conference room. He shook hands with Anatoly and Gourgen, but kept his attention on Anatoly. "How are you feeling?"

"Much better now, thank you. I still seem to fatigue more quickly, but nothing to worry about."

"So he says." added Gourgen.

"I am fine."

"He has lost weight and is quite pale."

"I can see that," said Tishchenko. "Are you sure you are all right?"

"Yes. I am fine. I will be much better when we get that damnable reactor covered up, so it stops polluting the land of my birth." All Soviets shared a devotion to the land – *Rodina* – the Motherland – that transcended governments, czars, premiers and potentates. The commitment to the land passed from generation to generation. They all shared it, and they did not need to talk about it.

Tishchenko turned to Gourgen. "I understand the testing has gone quite well."

"Yes, it has. We have rigged a set up of video cameras and developed a set of procedures Anatoly demonstrated for me at Gromov that seems to work. I am still quite concerned about the flying conditions over the reactor, but . . . we have to do, what we have to do."

"Good news, then," said Tishchenko. "I expect Mark shortly. It looks as if we can make some modifications to take the additional weight on the hook. You think you can fly it?"

"Yes, it appears so. We will not know until we actually fly the plate, and especially not until we have the actual load and ambient conditions."

Mark Vineberg entered the room with several rolled drawings and a stack of papers. Greetings were passed and dispensed with quickly. They all sat down around one end of the long table.

"Tell us about your work," Tishchenko said to Vineberg.

"We have completed all our analysis as well as modification sketches. The bottom line is, we believe we have a means to lift the 35 tons the engineers want." He rolled out a large, general assembly drawing of the Mi-26. "First, we cut a hole in the underside with peripheral reinforcement, then we must install a rigid strap through the hole," he said as he pointed to each element, "through the cargo compartment and another hole in the transmission deck. We developed a suspension apparatus that will attach to the main transmission mounts and hang beneath the transmission casing. We need to reroute several lubricant and electrical lines, but nothing spectacular."

"With those holes, there must be some additional flight limitations," Gourgen said.

"Yes. You will be restricted to 150 kilometers per hour forward speed, and we do not want more than 15 kilometers per hour in sideward flight or crosswind component. There are a few others as well, but we shall get to those later."

"Are the modifications reversible? Can we recover the aircraft?" asked Tishchenko.

"No."

"That is all right. If the aircraft gets contaminated over the reactor, it will not be allowed to leave the area," said Grishchenko.

"That says something right there, does it not?" Vineberg responded.

"There is no choice. There is no other way. It is up to us, and no amount of whining will change the facts. So, I would suggest we get on with things."

All of them stared at Anatoly Grishchenko. The middle-aged, veteran experimental test pilot of Ukrainian descent conveyed his frustration and anger. The emotions also did not change anything, and he knew it.

"I must apologize. I know we are doing everything we can. I keep thinking I may never be able to return to my childhood home because of what they have done to the land, and it makes me angry."

"We understand," answered Tishchenko. "It is just that we are about to lose an extremely valuable asset."

"Plus, you should not be going down there again anyway," added Gourgen.

"We have been through this too many times before. I am going."

Gourgen Karapetyan held up his hand in acceptance. There would be no arguing with the big Ukrainian.

"Have we heard anything from the engineers down there?" asked Tishchenko to change the subject and mood. "Have they completed their design for this plate, and do we know exactly what the final weight will be?"

"No," Gourgen answered. "I will call them when we are done here. I will let them know we think we can lift it, and I will make sure there are no last minute changes."

"Then, we should proceed?" asked Anatoly.

"Unless Gourgen hears something different – yes, we should proceed."

The two pilots nodded their heads in agreement. Vineberg looked grim as he rose from the table and simply walked out quietly. Gourgen knew Mark was not happy. He shook hands with the general designer, then followed Mark Vineberg. Anatoly followed Gourgen. Vineberg's small but bountiful office was four doors down from Tishchenko's conference room and office.

"What is bothering you?" asked Gourgen.

Mark turned to glare at Karapetyan. His eyes said, what a

stupid question. Gourgen waited for some type of verbal response. He could feel Anatoly behind him although Mark did not take his stare off Gourgen.

"I think you two are absolutely beyond insane."

"What choice do we have?"

"You can certify the configuration, the loads and the flying procedures, then let one of the Air Force pilots fly the mission. The country cannot afford to lose either one of you. Your knowledge is too important. With all this talk about openness and reform, we need the best talent we can find to compete with the West. Plus, I do not want to lose my friends."

Gourgen smiled. "Thank you, Mark. Neither of us has any intention of becoming casualties on this mission. The truth is, there is no one else. The Air Force pilots can be trained to do this task, but it would take too long. Both Anatoly and I are relying on decades of experience. It does not come easily."

"I understand, but . . . ."

"No, buts. There is no other way. This is simply something we must do for our country and the world, and we are going to do the best job that can be done."

"My birth village is near that plant," interjected Grishchenko.

"As you have said, Tolya. I guess I did not worry about this until now. I really did not want to think we could do it. Now that it looks like we can, I am worried for my friends and colleagues."

"Thank you for your concern, Mark, but this is our patriotic duty."

Mark Vineberg bowed his head not wanting to see their eyes and waved for them to leave. Gourgen knew what his friend was trying to say silently. The two pilots departed without another word.

Fortunately, Vineberg and Tishchenko had ordered some of the additional machined parts days before the approval meeting. Modifications began promptly. The necessary unique parts arrived within days of their need. Crews worked nearly around the clock to complete the rather extensive modifications.

The special, larger and heavier, practice blocks arrived over the span of several days. Military trailers designed to transport main battle tanks were used to move the blocks. They were offloaded by a heavy mobile crane next to the highway. The ground was too soft to take the heavy, dense loads. They would also have to temporarily close the highway when they lifted the weights. The downwash from the huge helicopter's main rotor would blow a passenger automobile off the roadway.

Within a week of the approval meeting, all was ready. Gourgen and Anatoly decided to start with a 20 ton flight to calibrate their procedures and techniques, and to evaluate the aircraft modifications with a known and familiar weight. With the flight test engineers watching their telemetry consoles, they prepared for the build up.

The actual, envelope expansion, flight test program began with the simple lifting of the 25 ton block. The engineers watched all the critical load and performance parameters to make sure the values were within the calculated and expected magnitudes. The next step involved simple translation of the block away from the highway. Translational speeds were increased in increments of 10 kilometers per hour until the characteristic shudder at about 55 kilometers per hour.

They worked completely through all the technical and operational elements of the testing with the 25 ton block before they returned for the 30 ton block. The initial lift of the heavier block reached the normal continuous operating limit of the two massive Soloviev engines. The remainder of the testing would be more difficult since they would be consuming engine life at progressively much faster rates. The unusually slow rate of change of velocity reduced the engine demands below what they would commonly see.

Several days were used to complete the 30 ton testing to minimize the abuse to the engines and the aircraft. The loads they measured on various critical parts of the aircraft were within their calculated values although a couple of parameters were near their analytical limits. The next higher load would undoubtedly push them over. The engineers feverishly worked their computers and calculators to determine what would happen at the next higher loads. The preliminary work done at the Mil Design Bureau indicated nothing would fail. Several parts would need to be thrown away. A couple would need to be changed after every attempt to lift 35 tons. The data collected told the engineers and especially Gourgen that slow, smooth movements were mandatory to prevent failures. The thought did not give Gourgen much comfort when he considered the flight conditions over the reactor.

When the next step was the 35 ton load, they collectively decided it was time to off-load the flight engineer. From now on, it would be just Anatoly and Gourgen inside the voluminous helicopter. They rehearsed their procedures several times before their next flight. The test team also ordered and accumulated some of the expendable parts they estimated they would need, to replace those consumed by the heavy load. Several sets of uniquely modified, Soloviev, 8,600 kilowatt – 11,500 horsepower – D-126X engines were staged at the facility.

While preparations were made for what they believed would be the final sequence of tests prior to the actual mission, Gourgen decided to call Colonel Nestrov to mutually update both elements of the team. Surprisingly, the connection came on the second try. Telephone connections often took many attempts.

"How is your progress?" asked Nestrov skipping the cordialities.

"We have completed the qualification testing up to 30 tons. We are collecting some additional parts to replace those that stretched beyond their useful limits plus several sets of engines."

"It is that much?"

"Yes."

"What about the world record?"

"Yes, 56 tons. Well, that flight was all internal, and just about everything was good for that one flight. They also used a rolling takeoff. They did not have to hover. We do. We are trying to not consume the whole aircraft before we get that plate in place."

"It will probably be quarantined here anyway."

"We figured that. Our concern is having sufficient margin for retries if we do not make it on the first attempt."

"Ah, yes. Wise move."

Gourgen knew he needed to ask the next set of questions, but he really did not want to know the answer. "What is the situation down there?"

"Well. The construction crews are making reasonable progress. We have ceased dropping sand and boron. The weight has caused the foundation structure to collapse several times." He hesitated probably thinking through the wisdom of explaining the results. Gourgen's curiosity wanted to know what happened, but it would not change their actions. "The engineers have completed the design of the cap cover. Construction of the plate should be finished in a week or so. They probably will not be ready for your placement for another few weeks."

"We should be finished before that, assuming we do not break something or run into a problem."

"Excellent. One other thing ... The plate is being constructed in Kiev. Can you lift it from there to Pripyat before you place it?"

Gourgen imagined the dangers associated with such a move as well as the cost in terms of aircraft life consumption. "You know what the risks are colonel. It would be a very long, slow flight. If the load picks up an oscillation, we would have to dump it. You know what a 35 ton load falling to earth would do. Plus, we would probably consume one or more of the specially modified aircraft in the process."

Silence told him the colonel had thought of the consequences, but something had persuaded him to ask the question. "I just thought I would ask. I will instruct Command to find a surface transport method, probably up the river. You are quite correct, of course ... too risky."

"Anything else?" asked Gourgen.

"No. Keep in communications. Let me know when you have completed your preparations."

"I will do that."

Gourgen's thoughts gripped the image of the massive enclosure being constructed around the damaged reactor crushing everything underneath it. Would this whole effort really work? Would they someday have to go back to tear down that structure? Gourgen shook his head in disbelief.

The preparations for the next and last phase of testing took three days to complete. Several parts had been changed. The maintenance crew collected the necessary spare parts the engineers calculated would be needed. Everything that was not absolutely essential to the heavy lift mission had been removed. The cavernous cargo compartment looked as if it was still under construction. Only load bearing – tension, compression, shear and torsion – structure remained. The large steel strap occupied the center of the compartment like some pillar holding up the overhead elements. The cockpit itself appeared like a large empty room. The navigator's and flight engineer's stations had been removed. Only the two pilot's stations along with some additional instrumentation to compensate for the missing flight engineer's position sat in the most forward portion of the cockpit compartment. They would use a chase aircraft to keep track of things until they arrived at the staging field in the Ukraine.

"This should be interesting," Anatoly said as they walked toward the stripped Mi-26.

"You are right there."

They received an understanding, empathic nod from the crew chief as they climbed into the huge machine. Both glanced around the cargo compartment before ascending the small ladder to the cockpit. Gourgen took the pilot's seat on the left since he would be flying the aircraft leaning toward the windscreen over the collective control.

"This really feels weird," commented Anatoly as they strapped into their seats.

"How so?"

"We normally fly the Mi-26 with a crew of five, six or seven. The minimum crew is four, and here we are . . . just you and me, brother."

Gourgen laughed. "How true . . . like no one wants to come with us on this little adventure."

Anatoly added his laughter as they completed the pre-start checks.

"Let's get this machine started," said Gourgen.

The process of starting the engines and bringing the rotor up to full speed took longer than normal as the two pilots worked cautiously with modified controls and instruments. Normally, the flight engineer would work the engines and monitor their performance parameters. From now on, Anatoly and Gourgen would have to perform the duties of the flight engineer.

"Control, Mil Zero One," Gourgen radioed when they were ready.

"Loud and clear, Gourgen. Everything looks good here. We are ready when you are."

There was some comfort in knowing a half dozen sets of eyes watched the telemetry to protect them.

"Here we go."

Gourgen slowly raised the collective. The increasing power of the huge engines could be clearly heard in the cockpit with all the insulation removed. The 42 meter diameter, main rotor coned upward as the lightened helicopter broke free of the ground. Gourgen moved the aircraft toward the highway. He waited for the militia to stop traffic on the highway in both directions before he repositioned over the 35 ton block of concrete and steel. The helicopter gently settled over the load. The video camera enabled him to precisely position the hook directly above the load attachment. The crewman grounded the substantial static charge from the helicopter before he attached the reinforced eye of the cable in the hook's latch. Gourgen waited for the crewman to clear the area. He scanned the area around the aircraft. Two lines of automobiles and trucks were parked on both the north and south sides of the highway. The helicopter's downwash blew everything flat except the stoutest trees.

"Guess we have quite an audience," Gourgen said.

"Do not screw it up," answered Anatoly.

"Not to worry, my friend."

Gourgen looked out his side window to find the ground crewman standing 100 meters away holding his right arm up signaling that everything was ready to lift.

"Control, Mil Zero One, we are ready to lift this beast."

"Take it slow, Zero One. We need to watch several critical load values," came the answer over the radio from the ground controller.

"We cannot take too long. Our downwash will be blowing everything pretty hard, and we have the highway completely blocked in both directions."

"Understood, but breaking something will not help the situation either."

"So be it, then."

"Control is ready."

"Here we go," Gourgen said, then slowly lifted the collective.

He adjusted the aircraft's controls to maintain the load position as he increased altitude picking up the snaked cable. As he had done many times in the last few weeks, Gourgen carefully drew the cable taught.

"We are on the load," he broadcast.

"We see it. Everything looks good."

"How does it look to you?" Gourgen asked over the intercom.

"Good to me," answered Anatoly.

"Mark torque and temps with the cable taut."

Anatoly read out the values although the ground telemetry displayed the same information. As Gourgen increased power to the engines, Anatoly continued to read out the performance measurements. They passed the maximum continuous power levels, and the load was still on the ground. With no alerts from Control, Gourgen pressed on. Even from 100 meters altitude, the rotorwash was blowing everything not deeply rooted, or heavy, into a big cloud. This is going to get worse before it gets better, Gourgen told himself. It felt like he was trying to lift the earth – nothing was moving other than the needles on the engine instruments.

Anatoly noted them passing the ten minute limit values, followed shortly thereafter by the 1 minute limits, and the load was still on the ground. Gourgen knew every moment was consuming significant life from more than one component in the large helicopter.

"This thing better come off the ground soon," Gourgen broadcast.

"Yeah," was the only response from Anatoly.

The engines strained against the massive weight. Exhaust gas temperatures continued to increase. The block pulled free of the ground causing the helicopter to jerk up. Gourgen lowered the collective slightly to arrest the climb and adjusted the cyclic stick to move away from the highway. As he tried to retrim the control forces, another jolt was felt. Gourgen instinctively focused on the video display looking down on the load. It was already swaying back and forth. He tried to slow the aircraft, so he could lower the load to the ground and start over.

"The load is oscillating," announced test controller as if the pilots did not know what was happening.

Gourgen's concentration remained completely focused on the load. The massive block weighed more than the helicopter. As the weight moved, it began to move the helicopter. Gourgen fought to make some control inputs to slow the motion. It got worse. The oscillation rapidly increased until the Mi-26 felt as if it was being thrashed about the sky.

"Let it go," shouted Anatoly.

Without another moment's hesitation, Gourgen hit the hook release button on cyclic control grip. The aircraft shot skyward like a rocket having been instantly relieved of the enormous extra weight. He gradually lowered the collective to stablize the helicopter. As he did so, he transitioned to forward flight.

"Well, that was certainly an event," Gourgen radioed.

"We need you to land and shutdown as soon as possible," responded Control.

Both Gourgen and Anatoly knew what that meant. The flight test engineers had seen something they did not like, something unexpected.

"No quick moves," added Control.

The two pilots concentrated on the instruments on the panel in front of them. Gourgen wished they still had the flight engineer on board. He might be able to tell them more than they suspected. He made his approach gracefully landing the big helicopter on the concrete pad. They completed the shutdown of the engines, but did not unstrap from their seats. Gourgen continued to hold the controls until the rotor was completely stopped contrary to their usual procedures.

"What do you think?" asked Gourgen.

"I think we broke something."

"Me too."

With the rotor motionless and all the power on the aircraft turned off, the pilots unstrapped and exited the helicopter. They quickly scanned the exterior. Nothing obvious came to them.

A small army of people walked toward the aircraft. They had either done something really good or something was dreadfully wrong. Mechanics and engineers began climbing up the outside and inside the aircraft, opening the engine cowlings and transmission panels.

Gourgen and Anatoly watched the flurry of activity wondering what could have happened. The senior flight test engineer joined them.

"We think you may have broken an engine mount," he said. "Maybe more."

"That damn block must have been stuck," Gourgen commented.

"Well, whatever it was, it did not look good."

"I think we are done for the day while we sort out the condition of the aircraft."

Gourgen nodded his head, then moved around the helicopter to get different views of the activity going on high above the ground on the top of the machine.

"It is broken," shouted down one of the mechanics.

Gourgen turned and walked away. There would be no more flying on this day. He called Mark Vineberg to give him a preliminary report of what happened. Mark was not surprised. He said he would gather up a few of the important design engineers and head down to the test center to help with the assessment and repairs. Gourgen then called Colonel Nestrov to let him know what had happened. It would take a day or more to determine the extent of damage, and what to do next.

The process actually took the better part of two days. The inspection revealed they had completely broken one engine mount, fractured two others and stressed several other parts beyond their elastic limits. Both engines would be replaced with new ones along with all new engine mounts. The other damaged parts were replaced. Several other parts were preemptively replaced with beefier items.

While the maintenance crews worked on the aircraft, Gourgen had evaluated the condition of the block they dropped. It probably fell from a height of 10-20 meters. It was more than half buried in the earth and tilted about 30° on one corner. Gourgen directed a crew to dig out the block and get some supports under it, so they would not have the same problem again. That process alone took two days to complete. He did not want to struggle with the load again.

The repairs were completed. The block's condition was checked several more times before they resumed the flight test program. The remainder of their effort passed as intended without further incident. The 35 ton load was qualified. The aircraft had actually done better than the engineering calculations indicated. There was still no question that each lift of that weight would cause progressively more damage until there was nothing left of the helicopter. Another set of engines had been consumed during the test. A third set was installed to prepare the aircraft for the transit down to Chernobyl and for the real lift mission. Now, the ultimate test would come.

The notifications were made. Another crew, using the test Mi-24, would escort them down to the staging area since virtually all of their navigation and non-essential instruments, and unnecessary equipment had been removed from the special Mi-26. The forward speed of the Mi-26, and thus its escort, was limited. They would need the Mi-24 configured with the large, internal, auxiliary fuel tank – the same configuration they flew the reconnaissance mission in a month ago. Even at that, their slow speed would place the Mi-24 at a more inefficient speed, and they would be pressing the useful flight duration for the attack helicopter. There were just too many compromises, deviations, alterations, modifications and other less desirable changes being made. This requirement was pressing the limit of everything they had available to them, or had been designed for that matter. Gourgen wanted this mission behind him as quickly as possible – too many things to go wrong.

Gourgen dialed the special number many times before he finally made the telephone connection. "Yes," the man said simply, not wanting to identify his affliation or location.

"Colonel Nestrov, please," Gourgen said.

There was no response other than the 'clack' of the handset hitting a wooden table. Gourgen could hear nothing in the background as he waited.

"Yes," came the recognizable voice of the senior Air Force officer.

"Colonel Nestrov, this is Gourgen Karapetyan."

"Are you ready?" Nestrov asked.

"We have completed the qualification testing. We can lift the 35 tons."

"Then, you are ready."

"No, not exactly. We need to gather up a variety of spare parts including at least one set of special engines to make sure we have everything with us for this mission."

"I will not go into the details, but we will not be ready for you until mid-July at the earliest. The plate is ready, but the locaton is not."

"That will give us plenty of time to make sure everything is as it should be for this lift."

"Good," responded Nestrov. "Is there anything you need us to do?"

"Just make sure the plate is on something that it will not stick to for the lift. We broke several parts when the 35 ton block got stuck in the dirt. We do not want that to happen again.

"There should be no problem there."

"So, you want us to wait here until you call us?"

"Yes. There is no need for you to be here until everything is ready for this lift. I will call you at the point. How long will it take you to arrive here and execute the required lift?"

"Half a day, unless something else comes up."

"Nothing else will have the priority of this mission. If anything appears to conflict, you are to get ahold of me immediately. I will take care of any obstacles. Understood?"

"Yes, precisely."

"Then, make ready all that you need and standby."

"We will be ready."

Colonel Nestrov hung up with no further words. Gourgen held the handset away from his head and looked at it as though something strange must have happened to it. He could only guess that progress at Chernobyl was not moving along as desired. The impression left him with a redoubled focus on readiness for the call that would send them to Northern Ukraine, again.

# 19

*08:45, Wednesday, 18.June.1986*
*Ministry of Interior Affairs*
*Stockholm, Sweden*

Evar Erickson hesitated on the sidewalk across the street from the old government building as the taxicab pulled away. A beehive of journalists and reporters along with their video cameramen were kept at bay by a half dozen armed guards. The attention of the hive fluttered to each new person who attempted to run the gauntlet. The hive quickly determined relative importance and lost interest only to return to their protest of being excluded from entering the building. He did not want to be subjected to the harassment of the largely American affiliated correspondents and their aggressive manners. Evar considered other possible avenues of entrance, but there were none. He swallowed hard, nearly forgot to check the busy street for traffic, then crossed the wide roadway, aiming for the left side of the expansive entry portico.

The beehive soon noticed him but did not recognize him as someone important. With the previous wasted effort, they quickly turned their attention back to the guards and other citizens trying to enter the building. One of the peripheral guards stopped him.

"Do you have business inside?" he asked.

Not wanting the say anything that might spark the curiosity of the journalists, Evar produced the letter directing him to appear. The guard scanned the papers, nodded his head, then waved him past the line. Evar made it into the building without a word being said. He felt a true sense of relief and took a deep breath to relieve the tension.

This was his first visit to the Ministry that employed him, so he sought the guidance of yet another guard sitting at a large console in the lobby of the building. "Where may I find the Board of Inquiry room?" he asked.

The man pointed to his left without a word. Evar walked through the double doors with large glass inserts and then quite tentatively down the hallway scanning both sides as people past him without acknowledging his presence.

A large wooden door in the only set of double doors along the high ceiling corridor on the ground floor of the old government building had a new professionally printed sign – Board of Inquiry – pasted over the normal conference room sign. Several people sat on benches on both sides of the corridor apparently waiting for their turn to be questioned. A young attractive woman stood at the door holding a clipboard. Evar again produced his letter to appear from an inside breast pocket of his suit coat. The woman glanced at the letter without grasping it.

"Mister Erickson, Evar Erickson, of Linstornborg?" she asked for confirmation.

"Yes."

"Please be seated, Mister Erickson. The Board is about to convene. You are schedule to be the third or fourth witness."

Evar nodded his head and found an open seat to the right of the door. Witness – that did not sound good. After all, he was just a simple weather observer who enjoyed his simple life. He did not care for all this excitement and officialness. He was perfectly comfortable leaving all that stuff to others. Evar wanted this to go away quickly so he could return to his small group of friends and his hilltop weather station.

One of the big doors opened just enough for a man to lean out and whisper something to the clipboard woman, then closed as the man retreated back into the room. The woman checked her clipboard, wrote several notes, then said, "Mister Sorenson." A young, disheveled man sitting on the far side of the room stood and walked toward the doors. She pulled the right door open for him to enter, then closed the door behind him. She checked her clipboard again and added, "Mister Evar Erickson, you have been called next, followed by Mister Pellsberg."

Evar nodded his head to acknowledge her announcement although she was not looking at him. As Mister Sorenson told the Board whatever it was he knew about this incident or situation or whatever they wanted to call it, Evar relived in his mind those horrifying moments that made him feel so alone, isolated and unprotected. He was not particularly excited about recounting that night, but perhaps they would not ask him about how he felt as he observed the first signs of a disaster. He wanted to simply state the facts, then leave, although he still questioned whether it was actually safe to live anywhere near Linstornborg. The Government experts that tested the dirt, the vegetation, the animals and some of the humans told them the radiation levels were elevated but still within acceptable limits. Acceptable to whom, he constantly asked himself.

There were eighteen people sitting or standing outside the Board room. Two thirds were males. The ages of the witnesses ranged from young to old. Some were well dressed. Others looked as if they had just come off the farm without changing clothes. Evar wondered what each of them did for a living and what brought them to this place and moment, in essence, what was their association or interest in this incident.

The first man, Mister Sorenson, walked out of the room and continued down the hall without looking at anyone. "Mister Erickson," the woman announced, motioned toward the door, then pulled the same door open for him and shut it behind him.

Evar entered the moderately lit, dark wood paneled room with portraits hung around the periphery who were probably past ministers, none of whom he recognized. A long table covered with an even larger green felt-looking cloth spanned the right side of the room. Eleven people, two women and nine men, sat behind the table with glasses of water or orange juices and papers scattered in front of them. A small, uncovered table was centered about two meters in front of the large table. Only two chairs were placed at the small table. Two human recorders sat at separate small desk at the far right of the long table.

The elderly man in the center of the long table spoke first.

"Mister Erickson?"

"Yes."

"Please be seated." He waited for Evar to take the right chair. "This is a Board of Inquiry chartered to investigate the events and facts associated with the elevated radiation levels detected since last month." He paused for an acknowledgment head nod from Evar. He also chose not to introduce the members of the Board, and Evar recognized none of them. "For the record, please state your name, residence and occupation."

"My name is Evar Erickson. I live in the little village of Linstornborg, and I am one of the duty weather observers at the Government weather station on the mountain north of town."

"Please recall the events of the late evening hours of Wednesday, the 30th of April, this year," the center man said.

Evar summarized the key elements in sequence, but did not feel it necessary to go into minute detail like what he had to eat and drink, or what he was doing to fill the time. He figured they would ask him what they wanted to know. Some of the board members listened intently without taking their eyes off him. While others, focused on their notepads and jotted down their impressions, doodled, or whatever it was they were doing.

"How did you know your instruments were accurate?" asked one of the women.

"We have procedures to verify any warning or abnormal indication. We also have various levels of reset procedures to start from scratch. I ran those procedures several times that night, some on my own and some at the request of the Ministry duty officer."

"And, you are confident those indications were accurate."

"Yes . . . as best I am able."

"Did you notify your successor of the situation?"

Evar thought the question to be rather strange. Did they not know about the special journal he opened that night in addition to his observation log? Did they really think he would not warn his colleagues of those very unusual indications? He decided to keep his answer as simple as possible. "Yes."

"How did you do that?"

"In addition to the normal observation log, I created a special journal to write down what I noticed or felt at the moment. I asked my relief to keep the journal and to pass the request along to each succeeding shift observer. We are still keeping that journal of thoughts in addition to our required observation log."

"Did they do that?"

"Yes."

One of the younger male board members held up a large, green, bound notebook. "Is this your journal?"

"It appears so, but may I examine it?"

The man handed the book to one of several clerks supporting the Board, who in turn handed it to Evar. He checked the first page and several subsequent pages, then handed the book back to the clerk.

"Yes, that is our journal."

The questioning continued as various board members inquired about several of his specific notations that night. They began to explore some of his impressions although they did not seem to be particularly relevant since they were not based on fact.

"Did you notify the community?"

Evar now began to worry about what they were really after. What did they expect him to do, call the town and start a panic? What did they want of him?

"Did you warn the community?" the man repeated.

"No."

"Did you not think the radiation warning and elevated readings were a threat to yourself and the community?"

"Yes, I did. I was very worried as my journal indicates. I took the correct actions," he said immediately regretting his defensive statement. "Once I confirmed the indications, I called the duty desk as our procedures dictate. I was just one lonely observer. The Ministry needed to decide what actions were warranted based on my observations, and perhaps those of others. I am just a weather observer. I am not a radiation expert."

"Indeed."

The central man interjected. "While this situation is troubling for all of us, I think we can all agree that Mister Erickson acted in a calm and responsible manner to what was clearly a very threatening situation." Not everyone nodded. "Are there any other questions for this witness?

When none came, Evar said, "I have one."

"This is rather unusual, but I do not see the harm," answered the central man, then nodded his head toward Evar.

"Are the news report accurate?"

"In what way?"

"They say the radiation I detected has come from a major nuclear accident in the Soviet Union."

The central man scanned his complete panel. He saw no objections. "It is impossible for me or any of us to establish the veracity of the news reports. However, let it suffice to say, we do have confirmation from the Soviet Government that a fire occured at a nuclear power station north of Kiev. With your readings on both the radiation levels as well as the prevailing winds from the various weather observations, we believe these indications are consistent with what you called a major nuclear accident."

"What are we going to do?" Evar asked, more as a worried citizen than a witness.

"That is one of the objectives of this Board of Inquiry. You have helped us establish the existence of these elevated radiation levels. We have subsequently determined the content of that radiation and narrowed the possible sources of such contaminants. They are consistent with other elements of information and fact. The Soviets are struggling with the greatest nuclear accident, or incident of any kind, in history. We have much work to do to protect our citizens and help the Soviets deal with this grievous situation, and so, if you would be so kind, we must proceed with our work."

"I am sorry," Evar said as he stood.

"No need to apologize. You have done your duty. Now, I must ask you not to talk to the press, and remain available should we need to recall you for further testimony."

"Yes, certainly."

"Thank you for your time," the leader said.

Evar followed the path of Mister Sorenson out of the room, down the hall and out of the building. The journalist group remained but seemed less frenzied. Since they did not know him going in, they did not bother him going out. Evar was thankful for the relief.

As he drove out of the capital city and into the forested countryside on his way back to Linstornborg. He worried about what was happening in the Soviet Union. The radiation detected in Sweden was a concern to his country. He knew the situation for the Soviets was monumentally worse. Evar Erickson cried silently as he saw unnamed people fighting to survive in the Soviet Union, and the innocence of the Swedes and others in the world as they grappled with the consequences of whatever it was that happened near Kiev.

# 20

*09:00, Wednesday, 9.July.1986*
*Between Buildings R4 and R5*
*Zhukovsky, Russia, USSR*

Gourgen heard his name called and turned to see Anatoly Kovatchur jogging toward him. It was going to be a warm day, and he was going to be in an unconditioned air cockpit for his one or more flights this day.

"I guess you have a late morning flight as well," Kovatchur said.

"You are correct," he answered as they turned together toward the parking lot.

"I just heard from a friend of mine – a fighter pilot from Afghanistan – just returned from Finland."

Gourgen thought that fact was a bit unusual but not particularly extraordinary. He motioned with his hands, eyes and head as if to say, so.

"He commanded a special detachment of Air Force MiG-29's to Kuopio-Rissala Airbase in Finland as part of some planned exchange program with the Finns. Longinenko is his name. Anyway, they took six aircraft from their regiment and a hand picked set of pilots and mechanics."

"All right, so a friend of yours got a tour of Finland, why is that so important?"

"Well, this is the first time the MiG-29 has been flown in the West."

"Finland is hardly the West."

"Yes, but, this one was different. The Finns allowed the Western press to visit the airbase several times. According to Longinenko, the interest in those aircraft was quite high, and, they wrote some very good things about the fighters."

"As they should."

"Certainly, but this is the Western press we have heard so many evil things about."

"Perhaps, they are not all that bad."

"Perhaps, but there is talk at Mikoyan that with all this political gibberish about openness and reform, several of us think we might get a shot at taking one of our aircraft to one of the big international airshows like Paris or Farnborough."

"Now, that would be nice, wouldn't it?"

"Indeed."

They stopped at the edge of the line of automobiles. They wanted to finish the conversation before Gourgen headed north and Anatoly Kovatchur went to the Mikoyan facility at Ramskoye.

"Do you think you might be able to go?" Gourgen asked.

"The talk is pretty misty. It is certainly not going to happen this year. Farnborough is held on the even year, and there has been no planning for such an endeavor."

"Maybe next year."

"Next year is Paris. We might be able to do that one. The other interesting thing that Longinenko told me was, he heard from the Finns as well as some of the questions shouted at them by the press that radiation from Chernobyl has contaminated parts of Finland, Sweden and Norway."

"We have heard some of the press reports. I imagine they are none too happy."

"Apparently, they are quite angry. There were protests of citizens outside the base. Colonel Longinenko had to confine his detachment to the base to avoid any confrontation. The press were able to get closer to our guys, and they asked more questions about Chernobyl than they did about the airplanes."

"I wonder if the Government agreed to this exchange to lessen the protests."

"Who knows. I am just thankful this exchange was allowed to happen. Many of us want to fly at the big airshows and meet other pilots."

"As do I."

"Before I go, I understand you and Anatoly Demjanovich are planning to fly a special mission at Chernobyl."

"We are complete with the extensive modifications and nearly complete with the preparation of our Mil Two Six for a very heavy external lift down there. This thing is apparently some huge steel plate to cover an access hole in the top of the sarcophagus they are constructing to cover up the damaged reactor . . . 35 tons worth."

"Thirty-five tons, that is some plate."

"We were not sure we would be able to lift it. It looks like we will make it."

"So, you and Tolya are going to fly the placement mission."

"Yes . . . somewhere after mid-month they tell me."

"Radiation is nasty stuff," added Kovatchur. "Didn't you two learn your lesson the last time you flew down there?"

Gourgen looked into his friend's eyes. "Yes, we did, but we are right on the fine edge on so many parts. We have broken the machine several times during testing. I have more experience with this machine and especially these modifications than anyone else. It would take too long to train someone else, and even then, it would be more risky that it already is."

"I see your point, but that stuff is really nasty," he repeated.

"I am not particularly exciting about going through that again, and neither is Anatoly, but as I said, there is no one else to do this task. The country needs us to do our duty."

"As you say."

They looked at each other. Neither had anything else to say, so they nodded and went to their respective automobiles. Anatoly Kovatchur stopped as he opened the driver's door, and shouted to his friend. "When do you go back down there?"

"We are nearly done. We are preparing the aircraft for the actual mission. The best I can say is probably sometime next week."

"Wouldn't it be better to wait for colder air . . . to get more lift?"

"Sure it would, but the task will not wait. They need this thing done as soon as we can complete our preparations, and they are finished with construction and ready for us to place the plate in its final position. The plate is ready and waiting. We understand the building is nearly ready. So, sometime next week, I guess."

"Does Milla know?"

Gourgen looked around to see if anyone else might be listening. "She knows something is going on, but no, she does not know I am going back to that place, again. Anatoly Demjanovich and I agreed we would take the wives to a nice dinner to tell them."

"They are not going to be pleased," Kovatchur observed.

Gourgen chuckled. "No, they are not."

"Good luck."

"Thank you."

# 21

*19:30, Monday, 14.July.1986*
*Kavkaz Restaurant*
*Moscow, Russia, USSR*

Gourgen and Anatoly reached the moment they both knew would come and neither looked forward to happening. The testing was complete. The preparations were complete. The anticipated telephone call came last Friday. The next step was the actual mission at Chernobyl. Both of them knew there would be less likelihood of a blow up or a scene at the public restaurant, and it would be easier together than separate.

Anatoly's automobile was a few years newer than Gourgen's, and in slightly better shape, so the two couples took his vehicle. The drive into the city was uneventful enough. Both women knew this was a little out of the ordinary and did not know what the special occasion was to elicit this response. Both men tried to find the humor in their surroundings making this just a pleasant night out. Since no one had any particular preferences, they agreed to go to Gourgen's favorite restaurant, located on the north side of the city. They all enjoyed the wide spectrum of tastes that came with every meal, almost like a treasure hunt of food among the meats, vegetables, tomatoes, breads and cheeses — a place where a meal became an intriguing journey.

The *maître d'hôtel* recognized Gourgen even without the gold star that often adorned his chest. They were ushered into a separate room off the crowded main dining room. It was always a very popular restaurant for Muscovites. The separate room enabled the owner to tend to dignitaries without causing any disruption to his regular business. The high-ceiling, square room with a circumferential mural depicting various panoramic scenes from the mountainous region that was the restaurant owner's and Gourgen's homeland of Armenia had only two other dining groups. Gourgen did not recognize any of the other patrons, but they were probably government officials.

"This is always an adventure," Galina said as they were seated at a corner table.

"That's why I like this place," added Ludmilla.

"Now, I know you two have cooked something up. Milla and I never get this treatment unless one or both of you have done some unspeakable act for which you need absolution."

"My aren't we getting religious," responded Gourgen. "Here I thought we were the only closet Christians."

"All this talk from Gorbachev about reform and openness has emboldened many," said Anatoly.

"Yes, now back to my statement." Galina looked at each man trying to find the chink in their armor.

Anatoly held up his hand. "Why don't we just enjoy a nice evening out with friends?"

"So, that is how you want it."

"Galya," protested Anatoly. "Let's just enjoy the evening."

She nodded her head and her expression conveyed her reluctant acquiescence. They began by ordering a sumptuous meal, then entered into the social dialogue common between close friends, parents, grandparents and colleagues. Laughter punctuated the conversation between courses as they shared the latest news from their children. All their offspring, with the exception of Dimitri Karapetyan, who had not yet entered the university, had completed or were immersed in a good university education. They were also creating their own success, and none of them followed in their fathers' footsteps as aviators, although Boris Grishchenko was a communications officer in the Air Force and occasionally flew long range bomber missions.

They finished their main course. All of them were quite sated, and they still had dessert to go. They asked their waiter to delay the sweets to let their supper settle.

"So, can we talk, now?" asked Galina.

"We have been talking," Gourgen responded.

"You know what she means," Ludmilla interjected.

Gourgen looked to Anatoly, who said with his eyes, maybe it is time. "We completed the big test project a few weeks ago."

"Excellent," said Ludmilla. "Now, what does that mean to us?"

"We were expanding the external load, hook lift capacity for the Mil Two Six."

"So."

"We were doing this work to lift a huge steel plate, about 35 metric tons worth." Both women just stared at him as if to say, what is next. "Anatoly and I leave tomorrow morning for Ukraine."

"Chernobyl," Ludmilla spat.

"Yes. They are nearly complete with the construction of a huge concrete building to seal in the remains of the damaged reactor. We must lift the close out, biological cover plate into place on the top of the building."

Galina looked at Anatoly. "Weren't you sick enough the last time?"

"It is our duty, Galya."

"Duty is for soldiers."

"No! Duty is for citizens" he said, probably more strongly than he wanted. "The country, if not the world, needs us to do our duty."

"So," Ludmilla said casting her icy glare upon Gourgen, "you are going back to that evil place."

Gourgen looked down at his cup of coffee, not wanting to see the anguish in her eyes that he felt coming from her. He told himself, this is what soldiers must feel when they tell their loved ones they are going off to battle. There was no easy way. There was no means to make this mission less serious or dangerous.

"Well," Ludmilla demanded.

"Yes."

"As Galya says, didn't you two get sick enough the first time?

You want to go back for more?"

"That is not it, Ludmilla. It is as Anatoly has said, this is our duty to the Motherland."

The waiter returned and stood patiently until he had the attention of the four diners. "Are you ready for your desert?"

"I am afraid I have lost my desire for dessert," said Ludmilla.

"Me too," added Galina.

Gourgen shook his head. There was no need for dessert.

"With your permission, sir, I shall bring you the bill."

Gourgen nodded his head in agreement.

"So, let me see here," said Ludmilla with a stern voice. "You two boys brought us into Moscow for a special supper, to make us feel better that you are bound and determined to sacrifice your lives for the Motherland."

"How many will have to die?" asked Galina before either of the men could answer.

"Look, Milla. Let me see if I can explain this."

"Please do."

"The maximum hook lift capacity for the Mil Two Six is 20 metric tons. There are pilots who can fly the aircraft but cannot fly a precision lift of a 20 ton load. This plate weighs something like 35 metric tons, nearly double the maximum hook capacity of the aircraft. We had to specially modify the aircraft, develop new equipment to help manage the load, and establish new procedures for how to lift this plate."

"So, if you have developed all this stuff, why not let one of the others of these few, highly skilled," she said with as much sarcasm as she could muster, "pilots do this final task?"

"We have been through this many times before. There is no one in the world more qualified to do this task. We developed the entire process. We have seen the mistakes. We know what to do, and what not to do."

"You were so sick the last time," Galina said to Anatoly. "Maybe this will be too much, and you will not come back home."

"Yes, I was sick. We all were, including Gourgen, but everyone recovered."

"Except Aleksandr Grigoryevich," Galina said.

"He was in the building with all the fires that night. This is not the same. We will have protection."

"Like you did last time," Ludmilla challenged.

"We did not have protective suits the last time. This time we will have them. We will have greater protection."

"Enough protection so that you will not get sick?" asked Galina.

"I do not know, but there is less radiation than that night amid the fires and compared to our first flight down there."

"I do not know why we keep talking about this," Ludmilla said. "You two – boys – are set upon doing this thing – for the Motherland – so, you go ahead. Just do not expect a blessing from me for your sacrificial spirit."

"Nor me."

"We just want you to understand," said Gourgen.

"Well, I do not think that is possible."

A strange silence occupied the space between them. The waiter returned with the bill. He must have waited for a lull in their conversation to return. He was probably smart enough to recognize a tense moment at the table. Gourgen nodded his head, checked the bill, not really caring if it was accurate or not, then pulled several large bills from his jacket wallet. He handed the bill folder along with the currency to the waiter, then waved his hand that he did not expect any change.

"Thank you, sir. Enjoy your evening."

"I am sure we will," mumbled Ludmilla.

"Shall we go?" Gourgen said, then stood to make the question rhetorical.

They walked silently to the car parked down the street a modest distance from the restaurant. None of them spoke until the city lights were behind them.

"I cannot speak for Milla, but I must tell you," she paused to gather her words, "it is not your flying or your sense of duty to aid the Motherland that bothers me. It is simply the risk you are taking, and the possibility I might lose you. You are not a young man."

"Thanks," Anatoly interjected trying for some levity.

Galina ignored the interjection. "Your body cannot recover from such abuse and wantonness as it once did. I just want to enjoy our retirement together, and you are risking our future."

"Are there choices?"

"Perhaps not, but that does not change the fact that I do not want to sacrifice you and our future. However, I also recognize it is not my choice. You are not giving us a set of options here. You are telling us what you are committed to do. Just do not expect us to be happy about it."

Gourgen wanted to respond, but chose to let Galina's comments rest. The silence remained until they arrived in Zhukovsky. Anatoly stopped in front of their apartment building. They said their good nights in a pleasant, friendly manner.

A stony silence between them blanketed the walk into the building and up the stairs to their apartment. Gourgen could feel Ludmilla's contained resentment, not of him, but of the situation. He wanted to be close to her, but he did not press her into what might become another set of harsh words. He believed he would be all right after the flight, and he would return to her in a few days or so. Gourgen waited through all the shuffling and normal preparation for bed as long as he could.

"Please do not be mad," he said softly.

"I am not mad, Gourgen. All this mess around that damnable power plant is wearing me out. It is consuming our country."

"Which is why we must fly this mission as soon as possible."

"I do not want to talk about this any more," she said, stopping her preparations and standing in front of him in her nightgown. "You are going to take Anatoly with you, and you are going to do what you believe to be the correct thing. I cannot change your mind. I am not going to try anymore. I just want you to come home to me."

"I will."

Ludmilla finished, then walked to her side of the bed and pulled the cover back and got into bed. "Then, there is nothing more I can ask," she mumbled.

"I will do my best."

Ludmilla just nodded as she lay her head on the pillow and pretended to be asleep. Gourgen finished his preparations for bed, shook his head in quiet frustration and turned out the lights. He found his side of the bed in the dark and lay down beside his wife. For a time that he could not determine, he thought about the evening's tension, the weeks of friction between him and his wife over the flying associated with Chernobyl, but more importantly, he thought about tomorrow and the events of the next few days. He wondered whether his words to her were correct. Would he really come home to his wife and the life they looked forward to as they approached retirement? These questions were too difficult to answer, and some of the answers lay far beyond his grasp or control. They would simply have to do the best they could do and hope for the good outcome.

# 22

*12:30, Tuesday, 15.July.1986*
*Military Response Team Camp*
*70 kilometers east of Chernobyl, Ukraine, USSR*

The flight to the Ukraine on the hot summer day had been uneventful. The Mi-24 attack helicopter flown by a pilot and navigator from Mil did a perfect job shepherding its behemoth cousin even at the significantly slower speeds.

The plate was ready. When they arrived, they learned the steel and concrete sarcophagus was not quite to the same state. The estimate of two more days convinced them to remain. The Mi-24 crew departed. They would return to pick up Gourgen Karapetyan and Anatoly Grishchenko when the mission was complete. Until then, the two veterans would be the guests of the Air Force.

"Where is the plate?" Gourgen asked Colonel Kalasnikov.

"Just south of Pripyat in an open field beside the main road."

"Can we see it?"

"Yes, but I would recommend you wear protective suits and respirators. Both of you have received large doses already, and you will receive more when you lift the plate into place."

"Agreed," Gourgen answered for both of them as if there had been a debate.

"See the equipment sergeant in the far tent. I will arrange transport for you."

As Anatoly and Gourgen were fitted for heavy, rubberized, environmental suits and high filtration respirators, an Air Force Mi-8 helicopter repositioned near the tent complex and remained turning.

"Have you taken a potassium iodine pill?" asked the sergeant.

"No. Why?" asked Anatoly.

He went to a table, found the container he was looking for, removed two, large, brown tablets, and gave one to each of them. "These pills will saturate your thyroid, so radioactive iodine cannot accumulate and cause cancer."

"They did not give us these before," said Gourgen.

The sergeant shook his head in disbelief. "I cannot fix the past. These will help you now."

They swallowed the tablets as recommended. They fitted and checked their respirators to make sure there were no leaks. The suits had built-in plugs for self-contained communications units or use in any armor or aviation vehicle including the Mi-8 and Mi-26 helicopters. The heavy, cumbersome suits made both men waddle to the waiting helicopter.

The flight to Pripyat took 20 minutes. The village remained deserted and dead. As they circled to land, Gourgen noticed the growing accumulation of contaminated, quarantined and abandoned helicopters, Mi-6's, Mi-8's, a couple Mi-10's and a half dozen Mi-26's, along with bulldozers, trucks and other assorted equipment. The cost of this accident in contaminated equipment alone was so incredibly high. He knew the price in human lives already lost defied comprehension. Gourgen could only wonder about the magnitude of damage beyond his immediate experience and knowledge.

Their transport helicopter landed in the field about 50 meters from the plate. The two, suited pilots disembarked and walked toward the object. The enormous, steel gray, plate sat on an array of railroad ties. As they approached the object, the size struck them. Massive plates of steel three or four centimeters thick had been welded together in a flat, bowl configuration with a grid of thick, reinforcement ribs connecting the various segments into the completed 20 meter diameter structure before them.

"Thankfully, they did not put this thing in the dirt," Gourgen said in the muffled tones through the respirator and over the noise of the helicopter still turning 50 meters away.

"Are these lifting eyes going to be strong enough to hold the cable and the weight of the plate when we lift it?"

"Good question. They look pretty strong. Perhaps we should have one of our engineers take a look at them before we lift this thing."

"Might be a good idea. All it will take is one of these to let go, and we will be in trouble."

Neither one needed any coaxing to leave without delay. They did not talk as they departed.

When they arrived back at the staging area, they went through the same decontamination wash they had done earlier after their reconnaissance flight. They were asked to step off the helicopter to be washed down individually. An Air Force man waved to them from some distance. He would drive them back to the tent complex.

As they removed the protective suits, Gourgen asked his friend, "How do you feel?"

"Not too bad considering what we experienced over the reactor last time. I have a bit of a headache, but other than that, I am all right."

"I have a headache, too. Do you think we should go to the medical tent?"

"No. I think we are fine."

Colonel Kalasnikov joined them. "What did you think?"

"Damn big plate."

They all laughed at the obvious observation.

"Yes, but can you lift it?"

"We can lift it," answered Gourgen. "The question will be whether we can place it in the proper position with the very short amount of fuel time we have available. Did they build in any guides?"

"They have had a very hard time building the crazy block house. To be honest, I do not know. If I was going to guess, I think not, knowing the problems they have had with the construction."

"Well, then, there is only one way we are going to find out."

The three pilots nodded their heads. Anatoly and Gourgen completed the process of changing out of their special equipment.

They asked Kalasnikov about the protective gear. The Air Force pilots who flew near the reactor still wore the various items. No more sand nor boron could be dumped. The engineers were already quite worried about the weight of the structure and all it contained. The Air Force helicopters had lifted large buckets of concrete to places the long, articulated, hose arms could not reach.

The warm, summer sun made the two day waiting period pass lazily. They watched and supervised the work of an Air Force and Army crew as they checked the various modifications of the big aircraft. The pronouncement of unsuitability for decontamination led to a vigorous discussion and a decision to delay the determination until after the lift. They also practiced ingress and egress as well as cockpit procedures while wearing the rubberized protective suits and masks they were encouraged to wear by the chemical corps specialists. The two test pilots asked various individuals numerous times why they had not been advised to wear the gear during their earlier flight. The answers came back the same every time – no one asked them.

"Anatoly Grishchenko," called a sergeant.

"Yes," he said.

"You have a telephone call."

Anatoly left Gourgen lying in the grass soaking up the warmth of the sun. The telephone call took long enough to allow Gourgen to doze off.

"Well," said Anatoly upon his return, "the toll goes up."

"Who?"

"Lelechenko." Gourgen sat up on one elbow and nodded his head. "He died this morning. This disaster has claimed another good life. That was his wife on the telephone. She said he died an agonizing death, and they could do little to help him through his suffering." Anatoly paused, staring at his best friend. "This must stop."

"It is up to us, Anatoly Demjanovich."

"It had better be soon, or we will lose more good people."

Gourgen lay back down in the grass and closed his eyes. "Yeah, soon," he mumbled.

They considered returning to Zhukovsky, however Colonel Kalasnikov insisted they remain. According to the senior Air Force officer, the construction crews would be ready for them to lift the cap plate any day now.

A large group of new people, most of whom wore civilian clothing or white coveralls, arrived the following morning. These were the design engineers and construction supervisors assigned to the unprecedented project.

They briefed the pilots on the status of the construction and more specifically the details of the close-out task of placing the cap plate on top of the sarcophagus. They allowed for nearly a meter variation in final placement, but they could not figure out how to install guides. The final placement would rest entirely upon the skills of the two test pilots. Gourgen and Anatoly wanted to fly a practice mission without the heavy plate, but everyone dissuaded them due to the continued radiation exposure. Adding more dosage counts proved to be a far greater cost than the lack of a trial run at the lift task. The four lifting eyes on the plate had been strengthened. As the design engineers reported, any two of the eyes could support the total weight of the plate. Also, special attachment cables had been prepared, tested and installed to enable a single point hook up for the primary lift cable.

After the general briefing, most of the visitors departed leaving one young engineer and a couple of the construction specialists. They used the remainder of the day to go over each step of the lift. They would take the 100 meter lift cable to Pripyat. It would be connected and deployed as they were instructed by Gourgen based on his experience during the test program. Once the cable was attached to the helicopter's belly hook, the two test pilots would be on their own for the lift. A Mi-8 helicopter with Colonel Kalasnikov at the controls and two key engineers on board would be orbiting well clear of the area just in case they needed some assistance seeing the placement. Once the plate was in place, they would land at

Pripyat and shutdown for the contamination evaluation by the chemical warfare troops. They expected the aircraft to be too contaminated to be allowed out of the area or successfully washed. If the Mi-26 was abandoned, the Mi-8 would land to pick up the two pilots.

They decided to make the attempt in the early morning just after dawn to minimize thermal convective currents beyond the reactor and winds. The weather forecast was good – clear skies with light winds from the southwest. As they finished their breakfast with other Air Force pilots assigned early missions, the call came in announcing the readiness of the plate and the lifting cable.

The start and preparations for flight took longer as the two pilots dealt with the annoyance of the cumbersome protective suits. They were already sweating when they took off from the staging area. Fortunately, the seal on their masks kept the moisture away from the transparent face plate. Without clear vision, the mission was impossible. The protective suit with its earphones and small microphone at least enabled them to talk on the interphone or use the radio.

As they circled the landing area where the plate rest, two men in yellow protective suits could be seen climbing down off the large plate. They retrieved the cable lifting eye and scurried back on to the plate as the large helicopter approached.

Gourgen came to a stable hover at 20 meters directly over the plate. He centered up the crosshairs on the hook video camera display. Very slowly, he lowered the helicopter until the two men could lift the eye and engage the hook. They watched the men check the latching of the hook then scramble down off the plate. As they had been briefed, the two men moved away from the helicopter on one side or the other.

"I do not have them," said Gourgen.

"I do. They are clear."

Gourgen twisted in his seat and suit to see the side of his friend's suited head and torso. "Well, this is it," he said. "Are you ready?"

"As I ever can be."

"Here we go."

Gourgen pulled up on the collective. The helicopter responded to the control inputs. Gourgen watched the details of the plate fall away on the positioning monitor.

"Eighty."

"Ninety."

Gourgen could see the final length of cable drawing taut. A slight jerk as the cable reached its limit defined the historic moment. They were about the lift the heaviest single object ever lifted on a single cable by any helicopter. It was also the longest cable length any of the pilots had ever used on an operational mission.

Looking out the windscreen before he lifted the plate, Gourgen found the red and white, trellised, exhaust stack rising next to the tomb of Unit No. 4. From a hover 100 meters above the ground, he could see the dark gray, buttressed walls of the sarcophagus. He adjusted his heading slightly so that he was pointed directly at his target. They could not quite see the hole that would be the final resting place for the plate, but it was there. The plate had to travel 1.2 kilometers and up 35 meters to the top of the sarcophagus.

"Everything look all right over there?" asked Gourgen.

"Ready."

"As well. Increasing power," Gourgen announced as he raised the collective.

The needles on the engine turbine speed and temperature instruments moved clockwise around the faces of the dials. They could hear the engine roaring at the higher power levels although the helicopter and its load did not move. Gourgen adjusted his position to remain directly over the plate. As they approached the calculated power values for the heavy load, still nothing was happening. Gourgen pulled in a little more power, past the expected lift values.

Gourgen dropped the collective lowering the temperatures on the engines below the maximum continuous power levels to avoid consuming too much engine life. "Do you think that thing is stuck somehow?"

"We both examined the support structure, Gourgen. There is no way it could be stuck unless they bolted it down during the last few days, and I doubt anyone has done that."

"Then, it must be heavier than they expected."

The two pilots considered the possibilities. Maybe it was now too heavy to lift even with the powerful Mi-26 helicopter. They were going to have to do something. They could not sit in a high hover all day long. They had fuel for several passes at the lift, but they were consuming their options.

"Dmitri Igorovich, we could not lift the plate within our calculated values," Gourgen radioed.

"Is it stuck?" came the radio voice of Colonel Kalasnikov.

"We do not think so. Can you ask the engineers if the plate is heavier than they calculated?"

"Sure."

Gourgen and Anatoly could not hear the conversation on board the Mi-8 circling above them in a large two kilometer diameter orbit. They waited patiently for the reply. As the minutes passed, Gourgen figured Colonel Kalasnikov did not get the answer he wanted from the engineers with him, and he was probably talking on another frequency to other engineers on the ground. Fifteen minutes passed before a reply came.

"Gourgen, this is Dmitri."

"Go ahead."

"We have discussed the situation with experts on the ground. No one knows the precise weight of the plate. You have several options. We can stop and require them to remove the plate and get a precise weight that you can balance against your performance data, or you can make an attempt at the lift. General Antoshkin wants you to make the attempt."

"We have a little margin, but if we fail to get the plate off the ground with sufficient excess power to maneuver the plate for the placement, we could fail the engines before we get the plate in place."

"Understood. Are the engines new?"

"They are. The only time they have on them is the flight down here."

"What do you think about an attempt?"

Gourgen switched his thumb to the intercom position. "What do you think, Tolya?"

"I did not feel any movement before you stopped."

"Neither did I. We could be close or a long way from breaking ground."

The two pilots instinctively twisted in their suits to see the other's eyes behind the masks.

"We are here, now, Gourgen. The Motherland needs us to put this plate on that hell-hole." Gourgen nodded his head instead of talking. "I say pull out the stops. If an engine quits, we will start over from that point. If we do not try now, we will not know if we were close, and that thing," he said nodding toward the powerplant, "will continue to poison the air and the land."

Gourgen stared at this friend. He knew Anatoly was correct. The hard part was the thought of an engine failure with such a heavy load. If they dropped the plate and it flipped over, they might not ever be able to turn it over to make another attempt, or it might be damaged sufficiently to render it inadequate as a complete biological cover. Gourgen told himself, there was no one else. He shifted his thumb to the radio position.

"We will give it a try."

"Good. We will move in to keep an eye on things," answered Kalasnikov.

"Not too close."

"Not too close," repeated the accomplished Air Force officer.

"Here we go," Gourgen radioed, then switched his thumb to the intercom. "Watch the engines closely, Tolya. If one of them starts to flicker, let me know. If I let go of the plate, I want it to land upright."

"As you say."

"Well, I hope Soloviev built this set well," Gourgen said as he increased power on the huge engines.

The speeds and temperatures wound up passing the normal and emergency values of operational engines. Within a handful of seconds, the engines roared beyond their maximum calculated values. Gourgen continued to demand more than ever before. The aircraft shuddered as the plate broke free of the supports.

Gourgen arrested the slight climb rate as he tried to press the cyclic forward to move in the direction of the sarcophagus. He watched the plate. The tell-tale oscillatory movement of the plate began slowly at first. He tried to slow the helicopter in an attempt to dampen the oscillation. The movement got worse.

"I have got to put it down," said Gourgen as he watched the oscillations increase.

"Your load is swaying," radioed Kalasnikov.

"I know," answered Gourgen. "I am going to put it down."

Gourgen looked up. The trees at the edge of the clearing were approaching rapidly. The helicopter began moving back and forth in reaction to the swinging massive plate. Gourgen lowered the collective. They could feel the weight hit the ground. He quickly stablized his position.

"That was fun, wasn't it?"

"Nobody said this was going to be easy," answered Anatoly.

"Now, isn't that an understatement."

"Are you going to try again?"

Gourgen scanned the instrument panel. The engines still looked acceptable. They had enough fuel. "Might as well. Everything still looks good to me."

"Agreed."

"We are going to make another attempt," radioed Gourgen.

"Good. Take it a little slower," Colonel Kalasnikov answered from the circling Mi-8 helicopter.

"Thank you, colonel expert," Gourgen said over the intercom.

"Right," chuckled Anatoly.

Fortunately, the ground was dry and relatively hard. The plate had not sunk into the earth. The second try worked better now that he knew how much power was needed to lift the plate free.

Gourgen lifted the plate straight up until it was above the nearby trees. Ever so slowly, he moved the helicopter toward the sarcophagus. Gourgen rapidly scanned the scene in front of them as he watched the hook display. Everything looked perfect, so far.

"How am I doing on line up?" Gourgen asked his copilot.

"Looks good to me. I can see the hole."

"You watch my line up," he said. "I am clear of the stack, so I am going to focus on the cameras."

"Got it."

"Am I high enough?"

"I think so," Anatoly answered.

A few seconds later, Colonel Kalasnikov radioed, "Yes. You have five to ten meters clearance."

Gourgen scanned quickly between the two displays. The load was stable. The edge of the sarcophagus passed down the forward camera. The plate was now at least partially on the roof of the structure. The temptation was, to quickly get the majority of the plate on the roof in case he had to let go of it. He stayed with his slow translation.

The edge of the hole came into view on the top display. An urge to study the interior distracted Gourgen. He could feel the rivers of sweat descending over his neck and entire body. The world for him narrowed down to two video displays.

The lower, inner opening was square. For weeks, he thought it was circular like the plate. He had never asked the question. As he saw the position, he was too far to the right.

"I think I need to come left."

"I agree."

He added a slight left pressure. He instinctively tried to trim the control forces. The helicopter shuddered as the control forces shifted. As had happened before, the load began to move relative to the crosshairs. He had to get the load stopped. He did not have much time.

Gourgen tried to position the load. As he fought to find the correct place, the plate hit the top edge of the upper hole. A cloud of concrete dust marked the impact as well as the shake in the aircraft. The plate seemed to bounce off the structure picking up a circular motion. It bounced a few more times raising even more concrete dust. Gourgen knew he had to get the plate either off the roof or firmly on it before the massive weight broke up the top of the building.

He lowered the collective. The plate descended into the hole. He had to get it down to stop the movement, then he could start over again to position it properly. The plate struck something several more times.

The sickening waves of nausea added to the intensity of the moment. Radiation was getting through all the protective items. Time was running out.

The load hit the inner roof structure and stopped moving. It was down.

Gourgen lowered the collective to relieve the tension of the cable and give the engines at little break.

"That was close."

"Yes," growled Anatoly.

"Are you all right?"

"No. But, the load is not in place. Let's finish this, so we can leave."

Gourgen wanted to see his friend, but knew that served no purpose. The best thing for both of them was to complete the positioning of the load. They could not leave now. There would be no way to reattach the cable if they let it go.

He repositioned the helicopter to evaluate how much he needed to shift the plate. Gourgen fought against his mounting nausea as he raised the collective and the thrust on the main rotor. He centered the crosshairs again as Anatoly choked out the power of the engines as turbine temperature readings. The veteran test pilot swallowed hard against his urge to vomit as he adjusted the position of the huge helicopter. The plate broke free of the concrete and steel shelf. Gradually, Gourgen shifted the position until the last of the darkened interior of the building disappeared from sight. He reduced power to lessen the tension on the cable. As he turned the helicopter, he made the control adjustment to remain directly over the plate.

"Let's make sure the plate is in position."

"Yes," came Anatoly's muffled response.

Gourgen wanted to help his friend. He watched the top display as the helicopter turned completely around over the plate. The hole was sealed. There were no openings. The huge plate was perfectly positioned. Gourgen moved his thumb to a red button half way down the side of the grip. As he depressed the button, an electrical signal was sent through the wiring of the helicopter to a powerful electromagnet. The current closed a relay that removed electrical power to the magnet retracting a latch and causing the huge hook beneath the helicopter to open. The cable fell away to remain permanently with the plate it had carried.

Gourgen smoothly added power to the engines as he pushed the nose over in the first aggressive maneuver he had made with the Mi-26 in many months. He quickly jockeyed the machine to the prescribed landing point for the inspection. Before he shutdown the engines, he reached for the radio button.

"Dmitri Igorovich, please land now. I need you to take Anatoly to the hospital. He is quite ill."

"On the way."

As Gourgen worked through the shutdown procedures, he glanced over to his friend. Anatoly slumped forward against his harness straps. The thought of Lelechenko came to him as he pulled Anatoly from the seat. He also remembered the doctors' explanation for Anatoly's greater sensitivity to ionizing radiation. Gourgen wanted his friend to be all right. Spatters of blood dotted the inside of his mask. The sounds of the Mi-8 landing brought some reassurance. Several men dressed in protective suits entered the large cockpit. They picked Anatoly up by the shoulders and legs to carry him to the waiting helicopter. Within seconds, the Air Force helicopter leapt into the air with another victim of the worst nuclear power disaster in history.

# 23

*17:30, Tuesday, 15.July.1986*
*Military Response Team Camp*
*70 kilometers east of Chernobyl, Ukraine, USSR*

"Good job," said Colonel Kalasnikov as Gourgen lay on the field hospital treatment table with two sets of intravenous tubes in his arms, once again.

"The engineers checked your final placement," added Colonel Nestrov. "They say the plate is perfectly located. Excellent work. How do you feel?"

Gourgen waved his hand as though he did not have time for the question. Everybody knew how he felt. He did not need to repeat the observations.

The two Air Force officers laughed.

"We know what you mean," Kalasnikov said.

"How is Anatoly Demjanovich?"

"They evaluated him when he arrived here. The doctors determined that he needed special treatment in Moscow. He was flown by helicopter to Kiev before you landed back here. He will be in Moscow within another hour or so," Nestrov said.

"Clinic Number Six."

"Yes," Colonel Kalasnikov responded with a puzzled expression. "How did you know?"

Gourgen smiled and glanced at Nestrov, who knew the answer. "The doctors ordered us to the clinic after our reconnaissance flight in May, and our good colonel here," he said nodding toward Nestrov, "insisted we follow the doctors' orders. Plus, if that was not enough, the firefighters and technicians from the night of the explosion were evacuated to Clinic Number Six. Just before we flew this mission, Anatoly heard that a friend of his died up there as a result of his exposure after the accident."

"I am sorry," said Kalasnikov.

"What about me?" asked Gourgen, as if he did not qualify for special treatment, which could be good or really bad.

"Let me get the surgeon," answered Colonel Nestrov. "He will know."

Nestrov returned with a young man in medium green surgical clothing with an open, white, laboratory coat. A black stethoscope hung around his neck.

"So, you want to know how you are doing," the doctor said as he checked the medical chart. "Our best estimate is, you received another fifty or so REM, that puts you in the acute poisoning range, as best we can estimate."

Nestrov and Kalasnikov left the curtained treatment space.

"What does that mean?"

"I suppose the first item would be the measurement. We measure radiation in REM, or Radiation Equivalent Man. In other words, we measure base radiation in *Roentgen* and adjust the values based on the body mass of an individual. Your life time REM is 270 per the table. Your measured dose of 50 REM coupled with your symptoms means you have received a sufficient dose of ionizing radiation to damage the lining of your stomach and intestines. The most vulnerable area is your bone marrow. Your critical blood counts have already fallen and will remain low for the next few days. We must support your immune system to allow the marrow time to regenerate. These are some of the reasons you have these drips in your arms. We are trying to stablize your medical situation."

"What else?"

"The nature of radiation poisoning, unfortunately, means we will not know precisely what effects you may experience beyond the acute phase. You should feel better each day, and you should be back to normal in a few weeks. Your accumulated exposure could cause problems, years down the road. The real damage is not likely to manifest itself symptomatically for 20 years."

"What kind of problems?"

"Statistically, you may develop one of many cancers within the next 20 years. The most likely is leukemia, a blood malignancy that can appear in many different forms."

"How will I know?"

"We will need to take blood tests periodically probably for the rest of your life to ensure we find any disease early, so it can be properly treated. If you develop an acute form, you will notice unusual and persistent fatigue as well as a susceptibility to infection and easy or persistent hematoma – bruises."

"Are these diseases treatable?" he asked, then looked sternly into the doctor's eyes, as if to say, you had better tell me the truth. "Will I survive?"

"The answer is generally, yes. The outcome is too difficult to predict. One thing is absolutely certain, you must avoid any radiation source, from now on. You do not want to add any more counts to your total body dose."

"Fine by me."

The doctor rechecked the chart, then put it down. He took Gourgen's blood pressure, temperature and heart rate as well as listened to his heart and lungs. He wrote everything down in the chart.

"You are recovering quite nicely. As an extra precaution, I think we will hold you here overnight, then evacuate you to Moscow."

Gourgen knew the destination. The image brought other thoughts. "What can you tell me about Anatoly Demjanovich?"

"Grishchenko?" Gourgen nodded his head. "Your copilot and I suspect your friend?" Again, Gourgen nodded his head. "To be honest, he is in more serious condition. Since he received essentially the same dose as you, there must be other factors. He has greater body mass, but I surmise he may be more susceptible, either by prior exposure or genetically. Perhaps he experienced some exposure earlier in his life. He was evacuated to Moscow for precise treatment. You can check on him once you arrive there tomorrow. You are going to the same place."

"Clinic Number Six," Gourgen repeated for the doctor.

"So, you are familiar with the facility. They specialize in the treatment of acute radiation poisoning, among other things. They have the best blood specialists in the country. You will be well taken care of up there – the best our medical profession can offer."

"I can't wait," Gourgen grumbled sarcastically.

"The two of you have done a very heroic thing," the doctor said as he stood at the foot of the treatment table. "They say you have saved the country."

"I doubt that, but thank you."

Gourgen took advantage of the time. He tried to sleep, but awoke several times with various images from the mission. Leaving the big helicopter at Pripyat, forever doomed to oblivion, offended his since of history. The prototype Mi-26 that set the many world records for lifting weight to altitude had been retired to an aviation museum to be marveled at by young children and aviation enthusiasts. Their Mi-26 had accomplished an equally significant feat. As far as Gourgen could remember, the machine lifted the heaviest external load in history and on one of the longest, if not the longest, cable ever. Sadly, the aircraft would never be appreciated as other historic aircraft were displayed. It now sat among a fleet of condemned Air Force helicopters and a mass of contaminated and abandoned construction equipment. He also remembered the sequence of events from the first suggestion to the final placement. The effort had been extraordinary in many ways, and so few people would ever know what had been accomplished. The most important element was mission completion. They successfully sealed the sarcophagus. No more radioactive isotopes would contaminate the air and the earth. Gourgen smiled despite his physical discomfort.

The following day, the Air Force flew Gourgen Karapetyan to the Northwest suburbs of Moscow. He underwent a variety of medical tests, many of which were repeats of those he received at the field hospital. Several days passed as his medical evaluation and treatment continued before they would let him see his friend. Ludmilla and Galina passed along information between the two pilots while they remained immobilized. As the field hospital doctor told him, he began to feel better every day. When they finally unplugged him from all the tubes, he began to move around the hospital. He found Anatoly.

"Hey, friend," Gourgen announced to wake up his copilot.

"Gourgen, good to see you."

"I have seen you look better. How are you feeling?"

"I probably feel as good as I look." They laughed. "So, they brought you up here as well."

"Yes."

"You must be doing better than me," Anatoly said.

"I suppose, but you are going to be fine as well."

"Perhaps." Anatoly stared at his friend. "We did it."

Gourgen smiled. "Yes, we did."

"What happened to the bird?"

"We had to leave it down there. We will probably never see it again . . . too much contamination from dust and other stuff."

"A pity . . . at least, that damn thing is covered up now."

"Yes, it is. They told me before I left that they would complete the tomb in another two weeks. The important thing is, the reactor is completely sealed, now."

"Right! And, it will only take several thousand years for the radioactive contamination of the surrounding land to decay away."

Gourgen knew the subject was a sensitive one, but there was nothing any of them could do to change what had happened. They had done their part to contain the disaster. Perhaps the world would be a little better for their efforts.

"What have the doctors told you?" asked Gourgen.

"They tell me all the pilots have been sick from the radiation. They also tell me they will not really know about me for several week or months, maybe even years. According to them, I have been the worst among the pilots."

"You will get better."

"Like Aleksandr Grigoryevich?"

"Tolya, that serves no purpose. We have all done our duty. The country . . . the world . . . needed us to do our job. Your friend, Lelechenko, did his job."

"And, I shall end up like him."

"Anatoly Demjanovich," shouted Gourgen, "we shall all pass in time. We do not need to hasten the arrival of our passing. Now, you rest, get back to health, so we can go fly."

"What we do best."

"Yes. Exactly. What we do best."

Anatoly finally smiled and nodded his head. "As you say, then. Now, get out of here. I am tired. I need a nap."

Gourgen chuckled at his dismissal, then touched Anatoly's shoulder as his eyes closed. He took one last look back at his friend and colleague as if to make sure he was truly resting.

The nurse in his ward told him which doctor he wanted to talk to about Anatoly. He considered going directly to Doctor Vorobiev, the Director of the All Union Center for Hematology, but knew the important man would be very busy. The search took the better part of 30 minutes with several redirections.

"I want to know how my friend, Anatoly Grishchenko, is regarding his recovery," he said to the young doctor.

"Who are you?"

"I am Gourgen Karapetyan."

"Oh, yes sir," said the doctor probably connecting the person standing before him with the other information about their patients. "Mister Grishchenko is suffering from acute radiation poisoning. His blood counts are dangerously low. We are supporting him now with special blood products."

"Yes, but will he recover?"

"That is very hard to say. We have seen many patients from Chernobyl. The biological damage has been significant, but in the end, it comes down to each individual. There is no way to tell at this stage, what Mister Grishchenko's prognosis is. It will take some time for his situation to stablize enough for us to have a clear view."

"Is he in danger?"

"For the moment, I suspect not. However, like I said, we will not know about his full recovery for probably many months. The human body is a very resilient organism. It can tolerate much abuse, but when it comes to radiation poisoning, there are fragile boundaries. Whether he crosses over onto the downhill slope depends on what is going on inside him."

"Is there anything I can do?"

"Encourage him."

"Can anyone do more?"

"That depends upon his medical condition."

"Such as."

The doctor looked around the large treatment room. Gourgen did the same. No one seemed to be listening and most of the others were beyond reasonable hearing distance.

"First, there are no solid indications Grishchenko warrants such treatment. My best guess at this stage is, he will most likely respond to conventional treatments for months, perhaps years. He may even fully recover. There is no way to predict such outcomes. However, I suspect, based on his symptoms, he will probably deteriorate over time. Now, given that and with the condition . . . you did not hear this from me," he said as he looked around again, "there are some treatments that can only be administered in the West. Hopefully, it will not come to that," he added as if his preface had not placed enough ambiguity on the words.

Gourgen wondered why the young doctor might be concerned about who could be listening. The information seemed relatively innocuous. He decided to press for more information.

"What treatments?"

"The most common disease associated with radiation poisoning is leukemia. The bone marrow, which produces all the blood cells and because it regenerates at a relatively high rate, is the most susceptible to damage from ionizing radiation. Leukemia, simply, is a failure of the marrow to produce normal blood cells. The only known treatment is a bone marrow transplant . . . extracting good marrow from a healthy donor and transfusing it into the patient once his damaged marrow has been completely destroyed."

"Bone marrow transplant?"

"Yes."

"Do they use a dead donor like a heart transplant?"

The doctor laughed softly. "No. The extraction is more complicated than drawing blood, but the marrow is a renewable resource like blood itself."

"When will you know if he needs one of these bone marrow transplants?"

"As I said earlier, it may be many months. He may fully recover. We just do not know what to expect."

"Why are you so worried about who will hear?" Gourgen asked going directly to the point.

The doctor glared back at Gourgen. "We have instructions to contain the treatment of the Chernobyl victims. The government does not want us stirring things up with demands for medical treatments in the West."

"Can't we do these bone marrow transplants in Russia?"

"Yes, but our success is not as good, and we can only do transplants from related donors, meaning direct, blood, family members. Unrelated donor transplants can only be performed in the West, today. They have special medicines for treatment of the side effects. They have done most of the research. The doctor who developed the procedure works in Seattle in America."

"So, if you needed a bone marrow transplant, you would go to the West?"

"Yes, but I would be more likely to be able to go."

"What do you mean?"

"The other doctors, the older doctors, have told me who you two are. They told me you are a Hero of the Soviet Union. You are both very important test pilots. They say, the Government will not admit that it cannot treat men of such stature."

"We shall see."

"I wish you luck."

"What is so special about this procedure?"

"It is very complicated, but like any transplant, the compatibility of the donor and the recipient is the key. The highest probability of success is with a genetically matched donor, like a sibling."

"Anatoly has no brothers or sisters."

"Then, if he needs a transplant, he will probably need what is called an unrelated or allogeneic donor. The American doctors have just begun unrelated donor transplants. Far too early for any appreciation of results or success, but the concept is very promising if they can sort out the tissue rejection problems."

"That is beyond my level of understanding," Gourgen chuckled waving his hand as if swatting a fly.

"Yes . . . well . . . we have much before us."

"Should I start finding a way to get Anatoly to America for treatment?"

Shock drained the color from the doctor's face. "No! Please do not do that. If you make official inquiries, they will soon figure out that it was me who told you this information. Also, it is too early to determine the best course. You asked me some hypothetical questions. I have tried to answer them truthfully. Anatoly may fully recover. We cannot know at this stage."

"I will respect your concerns, comrade doctor," Gourgen said as if to remind the physician of his own status and influence, and conjure up tones of Stalinist absolutism. "We shall wait, then."

"Good."

"You must take the best care of Anatoly Demjanovich. He is a very special pilot and a friend of more years than I care to count."

"We will do our best. I promise."

# 24

*17:30, Tuesday, 15.May.1987*
*All Union Center for Hematology*
*Moscow, Russia, USSR*

The year since the reactor accident and their exposure added to the seriousness of Anatoly's illness as Gourgen understood it. His friend would have good days and bad days. The doctors seemed to worry far more than either of them. This was now Anatoly's fourth return to Moscow's All Union Center for Hematology. Without making a calendar calculation, Gourgen believed the frequency of his friend's admissions was increasing. He tried to find a nurse or one of the doctors he recognized, but could not do so within a few minutes. He did find Anatoly's private room.

The usually warm spring day made the hospital room feel like a steam room. There was no breeze coming through the open windows. Gourgen Karapetyan did not want to be there for any one of a host of reasons, but Anatoly's re-admittance caught their immediate attention.

"What happened?" asked Gourgen as he entered the room.

Anatoly lay in the bed with fresh white sheets and a cover sheet pulled up between his legs covering only his hips. He had an unusual pink tint to his skin, not the normal brownish color, like he was as white as the sheets, but something flushed his skin.

"Some type of infection, they say."

"How do you feel?"

"Not the best, actually. I feel weak. I seem to fatigue much quicker than I used to."

"What does all of this mean?"

"The doctors do not tell me much. But, from what I can gather, my bones are not producing the number of white cells I need, so I am more susceptible to infections. I have a simple cold, but the doctors worry about it."

"Maybe I should go talk to them."

"Perhaps. You seem to get more out of them than I do. Why don't you see what they will tell you?"

"I will do it. So, you are going to be all right?"

"That is what they tell me. I think so. I do not feel that bad, just tired."

"All right. I shall go find the correct doctor to get some answers for us."

Anatoly nodded his head and smiled before Gourgen left his friend's hospital room.

The search for the correct doctor took much longer than he anticipated, compounding his frustration. Several of the interim attempts yielded nothing he did not already know. Eventually, he managed to track down the same young doctor he had learned so much from last year. With the usual professional greetings completed, Gourgen jumped directly to the point.

"What is Anatoly Grishchenko's condition?" he asked.

"Serious."

"How so?"

"He has a blood disorder called, aplastic anemia. It means his bone marrow is not producing the normal amounts of cellular products. He has developed a serious infection from a virus that would not be much consequence to you or me. He also appears to be exhibiting the early stages of leukemia."

"Is this from the radiation?"

The doctor began looking around again. The topic was obviously sensitive. They found a small office and closed the door.

"We have been directed to not speculate about the cause factors for anyone who might have been near Chernobyl. The Government is very sensitive to such speculation."

"So, answer my question," Gourgen said with mounting impatience. He did not care for any of the politics. He just wanted to help his friend.

"I believe the answer is, yes."

"And, the Government does not want to help us treat his

illness?"

"I would not say that. We are treating his illness as an incidental occurrence, rather than radiation induced."

"What is the difference?"

"To him, probably nothing, but it does change how we report our findings and treatment."

"What can I do?"

The doctor thought about his answer as he held Gourgen's eyes. "Both of you flew over the reactor at the same time, did you not?"

"Yes. We were together on each flight."

"I would like to do the same tests on you. Perhaps, your data will give us more information regarding his condition."

"How?"

"Well, I am not sure. It depends on the results. Both of you were exposed to approximately the same levels of ionizing radiation, for about the same time. You are also smaller than him, thus your equivalent dosage would be higher, and there should be more damage to your biological systems. But, if your blood counts are perfectly normal . . . mid-range or so . . . then, perhaps his illness is incidental."

"Why does that matter? If he is sick, he needs treatment. The cause has no meaning to me. I just want him to get the best treatment whether it is here, in Mother Russia, or in America."

The doctor's eyes narrowed slightly. "I would be careful with that line of reasoning."

"Bullshit!" barked Gourgen. "He will get the help he needs."

"I just caution you, there are some very powerful people who do not want to recognize the injury done by that accident."

"I am not concerned about their feelings. I am only concerned about my friend."

"You recognize, I am sure, I cannot openly associate Anatoly's illness with his exposure at Chernobyl."

Gourgen felt that grating frustration commonly experienced around professional bureaucrats just trying to protect their jobs rather than doing the right thing. "I understand. Now, let us get on with these blood tests you want to do. Perhaps, my results will help Anatoly."

The medical technician assigned by the doctor took a half dozen vials of blood from his left arm without saying a word. They also scanned his body with some special instruments he had never seen before. The technician would only say it was standard procedure for patients exposed at Chernobyl. The result would take a little more than a week to process and analyze.

Gourgen returned to Anatoly's room to report what little information he had gathered, and what the doctors wanted to learn from his blood tests as comparisons to Anatoly's data. He felt sorry for his friend, but in his heart, he knew they would find a way to help Anatoly.

The visits were not every day, although they were as often as Gourgen could get away from his duties. He was spending more time with Anatoly than Galina or anyone else other than the medical personnel. The observation quietly bothered him. Anatoly held his frustration regarding the extra burden his illnesses placed on everyone around him. Galina's aversion to the hospital and Anatoly's condition added a little more weight to Anatoly's burden, each day.

Gourgen received a message at the conclusion of a long series of flights testing the new Mi-28 advanced attack helicopter for the Government. He was tired when he read the message asking him to come up to the All Union Center for Hematology as soon as he could. They had another long series of flights scheduled for the next day, but he made arrangements to postpone the afternoon flights. His colleagues understood.

Gourgen did not like the familiarity growing on him regarding the famous medical establishment. None of the pilots liked hospitals; it was physical proof and a reminder they were all too vulnerable. Nonetheless, he found the appointed room.

He located the same doctor whose name he could never

remember. The man shuffled through a small stack of papers in the folder.

"Well, from these tests, we know you have not developed any leukemia. Several of your counts are on the low end of the range which might indicate a slow deterioration due to your exposure, however today, they are within the acceptable boundaries."

"That is reassuring."

"Yes, well, there is more. We made an attempt to determine your background emission levels."

"What!"

"You have been exposed to ionizing radiation. You have also suffered acute symptoms of radiation poisoning. Your radiation counts are similar to those of Anatoly and other pilots we have evaluated."

"So, that proves it."

"Although I cannot admit so outside this room, I would say, yes."

"Then, why aren't I as sick as Anatoly Demjanovich."

"For the same reason some people develop symptoms from the common cold virus and others do not. It depends upon many factors some of which we understand, many we do not. He was just more susceptible."

"How does that help him, or help us help him?"

"To me, it confirms my suspicions."

"And?"

"We do not have the ability to treat him properly in this country."

"We need to get him to America."

"I cannot even suggest that . . . ."

"Look, doctor," barked Gourgen interrupting the physician. "You have told me too many times about the Government's coverup. You tell me the best thing to do, stop giving me all this crap, and I will take care of the rest. I will not expose you."

The doctor sat in his chair behind his little desk somewhat stunned. Gourgen wondered if the man had never been confronted before now. Maybe he was too young to have developed the calluses Gourgen and others had grown over the years of living in this environment.

"I am sorry," Gourgen said finally. "I did not mean to shock you. I just want Anatoly healthy again and able to fly with us."

The doctor nodded his head in agreement. "I understand your impatience. I will do my best to assist you with information. The answer to your question is, yes. I believe that is the only place for proper treatment of Anatoly Demjanovich."

"When you first mentioned this treatment, you said the Americans had only done a few of these bone transplants."

"Not bone transplants," the doctor corrected. "Bone marrow transplants. It is a much more complex version of a blood transfusion, but it works."

"Whatever. Can this really save Anatoly?"

"Just in the last year, they have done a few hundred more unrelated transplants. While it is still too early to tell whether this is a permanent cure, the results appear to be very promising. The long and short of it . . . this treatment is probably his only hope. It is the possibility of a true cure of his illness."

"Then, that is what we will do."

"It will not be easy."

"Doctor, in our profession, we are quite accustomed to doing the impossible. I will get this done. How much time do I have?"

"It is difficult to say. If he takes care of himself and minimizes his exposure to infection, he should survive for another year or two. If not, he might not last more than a few months. He must take care of himself and avoid infections or other afflictions that might deplete his weakened immune system."

"I will ensure that he understands this. Then, I have a year or two to make the arrangements for his treatment in America."

"Yes."

"Then, so it shall be. I will start working on this immediately."

Gourgen stood to leave the doctor's small office.

"Wait. One more thing," said the doctor. Gourgen paused.

"Please be seated." Gourgen did as he was requested. "The tests found something else." The veteran pilot nodded his head. "You have chronic hepatitis. You must have been exposed one or more times in your past. It appears to be asymptomatic at this point, but it is a disease you must pay attention to for the rest of your life."

Gourgen had heard of the disease, but knew little about it. From the doctor's tone of voice, it was serious. He wondered if this was his form of injury from the Chernobyl flights.

"What is it?"

"Hepatitis is a degenerative disease of the liver. You appear to have the chronic form which is more difficult to diagnose and treat. It is a disease we will have to watch closely."

"Isn't that grand."

"I am sorry."

"Is there anything I need to do, now?"

"No. We simply monitor the disease. If you develop symptoms like joint pain, fever, fatigue, nausea or jaundice, you must return to the hospital immediately. The key for you will be prompt treatment."

"Anything else?"

"No."

"Is this from Chernobyl?" he asked, although the answer really did not matter or change anything.

"No. This disease is thought to be viral. It cannot be induced by exposure to ionizing radiation. So, no, there is no way it could have come from your flights over the power plant. You were exposed one or more times, to one virus or another, probably many years ago. Granted, your radiation exposure will probably not help your condition, but it certainly was not induced by that exposure."

Gourgen thought about the senselessness of all this medical dialogue. This is just one more reason I do not like hospitals, he said to himself. "Thank you for your help . . . and this additional information."

"I will do my best to help."

"Thank you."

Gourgen departed for Anatoly's room. He found his friend alert, sitting up and reading a book. He looked much better than the week prior.

"Ah, good to see you, Gourgen. Have you come to get me out of this place?"

"How are you feeling?" Gourgen asked, repeating the all too prevalent question.

"Like a caged animal. I feel fine, but the doctors say they are not quite ready for me to leave."

"What have they told you?"

"I have a blood disorder," Anatoly said as he turned his eyes to the window. "They say it is from natural causes, but I know it is from that damnable reactor."

"What else did they tell you?"

"There is no treatment for my illness, and I must take care of myself to live longer."

"That was rather blunt, wasn't it?" Anatoly nodded. "Well, my friend, we have work to do."

"What do you mean?"

"I have learned that a treatment does exist that will cure you. The only problem is, we must get you to America."

Anatoly laughed loudly. "Well, now, isn't that encouraging. My cure might as well be on the Moon."

Gourgen felt the urge to chastise his friend. Neither one of them had ever given up on any situation despite the odds. They were alive today because of their 'never-say-die' attitude. He chose to let the challenge pass for the moment. "Perhaps . . . but, we shall begin the process today."

"Whatever you say."

"Anatoly Demjanovich, what is with you? Are you ready to die? Have you given up on this already?"

"No."

"Then, what do you want to do?"

"I want to get back to what we do best . . . fly."

"If you do not fight this disease, you will not return to flying."

"So, what is this cure."

"A bone marrow transplant in America. They have developed the procedure."

"Now, doesn't that sound like a great idea. You want them to crack open my bones to transplant someone else's marrow. What a delightful idea?"

"I am getting tired of your attitude."

"It is not your life that is in jeopardy, Gourgen. I do not want false hope. I simply want to return to what I was."

"Then, let me make the arrangements. You just fight this sickness."

"All right. You have a deal."

For Gourgen, the exchange with Anatoly set his course. He was more determined than ever to find the path. Gorbachev's initiatives for governmental and societal reform as well as the openness he called for, grew in strength and tempo. Gourgen remembered the visit of the Soviet Air Force fighters to Finland last year and Anatoly Kovatchur's efforts to translate the opening to the West. The pilots thought that they might be allowed to attend the great international airshow in Farnborough, England, next year, along as the Western press continued to play up the new openness.

Gourgen started to leave Anatoly. "One more thing," said Anatoly. Gourgen stopped at the door and faced his friend. "Would you go see Galina? She is having so much trouble with this sickness. She does not come to see me like she used to, and I am not sure I blame her; but, I am worried about her."

"As soon as I get back to Zhukovsky. Well, maybe not quite as soon as I get back."

"What do you mean?" asked Anatoly with a stiff inquisitiveness in his voice.

"I want to talk to Anatoly Kovatchur, first, as soon as possible. I remember him telling me about a flight demonstration of the MiG-29 in Finland, last year. As a result of that, they are making plans for participation in one of the international airshows, I think Farnborough, England, next year. He might be the designated pilot.

It may be our best chance to make contact with one of the American pilots to help us get you to America."

"Really?"

"Yes, it was apparently decided a few weeks ago, so I hear, but I have not had an opportunity to talk to him. Now, I have a reason."

"Good luck, then. But, please talk to Galya."

"I will try to do that tonight. I will asked Ludmilla to come with me."

"Excellent. I hope you can help her."

"I will. Now, you rest and get better."

Anatoly nodded his head in agreement. Gourgen turned and departed. He stopped to say good-bye to the nurses he recognized and admonished them to take the best care of his friend Anatoly Demjanovich.

As Gourgen learned of the governmental constraints on the handling of the medical consequences of the accident, he also decided to take a different parallel path around the roadblocks.

He sought friend and fellow test pilot, Anatoly Kovatchur. After a few telephone calls, he located Kovatchur – Ramskoye Aerodrome.

Gourgen waited for Anatoly's return from a test flight at the Mikoyan flight test facility on the enormous government airfield at Zhukovsky.

"What are you doing here, Gourgen?" said Kovatchur, carrying his white flight helmet and looking like some spaceman in his high altitude suit.

"We need to talk."

"Is it Anatoly Demjanovich?"

"Yes."

"Did he die?"

"No, but he needs our help."

Anatoly nodded his head. "Let me debrief this flight and get out of the monkey suit, then we shall talk."

Gourgen waited. He wandered around the main lobby studying

the various memorabilia collected over the 50 years of aviation experience within the Mikoyan-Gurevich Design Bureau. They had a proud history as all the aviation companies did regardless of nationality. Mikoyan was the premier fighter organization just as Mil was the most renown helicopter group.

Anatoly returned without all the flight regalia. "So, what do we do, Gourgen?" he asked as he waved for Gourgen to follow him. They walked toward the apartment buildings where they all lived.

"Anatoly Demjanovich is recovering from his latest infection, but the doctors tell me he has a serious disease that may soon kill him, if he is not careful." Anatoly nodded, not wanting to interrupt Gourgen's train of thought. "His only cure is apparently something called a bone marrow transplant."

"That sounds bad."

"I suppose, but the doctors think it is his only hope."

"Then, we get him one."

"The only place is in the West – England, France. But, they developed the procedure in America. They have the most experience with this."

"Ah ha, and so the story thickens. How do we do that?"

"Well, I understand you are preparing for the possibility of displaying the MiG-29 at Farnborough, England, next year."

"Yes."

"Do you think the Americans will be there?"

"Yes, well, there will certainly be Americans there."

"Are you going to go?"

"That depends. We have talked about it. There seems to be some government encouragement with all this openness stuff going on around us. They like my work. Menitsky says I am the likely primary pilot since I learned English is school."

"Would you be agreeable to finding an American pilot you think would help us overcome some of the obstacles over there?"

"Like what obstacles?"

"They tell me that without an invitation and specific

arrangements in America, the Government will not grant an entry visa. And, without an entry visa, he gets no exit permission from this country. Without that, he goes nowhere."

"So, if I go to Farnborough next year, you want me to find an American to help us?"

"Yes."

"Do you want a helicopter pilot or a fixed wing pilot?"

"I do not think it really matters, but I guess a helicopter pilot if you can find the right person to help us."

"Gourgen, you know you can count on me. We have to show the Government we need to go to Farnborough."

"Then, you must fly the piss out of your machine, so there will be no doubt about it. With that, the demand to go should be great."

"Should be. I will do my best."

"We can ask for no more."

"Are we going to have a get-together tonight?" asked Anatoly. "We have not had one in several weeks."

"I doubt it. Anatoly has asked me to talk to Galya. She has not been up to much of anything in the last few months. When Anatoly went back into the hospital this time, she virtually withdrew from life. She just stays in her apartment."

"Is there anything I can do?"

"I do not know, Anatoly Sergeiyevich. I am going to see what I can do. I will leave you, now. I want to pick up Milla, and the two of us will go talk to Galya."

"Good luck."

"Right. Thanks. I suppose we need to decide on another place for our Friday night parties."

"We can use my place, but it is quite a bit smaller, no family yet, and all."

Gourgen laughed at the thought of everyone crowding into Anatoly's small apartment. "We can find a better place. Perhaps I can convince Milla to host the party at our place."

"Whatever you decide, Gourgen."

Gourgen took a deep breath and let it out in a near whistle. "I am not looking forward to this conversation, but I promised Anatoly, so I had better get on with it."

"Good luck, and again, if there is anything I can do, just let me know."

"You have already agreed to take the biggest step for all of us. We need things to fall into place quickly. The doctors say, he does not have a great deal of time."

"Understood. Again, good luck tonight."

"Thank you."

# 25

*19:30, Tuesday, 15.May.1987*
*Building R4, Apartment 44*
*Zhukovsky, Russia, USSR*

The thought of facing Galina alone did not give Gourgen a
sense of joyous anticipation. She was not happy, nor was Ludmilla
for that matter. They had not been given a choice; actually, neither
had he and Anatoly, although many said they made the choice to
fly the mission. The flights over or near the disaster site were
completed. The best they knew, they would never have to go back
to that place again. Unfortunately, as is the case in war or any other
situation of national sacrifice, the participants and their loved ones
would pay a much longer and deeper price. Anatoly's medical
condition crossed over the line, and they did not have a great deal
of time. Galina would simply have to put aside her resentment and
help her husband.

Gourgen found Ludmilla in the kitchen.

"Galya says you went to see Anatoly today," she said without
looking up from the vegetables she was chopping on the cutting
board.

"Yes, I did."

"How is he?"

"Milla, I need your help."

She stopped her work to look at him. "What for?"

"We need to talk to Galya. Anatoly asked us to talk to her."

"Us or you?"

"Well, me, but you can help her understand."

With the large knife still clenched in her hand, she placed her
knuckles on her hip and faced Gourgen. "Now, how do you suppose
I can do that when I do not understand it myself?"

"Milla, please. We have been through this too many times. I need your help. Tolya and Galya need our help."

She remained frozen in time, without even a blink of her eyes. Gourgen shrugged his shoulders and held his hands out, palms up, as if to say, well, what is your answer.

"All right," she said as the trance broke. "Can we eat supper, first? Or, is this something that must be done this instant?"

"It can wait."

Gourgen washed his hands and helped Ludmilla prepare the simple meal. He removed three plates from the cupboard.

"Dimitri will not be here. It is just us," she said.

"That boy has not yet finished school, and he is already gone."

"He is the last, and he is trying to grow up faster than his brothers and sisters."

"It would be nice to have a meal with him once in a while," Gourgen lamented.

"You are the one who is gone. I have breakfast with him just about every morning, and lunch on the weekends. So, it is you, Gourgen, who is not here."

Gourgen nodded his head in quiet acquiescence. He knew when the topic was lost.

Sausage, cheese and black bread along with early tomatoes comprised the meal. They completed the preparation. The mixture of aromas from the various elements of the meal produced an anticipation Gourgen liked. He swallowed several times to control his salivation. Several bites were needed to settle his senses down to a routine.

"So, tell me about Anatoly Demjanovich, and what we must tell Galya," she said as she took another bite.

Gourgen finished chewing and swallowed. He put his fork down, rested his elbows on either side of his plate and clasped his hands. "You asked me earlier how Anatoly is. The plain and simple of it is, he is not well. I had to practically beat one of the doctors to get any real information. The Government is trying to eliminate or avoid any connection between Anatoly's illness and Chernobyl, but he has some type of blood disease that will be fatal if he does not get proper treatment."

"Then, why don't they give him this proper treatment."

"The best place for this treatment is America."

The sound of incredulity burst from her as if she had caught her husband pulling her leg. When his expression remained stoic, the humor vanished from her eyes. She thought about what Gourgen had just said. "There is no other place?"

"The doctor tells me, it is a procedure that cannot be done in this country. They can do it in England or France, but the best place is America."

"Would not France be better?"

"In some respects, yes, but the doctors who developed this procedure, who have perfected it, are in America. We need to get him to America."

"And, Galya does not want him to go?"

"No, that is not it. She does not know about the American treatment. I just learned that this afternoon." He looked at the food still on his plate and considered whether he should take another bite to produce a longer pause. "Anatoly is worried about her. He thinks she is so angry over his illness that she will not come to see him."

"Yes, she is angry," barked Ludmilla with defiance in her eyes. "You two went off to do some heroic thing, and now Anatoly is slowly dying."

"He does not have to die. He can be cured if we can get him to America soon enough."

"Then, we must get him to America."

"Sure, but Anatoly needs Galina's support. He needs to know that his illness is not destroying her, too."

"She will overcome her aversion. She is a strong woman."

"You will help me?"

"I will help Galya. I am not sure what help you need from me, unless you think Galina might become hysterical . . . which I do not . . . and, you want me to deal with it."

She was partially correct. Gourgen started to tell her about the other news he received this day. The distraction would not help Galina or Tolya. He would wait until later. "Just be there," he answered simply as he returned to his meal. Ludmilla followed.

They finished, cleaned the few dishes and utensils they used and wrote a short message for Dimitri, just in case he came home while they were with Galina. The cool evening air now smelled of rain. Gourgen knocked on the Grishchenko's apartment door, then put his arm around Ludmilla's waist which he rarely did these days. Gourgen tried to smile as she opened the door.

Their expressions told Galina the wrong thing. She started shaking her head and staggering backward.

"No, Galya," protested Gourgen as he held his hand up. "Tolya is all right. Everything is OK," he lied to avoid her total breakdown. The wives of aviators had become all too aware of the odd knock at the door and the heavy expression of a friend, colleague or neighbor standing before them – the harbinger of bad news. She had seen the worst.

She regained partial control. "Are you sure?"

Gourgen nodded his head. Galina motioned for them to come in, then led them into the kitchen. She placed a small tea kettle on the stove. Ludmilla helped her friend gather some cookies and crackers. Gourgen stood in the doorway with his hands high on the sides of the doorjamb as if he was Atlas holding the world on his shoulders. He listened to the pattering of the women until they sat down in the living room with a cup of tea and a cookie each. Galina looked at Gourgen as if to say she was now ready to talk.

"I visited Tolya at the clinic today."

"How is he?"

"He is doing reasonably well, Galya, but he needs your support."

"I know he does," she said lowering her chin to her chest. "I just get so angry when I see him. He was a big, strong man until he went to that place. They made him sick. They are killing him."

"Galina, that thinking does not help him. It hurts him. He can feel your revulsion. He knows what you are thinking."

"Why?" she shouted. "Why have they done this to him?"

"No one did this. It was an accident. It was a most unfortunate accident. Many others have died from this accident. Tolya does not have to die, too. He can be cured."

"They . . . cure him," she spat.

"It is not so simple."

"Why didn't you get sick?" Galina growled.

Gourgen stared at her, then looked to Ludmilla who could only look back at him. He was on his own and would not get much help from his wife. "Everyone is different. Some people get colds; some people don't," he said, repeating the doctor's words.

"This is not a cold."

"I know that, but I cannot explain this. We were both in the same aircraft, for the same time, at the same place."

"He was sick, too, Galya," Ludmilla said finally.

"Yes, but, he is fine, now," she protested.

"If you call hepatitis fine," he blurted out, then instantly regretted his lapse of control.

"What?" Ludmilla said.

"Never mind."

"No, I want to know."

"I am sorry I said anything. I am not the topic here – Anatoly is."

"Gourgen . . . ," Ludmilla began, then stopped when he held up his hand.

"We need to help Tolya."

"So, what do you want me to do?" Galina asked.

Ludmilla leaned forward in anticipation of whatever Gourgen was going to tell her.

"When was the last time you made love to him?" Ludmilla asked, interjecting her own thoughts.

Gourgen looked at his wife with incredulity. They did not talk about these things with other people. He started to interrupt, but decided to let her run with it.

"That is rather personal, Milla."

"Yes, but I will bet it was before the disaster." Galina lowered her head to avert her eyes, then nodded her head slightly. "He needs you, Galya. You need him. You are not going to get this disease from him." She stopped to look at Gourgen. "Is she?" Gourgen shook his head. "See. There you have it. He needs to be reminded there is something worth living for, beyond that hospital bed."

Galina meekly nodded her head, again.

Gourgen leaned forward to take control of the conversation. "I will work to get him to America as soon as we possibly can, but that may take a while. In the interim, he needs your support. He needs to feel your love; that will sustain him for however long it takes us to accomplish this." The stunned expression and open, speechless mouth told him he had jumped too many steps.

"America! Are you crazy?" she sneered.

Gourgen held up his hand. "Wait, Galya. It is not as bad as it sounds. The treatment to cure Tolya can only be done in the West."

"America?" she said more softly.

"My apologies. I forgot that you did not know about this. Trust me. It is the appropriate action from everything I have learned. But, only you can give him the attention he needs today."

Galina just stared at him as if she was waiting for him to flinch or blink. The urge to say more mounted within his thoughts. He resisted the temptation. She needed to feel his strength, his commitment, his determination. His patience paid off.

"You are right. I will go see him tomorrow. I will do my best to be happy, to make him feel better."

"Good, and I will do my part."

"I am so scared," Galina added.

"I know," responded Ludmilla as she must have finally felt it was her turn. "We all feel threatened by this. I worry all the time. Before this thing down there, I really did not worry about Gourgen. I just knew he would always come home. But, now, I worry about everything. It is not easy."

"You need to think of the future."

"That is precisely what worries me – the future. What future will I have if Tolya dies? I have seen what happens to the wives when their husbands are killed. I do not want that to happen to me. I need Tolya for many reasons."

"I know, Galya, I know."

"Then, we must work to make this successful, to get him the treatment he needs."

"If anyone can do it, I know you can, Gourgen. I know you can. I will do my part, and I know you will do yours."

"You can count on it," Gourgen said, then took a sip of his cold tea. "We must go."

"Do you want us to stay, Galya?" interjected Ludmilla.

She smiled. "No, that is not necessary. I am fine. I will go to Tolya tomorrow morning."

"Excellent." Gourgen stood, holding his hand out to Ludmilla. She rose along with Galina, and gave her a long hug. Gourgen embraced her, then kissed her on both cheeks. "We will whip this thing," he said.

"I hope so."

They left the Grishchenko apartment and walked in cool silence to their building. Ludmilla waited until they were completely inside their apartment.

"So, when were you going to tell me you are sick, also?

"I am not sick."

"Well, I am no surgeon, but as I recall, hepatitis is a serious disease."

"Perhaps. The doctors found this when they were doing tests on my blood for Anatoly. They called it, chronic hepatitis."

"What is it?"

"They told me it is a liver disease."

"Did you get this at Chernobyl as well?"

"No. The surgeon said I was probably exposed to the virus years ago, and it has slowly built up."

"What happens now? What do we do?"

Gourgen looked into her eyes as if to ask, do you really want to know this? She returned a determined expression. "We watch things. He said we watch and wait, and deal with the symptoms when they occur."

"Is there any cure?"

"No."

Tears began to form in her eyes. "Oh, Gourgen. What are we going to do?"

He reached for her, pulling her into his firm embrace. "We are going to do exactly what the doctors have said. We live our lives and stay ahead of this disease."

She began sobbing with her face buried against his chest. In a muffled voice, she said, "You have done so much for the Motherland. Why is this happening to you and Anatoly? You have been such good pilots."

"Things happen, Milla. This is not something the State has done to us. This is just something that happened."

Ludmilla pulled back slightly and wiped the tears from her cheeks. "Maybe so, but it seems so odd that both you and Anatoly are ill."

"For different reasons."

"But, sick nonetheless."

"Yes."

She extricated herself from his arms. Then, as if some demon possessed her soul, she smiled in the most devious way, and reached for his hand. "Perhaps I should give you some of the medicine I prescribed for Galya and Anatoly."

To his private embarrassment, it took Gourgen a few extra seconds to realize what she was talking about. He smiled and followed her to the bedroom. He knew it was good medicine. They would enjoy the familiarity, the comfort, the love for each other. This was good.

# 26

*09:00, Saturday, 20.February.1988*
*Building R4, Apartment 44*
*Zhukovsky, Russia, USSR*

Gourgen dialed the telephone number from memory. The clicking in his earpiece told him the system was working. He heard three rings before an answer.

"Kovatchur."

"Anatoly, this is Gourgen."

"And, a good morning to you, my friend."

"Good morning to you. Are you busy?"

"No."

"May I come over? There are a few things we need to talk about, and I need your help."

"Sure."

Gourgen hung up the telephone, then told Ludmilla where is was going. The walk to the apartment building, R2, two places to the north in the bitter Russian winter brought the usual invigoration and quickness to his movements. He ascended the four flights of stairs to Anatoly's floor. He stood in front of the proper door and knocked.

Anatoly opened the door. They embraced, then he closed door behind his friend and colleague. Anatoly lived alone in a smaller, simply furnished, apartment.

"So, to what do I owe this honor?"

"Anatoly is back in the hospital."

"So I heard."

"He is getting progressively worse with each infection. The doctors are worried about him."

"What can we do?"

"The doctors have only a few tricks left. I think we are

approaching the time when we must admit our doctors are not going to be able to help him. We need to get Tolya to America."

"As you say."

"The Government people I have talked to say that Tolya cannot obtain an entry visa without a sponsor in America." Anatoly nodded his head. "I remember our chat eighteen or so months ago about the Air Force crew that went to Finland."

"Yes."

"Has there been any progress on attending an international airshow? Farnborough is this coming September."

Anatoly smiled. "As a matter of fact, yes, there has been a decision. I am not sure who approved it, but the Government has approved the mission. The applications have gone in. As of a few weeks ago, we are taking an Antonov One Two Four . . . partly to demonstrate, partly as a flying maintenance hangar . . . and, we are taking two MiG Two Nines . . . a single seat demonstration bird and a two seat back-up." A bubbly animation washed over him. "Menitsky and I are going to fly them."

"Fantastic."

"In another month or so, we will begin to construct our flight routines, then everyone will know."

"So, you are going to fly the show at Farnborough?" Gourgen asked as if to confirm what he had just heard.

"It looks like it."

"This will be the first time we have flown at one of the big international airshows."

"As you say," Kovatchur said. Gourgen stared at him. "What is on your mind, Gourgen?"

"Anatoly Demjanovich seems to be on a down hill slope."

"What about you and the other pilots?"

"I have my days, but I think most of the pilots have recovered fairly well, considering what we have been through. The doctors say Tolya still might recover as well, but he has been hospitalized quite a few times since the accident, and it sure does seem like each time he goes back in that place, he is a little worse and his recover is a little slower."

"Hopefully, they are correct."

"Yes," Gourgen responded with a pensive expression in his eyes.

Anatoly smiled again. "Why is it I sense there is a connection?"

"The doctors tell me that Anatoly's blood disease may degenerate. They have already suggested the treatment for him can only be delivered in the West – the best place is in America."

"And?"

"The Government experts tell me we must find a sponsor for Anatoly's treatment, as I said, in America. As we discussed before, I think our best chance is finding an American pilot who is close to what we do."

"A helicopter pilot."

"Yes, so he will be more interested in helping us."

"And, you want me to find us one of these American pilots?"

"Yes, just in case we really do actually need to do this."

"I can do that if I am the final pilot who goes."

"Is there much risk?"

"Sure. You know that. Things change. There are many pilots who are capable of doing this flying. Who knows what is going to happen when it comes time to leave for England."

Gourgen stood, walked to the window and pulled the curtain back. The sky had darkened, and snow was falling. The trodden paths and cleared walkways were covered again. Only a few strings of footprints appeared in the fresh snow below him. He considered the situation and options, then turned to his friend. "As I said, the doctors are not certain Anatoly Demjanovich should do this bone marrow transplant procedure. So, we may not need the sponsor, but we need to prepare just in case. If you do not go to England, hopefully someone will go, and I am asking you to help me enlist the pilot for this task."

"You can count on me for anything that well help Anatoly Demjanovich."

"I do not doubt that."

"But . . . ?"

"For selfish reasons, I suppose, we need you to be the pilot. I know you will be the best one if we are really going to do this for Anatoly Demjanovich."

"As I am sure you know, I need to be careful not to appear too eager or aggressive in being the show pilot. Let me think about this. Right now, I am the pilot scheduled to prepare the routine, and thus, should fly the demonstration. I will talk to Menitsky to see if he can help us."

"Good."

"I will not burden you with all the coordination. I will do that. I just need the introduction, if it should come to that."

"Understood."

Gourgen walked toward his friend. They embraced as friends.

"Thank you for your help, Anatoly."

"My pleasure."

# 27

*14:10, Tuesday, 30.August.1988*
*Royal Aeronautical Establishment*
*Farnborough, England, UK*

Only the needles on the navigation instruments told Anatoly Kovatchur his MiG-29 fighter was still headed toward the correct destination. The blanket overcast layer covered most of England as well as the sky and sun above him. The excitement of actually seeing the countryside of a region he had only read about had been dampened by the weather forecast predicting this cloud cover. Unfortunately, he now told himself, the weather reports were precisely correct. The cloud ceiling reports at 700 meters offered at least minimal opportunity for an impressive arrival.

The cloud blanket below him lay like a silk sheet on a grassy knoll. They were just 500 meters above the last layer, after descending from their cruising altitude of 12,000 meters. Anatoly moved his fighter closer to the 2 seat trainer version piloted by Valery Menitsky, the Mikoyan chief pilot, and the English speaking, Aeroflot navigator, Yuri Ermakov, in the back seat. They would soon penetrate the cloud layer reported to be about 500 meters thick.

As he looked down on the clouds, Anatoly imagined the squadrons of Spitfires and Hurricanes rising up to meet the hordes of German bombers and fighters during the early part of the war. While they fought the Germans, the Russians sat safely in their homes without the slightest knowledge of what lay ahead of them in that fateful Summer of 1941. So much history existed all around them.

The penetration of the cloud deck proceeded routinely as it usually did. Kovatchur concentrated on the position checkpoints on Menitsky's fighter-trainer and listened to the Ermakov's English radio calls to and from the British ground controllers. He mentally rehearsed his short, low-ceiling, arrival routine to let the world know Soviet aviation was coming out from behind the Iron Curtain in a big way.

The shades of green covered the Earth as they broke through the cloud cover. Anatoly moved away from the tandem seated, lead fighter to scan his map and quickly orient himself geographically. They were aligned perfectly for Runway 24 at the Royal Aeronautical Establishment Farnborough, the site of the even-year international airshow.

Ermakov made the appropriate radio calls for the two seater to proceed straight in for landing, and Anatoly was permitted to make a break into the landing pattern. There was no other traffic in the pattern, nor any other aircraft behind them coming in for landing. He shifted his position from the left wing to the right wing position. He knew it would probably be a little different from what the British controllers were probably accustomed to seeing, but they wanted to make sure everyone knew the Soviets had arrived.

"*Ni pukha, ni pera,*" Menitsky broadcast in Russian.

"*Da.*"

Anatoly Kovatchur pushed the throttles forward to accelerate past his leader. As he reached the threshold of the runway, he rolled sharply to the right into a steep turn to the downwind leg. They had studied the American Navy and Marine pilots in their landing patterns for carrier operations at sea, and noted the use of the same patterns at land bases as well.

He throttled back, lowered the landing gear, and when he was abeam the threshold, he began a descending turn. Anatoly made it look like a routine landing until the wheels touched the runway.

The throttles went forward into full afterburner, or reheat as the British called it. Huge special pumps dumped a large volume of fuel into the spray grid in the engine exhaust. The powerful Isotov engines shot the fighter forward. As soon as he felt the wheels lift off the runway, Anatoly sucked up the landing gear keeping the fighter just off the runway surface. The significantly lighter weight fighter accelerated like a scared rabbit.

The two blue-white flame tails gave visual dimension to the enormous noise of the engines. No one in aviation could mistake the sound. As he reached the upwind end of the runway, he pulled the nose up, then rolled the fighter onto its right wing. As he attained 150 meters height above the ground, Anatoly leveled the nose, then leveled the wings as he paralleled the runway. About mid-field with the afterburners still lit and the aircraft gaining speed rapidly, he rolled the aircraft again into a 90° angle of bank, and pulled back hard. He strained his abdominal muscles and felt the squeeze of his g-suit as the g-meter climbed quickly to 9 g's. Anatoly kept the aircraft in a level, high energy turn through two full circles adjacent to the runway. Halfway through the last circle, he pulled the throttles back out of afterburner all the way to idle. The aircraft decelerated sharply without the high thrust needed to sustain the turn. He waited for the right moment to level the wings straight downwind and level the nose. He pushed the stick hard left rolling the aircraft through two consecutive, 360° rolls to the left, before returning the machine to a level state.

Anatoly glanced at the airspeed indicator, recognized he was too fast for landing, so he maneuvered the MiG-29 a quick series of sharp S-turns to decelerate the aircraft even more. As the airspeed came down quickly, he lowered the landing gear, started his landing turn, then pushed the throttles up slightly to hold his approach speed. This time he kept the aircraft on the runway and deployed his drag chute.

As at most airfields throughout the world, a 'follow-me' truck waited for him at the far end of the runway. He followed the truck down the taxiway through a break in the trees to an open area. Several other aircraft were already parked there. A Canadian Forces CF-18. An RAF Tornado. His two seat MiG-29UB sister aircraft. The other aircraft he recognized from the photographs as a US Army AH-64 Apache attack helicopter. It was not a very attractive machine; it looked rather brutish. The American helicopter reminded him of Gourgen Karapetyan's Mi-28 attack helicopter, his friend had been working on for several years now.

He positioned the fighter next to Menitsky's fighter-trainer, set the brakes, and secured both engines. Everything looked normal as he raised the canopy, then switched off all the electric power.

His ground crew waited for him having arrived earlier in the massive, four engine, Antonov, An-124, heavy lift transport. As he descended the ladder, two, blue, flight-suited, pilots preflighted the Apache. They looked over to give him a prominent thumbs up sign – a pilot's universal sign of approval. His brief 'I've arrived' show had made the desired impression. Anatoly gave the American pilots an acknowledging salute.

As he completed his aircraft status report to his crew chief, a small, military, Land Rover came to an abrupt stop in front of his fighter. An RAF officer got out and walked directly toward him. The man pointed to his MiG-29 and asked, "Are you the pilot?"

Anatoly recognized the tone, knew he was about to receive a lecture, and although he understood the English, he shook his head and motioned for the navigator-interpreter.

Through the interpreter, the man repeated the question. Anatoly nodded his head.

"I am Wing Commander Henderson, the aerodrome operations officer."

The appropriate translations and introductions were completed.

"I know this is your first time in England, so I shall be reasonably tolerant. In short, that little display was an unauthorized aerobatic routine in a controlled air space. I must ask you to refrain from such displays except during scheduled rehearsal and airshow periods."

Although Anatoly understood most of the wing commander's admonition, he waited for the interpreter to complete his translation, then he smiled and nodded his head in agreement.

Henderson motioned toward the cockpit. "Would you mind?"

Kovatchur again waited for the translation, and once more nodded his head. He then motioned for the interpreter to follow him up the ladder to assist the RAF officer in a brief tour of the

MiG-29's cockpit. Anatoly watched and assisted with bits of information the interpreter could not answer for Wing Commander Henderson. Ermakov performed his public relations task admirably as Anatoly continued to glance across the concrete parking pad at the crew preparing the Apache for flight. They probably had a rehearsal period.

The Apache's Auxiliary Power Unit made casual conversation more difficult. Several minutes passed as the American's proceeded through their systems initialization procedures. The Apache had gained a very serious reputation in the Soviet Union as a complex, highly capable, hardened, anti-armor, helicopter capable of firing laser guided missiles that could reportedly eliminate any main battle tank in the world. The Apache commanded respect by everyone despite the fact it was a helicopter. As the engines were started, Wing Commander Henderson scurried from the MiG-29's cockpit.

"Thank you," he said. "I must return to the control tower."

Henderson drove his Land Rover away as the pilot engaged the Apache's main rotor. As the Apache taxied away, the crew returned to the task of readying the fighter for the next day's airshow rehearsal. The 20 minutes slipped quickly until they heard the peculiar beat of a high speed helicopter. They turned their attention toward the sound.

The Apache entered the show area at high speed. The pilot started his show routine with a 360° roll, then he pulled the nose straight up into what looked like a Hammerhead Stall. As the airspeed decayed near the top, he did a pedal turn much like the competition aerobatic pilots used their propeller wash and rudder to kick out, as they say, rather than fall on the tail. The helicopter accelerated quickly straight down.

The Soviet crew watched with some fascination. None of them had seen a helicopter and especially a fairly large helicopter with full wing stores and a complete crew do such maneuvers. The deep pulsing sounds of the rotor biting through the air added to the rugged image associated with this aircraft.

He pulled up to about 45° nose up, then rolled inverted and

pulled through what looked like a reverse Half Cuban Eight, another classic aerobatic maneuver. Another Hammerhead Stall and turn changed his direction.

"This is amazing," said one of the mechanics.

"Yes, indeed," responded Kovatchur without taking his eyes off the American helicopter.

"Have you seen anything like this before?"

"Never. I have never even heard of helicopters doing these things."

Just then, the Apache performed what the fighter pilots called a Tuck Under Roll – a 270° roll into a 90° bank turn. The aircraft groaned heavily under the g load as it turned through a descending 270° of heading change directly into what would be the crowd center. He pulled the nose up sharply to arrest his forward speed and transition to a level climb straight up – a maneuver helicopters were built to do. As he climbed, he turned about his vertical axis several times before stopping to face what would be the crowd in a few days. He hesitated for an instant, then dropped the nose into a maneuver the fixed wing pilots would call, an Upright Spin. He held the spin descending much lower below the treeline that separated the parking area from the runway. Anatoly and the other Soviets walked toward the trees to find at least a broken view of the flying area. When they regained sight of the Apache, the aircraft was flying sideways very fast, then banked sharply back in the opposite direction to arrest his speed. He turned quickly to be broadside to the viewing area, then dropped the tail to accelerate backward. Smoothly, the tail rose straight up in an odd maneuver that looked like the reverse of a Hammerhead Stall except this time he did not spin the nose around. He let the aircraft accelerate straight down, then amazingly he rolled the aircraft 180° with the nose straight down. As he pulled up to avoid the ground, he accelerated and departed back out the way he came.

"I do not think anyone would believe us if we told our friends back home what we have just seen," said the crew chief.

"You are probably correct," answered Kovatchur. "I simply

must meet this pilot."

The Apache helicopter performed his routine several more times as he continued to practice over the show area. He was doing what all the pilots had to do, performing his routine and finding those ground marks to ensure he kept the maneuvers positioned in three dimensional space properly for the crowd. After all, the Americans were here for the same reason they were all here, to show off what their aircraft could do in an effort to attract buyers from the world aviation community.

They watched the American pilot perform his routine four times that afternoon, and it was just as fascinating as it was the first time. The repeated routines without stopping for fuel and a full set of wing stores meant the Apache pilot was performing his show routine at a heavier weight. Most, if not all, fighters carried just enough fuel for their routine and a little spare for landing. The brute force demonstration by the Apache made its performance all the more remarkable.

The ground crews completed the preparation of the Mikoyan fighter for the next day's rehearsal period. Anatoly Kovatchur decided to wait for the Apache to return. He wanted to meet the man who made that helicopter do those things. What they saw would certainly change the impression they all had of the American helicopter. None of them expected an aircraft of that type to do such maneuvers, and yet, the machine appeared to be very graceful like it was intended to fly like that. Anatoly wondered what Gourgen Karapetyan and the others would do when they heard about this airshow routine.

This time it was Kovatchur's turn to give the American pilot a thumbs-up approval sign as he taxied his aircraft back to his parking spot. He waited for the aircraft to be secured, and the normal post-flight routine to be completed. Anatoly walked toward the Apache with a smile on his face. As soon as he caught the pilot's eye, Anatoly gave him another thumbs-up and broad smile. The American returned the smile and began to walk toward him. They met in the middle between the two combat aircraft.

Anatoly extended his right hand still several meters away. "Good show," he said waving to the sky with his left arm.

The two men clasped hands in a hard squeeze. Anatoly reached to grasp the American's right elbow and pumped his right hand in a vigorous, exaggerated way.

"Thank you."

"My name is Anatoly Kovatchur."

"Great to meet you. My name is Cap Parlier." He motioned toward his comparably sized copilot with a salt and pepper full beard. "This is my colleague, Ed Wilson."

"Great to meet you, Cap Parlier and Ed Wilson. Very good flying."

The three pilots talked about flying, and their mutual appreciation of each other's aircraft performance. The American, Parlier, asked to inspect the MiG-29. Anatoly obliged, then received an expertly guided tour of the AH-64. He learned, as he suspected, they were both company experimental test pilots with McDonnell Douglas Helicopter Company, the manufacturer of the Apache. Both of them had significant military flying experience. Each of them had combat time – his in Afghanistan, and Parlier's and Wilson's in Vietnam – both traumatic, wasted and losing propositions. It was amazing how much they shared in common.

While they talked about aircraft, Anatoly's crew arrived to tow the Soviet fighter to their mobile service station – the massive An-124, parked near the control tower. Anatoly motioned for the Americans to walk with him as they towed the MiG-29. Parlier told his ground crew where he was going. The servicing was underway when they arrived.

"What are they doing?" asked Parlier motioning toward the single and dual seat fighters, one under each wing of the An-124 with large diameter hoses connecting the fighters to the transport's wing.

"Refueling."

"No."

Anatoly smiled. "Yes."

"Is this normal?"

"When we are not at home, yes."

"All aircraft can do this?"

"All Soviet aircraft have common fuel fittings. We refuel fighters, helicopters, any aircraft from the Antonov One Two Four, Ilyushin Nine Six, or any other transport aircraft, even Mil Two Six."

"I'll be damned. That's ingenious."

"No. Just standard," responded Anatoly wondering why the American was so impressed with something so simple. The sensors on his Apache helicopter were some of the most sophisticated systems Kovatchur had ever seen on any aircraft beyond his fighter's radar and infrared targeting systems, and yet, they apparently could not refuel from other aircraft. Anatoly wondered if the American was telling him the truth. Surely, the Americans had simple field operations capabilities like the Soviets.

Anatoly arranged for the pilot of the An-124, who still happened to be around the large aircraft, to give Parlier and Wilson a tour of his aircraft. It seemed so routine for Kovatchur. It was hard to understand the almost wide eyed amazement of the Americans. They showed him the cockpit, the in-flight accessible electronics cabinets, the flight crews galley and berthing compartment behind the cockpit and forward of the wing. Parlier continued to marvel at the two mobile vans secured in the cargo compartment and the maintenance crews quarters above the cargo compartment aft of the wing. The An-124 was virtually a self-contained maintenance hangar which is why they brought the big aircraft.

The Farnborough Airshow lasted two and a half weeks – a week of rehearsal flying and coordination, then ten days of the actual industry and public airshows. Anatoly Kovatchur and the other pilots had to endure many press conferences. This was the very first time Soviet aviation had joined the rest of the world's aviation companies at RAE Farnborough. They were quite the attraction.

Sometimes Anatoly felt like one of the trained bears in the Moscow Circus.

Several social and semi-professional events allowed them to join the other pilots. As he believed over the years, pilots were just pilots around the world. They shared a common heritage and avocation although they spoke different languages, and yet some of their languages were common – the language of aviation.

They enjoyed the exposure and spectacle of participation in one of the world's two, oldest and most prestigious airshows. They watched aircraft fly impressive routines and could feel the thunder – before they only had intelligence photographs. Most importantly, Anatoly Kovatchur believed he had accomplished his primary task.

# 28

*17:00, Wednesday, 14.September.1988*
*Building R5, Apartment 1*
*Zhukovsky, Russia, USSR*

"How was it?" asked Gourgen.

Anatoly Kovatchur grinned and held out his arms to his side with his palms up. "If there is a God, he has blessed us."

"What happened?" asked Anatoly in anticipation.

Kovatchur looked into the eyes of his friends. "First, how have you been? What do the doctors say?" he asked as he turned the straight chair around and sat down leaning forward against the back. The Grishchenko living room served as their meeting place, once again.

"Never mind me."

Anatoly held up his hand to stop. "Nonsense, my friend. I must first know how you are doing."

"I am well," he lied. "The doctors in Moscow tell me it was only the flu virus."

"Damn them. You do not get the flu several times in the year. It was that radiation."

"The other pilots who were ill appear to have recovered," Gourgen added.

"So, does that mean Anatoly is not ill from the radiation," barked Kovatchur.

Gourgen shook his head. "No, it just means Anatoly is apparently the worst hit so far."

"And?"

"And, I think we all feel he is not going to receive the treatment he deserves here in Russia . . . as long as the Government is trying to pretend the disaster was not so bad."

Galina Grishchenko joined the group of pilots carrying a tea service tray. "Have you found us this help?" asked Galina as she poured tea for the three men.

"I think so. He is a rather young American, but he is quite friendly and open, plus he can fly like the falcon."

"How young?" asked Gourgen.

"Late thirties, early forties, I would say."

"Your age, then."

They laughed and poked at the youngest among them, and certainly the youngest of the government certified test pilots. The habit of teasing Anatoly Kovatchur about his age remained a favorite activity among the relatively small group of government test pilots at the various design bureaus and the flight research center.

"Tell us what happened in England," Galina commanded, to bring them back the topic she was most interested to discuss.

"Yes, well. It was an experience I shall never forget." Kovatchur paused to allow comment. Three sets of eyes remained transfixed upon him. "Some very impressive flying. The world's best aircraft and pilots. We commanded the attention of the show."

"You are just saying that."

"No. It is true. The press, the other pilots, even the business men from every company wanted to meet us and talk to us."

"Good. Then, we have taken our place in the aviation world," added Grishchenko.

Kovatchur smiled. "I would say we have."

"Good."

"Yes, but help for Tolya?"

"Galya," protested Anatoly, as if his wife were interrupting the pilot talk.

She nodded her head, but did not deflect her gaze from their friend.

"I think the American is the one."

"What is his name?" asked Anatoly.

"Cap Parlier."

"Do you really think he can help Tolya?" asked Galina.

"We will never know unless we try, but yes, I do believe he

can help."

"Maybe the American government will stop him like our government has told us, there is nothing they can do, and there was no injury from that damn radiation." Galina nearly spat the words turning the living room into a morgue.

None of them disagreed with her feelings about the medical treatment Anatoly Grishchenko received. At least the men agreed, the Soviet doctors were doing everything thing they could. It was one of the young hematologists that had told them about the new treatment developed in the United States. The thought of a bone marrow transplant did not have any appealing aspects other than it was a potential cure. None of the Soviet hospitals could perform the procedure using unrelated donor marrow, yet. Their only hope now was the transplant in America.

"We will not know unless we try," added Gourgen, again.

"What do we do next?" Anatoly asked.

Gourgen Karapetyan looked first to Tolya, then Anatoly. "Your success at Farnborough started many things happening, also the American Apache demonstration has pushed Mil to petition for government approval to take the Mil Two Eight to Paris. Tishchenko has asked me to prepare an airshow routine for next year. So, maybe between us, we can convince the American to help us."

"When is Paris?" asked Galina.

"Next June."

"That is a year away," she snapped. "Tolya needs help now."

The room fell silent again as the three men lowered their heads rather than see the fire in Galina's eyes. She charged from the room and out of the apartment in disgust. A walk would help calm her.

"She is correct, you know," Anatoly finally said solemnly.

"Are there any other opportunities to talk to the American Parlier? Are there any other contacts?" Gourgen asked Kovatchur.

Anatoly considered the question carefully, going back over all the people he met at Farnborough. "Many were military, so those are probably out. There were a few other company pilots, but none of them seemed as approachable as Parlier."

"Then, let us see what happens at Paris. If either of us can talk to him, maybe he will feel support to the helicopter pilots. If so, we will press for his help." Gourgen looked his long-time friend in the eyes. "Are you ready for this?"

"Yes. They are not going to help me here. I have much more flying to do, so yes, I am ready."

Contemplation filled the few moments as the three pilots looked to each other several times, then nodded their agreement and smiled.

"We must talk to Doctor Vorobiev," Gourgen said, thinking out loud. "He will support our efforts to get special treatment in America, and we will need his help to sustain you while we work out the details."

"Do not worry about Galya," added Anatoly. "She is only worried about me. She seems to only think of what the government medical doctors cannot or are not doing to help me and the others. She only sees the negative."

"All women are the same in that regard," said Gourgen. "That is why we love them so much. Our mothers nursed us as infants and trained us as children. Our wives sustain us in life."

"Those of us who have wives," grumbled Kovatchur.

"You must seek if you are to find," Gourgen said. "You need to find a good woman who will take care of you."

"Ah, it is no life for a good woman. I see what our flying does to the other women, and I would not wish that pain on anyone."

"So, you intend to go into later life alone?" Grishchenko asked.

"No. I just do not know what I can do. I am happy flying. I have the perfect assignment. I will enjoy that for the time being."

"Our job, then," Gourgen said nodding to Kovatchur, "is to prepare for next spring and Paris."

"Yes."

"Your job," he said looking directly at Grishchenko, "is to take very good care of yourself."

"The doctors will not let me fly."

"Then, you will not fly until you are cured of this illness. It is unfortunate we must wait until next spring, but the government has made it impossible for us to proceed without American assistance. We will overcome the obstacles, Anatoly Demjanovich, but you must help us, and if that means no flying for you, then so be it."

"I do not like it."

"The only way you can return to flying is for you to get cured in America."

"As you say, then."

"Anatoly, you work on Mikoyan and the fighter side. I will work on Mil and the helicopter side."

"Maybe, by Paris," Anatoly observed, "we will not have those KGB shepherds, and it will be easier for us to talk privately with the American, Parlier."

"What if Parlier is not at Paris?" asked Grishchenko.

"Then, we will find another suitable American pilot to help us."

# 29

*09:00, Tuesday, 24.January.1989*
*Building R5*
*Zhukovsky, Russia, USSR*

"Good to see you up and about, Anatoly Demjanovich," Gourgen said as they met outside his apartment in the cold, crisp air of winter.

The sun shown brightly in the crystal clear, blue sky and reflected sharply off the week old snow accumulation. This was a good day. They were both dressed for the cold. Anatoly was not wearing the surgical mask that had become so common for him in the preceding months.

"I certainly feel much better, Gourgen."

"That is a good sign. Have the doctors pronounced you healthy?"

"In a manner speaking, I suppose so. They indicated most of my blood chemistry has returned to some normal range although I still have this anemia as they call it."

"They will not say you are cured?"

"No."

They walked toward the car park and greeted several neighbors on their way. Gourgen considered Anatoly's words wondering what the real story was. Were the doctors actually telling him the full truth about his medical condition?

"Where are you going?" asked Gourgen.

"Where are you going?"

"I have several test flights to fly today at the Mil facility."

"Then, I am going to the Mil facility. Perhaps, I can talk my friend into letting me fly with him."

Gourgen swung his left hand to backhand Anatoly's shoulder.

"So, this is a conspiracy."

"Oh no," Anatoly chuckled with an air of sarcasm. "What would ever give you that idea?"

"Well, let me see. You were grounded by the doctors two and a half years ago. Have they released you back to flight status?"

"No, but . . . ," Anatoly said and stopped when Gourgen raised his hand.

"Are you trying to get me grounded to?"

"No, Gourgen," Anatoly answered with some indignation. "I am not. I just want to fly, again."

"So, you think we can do this?"

"Yes, if we do not tell anyone what we are doing."

"That may be rather difficult since both of these planned flights are full test flights," Gourgen answered, referring to the use of a ground crew to monitor the aircraft's on-board instrumentation.

"We will not refer to my medical condition. We will act like everything is completely back to normal, then no one will feel the need to ask questions."

Gourgen stopped and turned to his friend. Looking into Anatoly's eyes for answers, Gourgen responded, "Are you really sure this is a good idea?"

"Gourgen, how would you feel if you had not flown in two years? I just want to look down on the earth, again. It will make me feel much better."

"What about exposure to more people who might infect you?"

"That is a possibility these days, but the doctors say I am in reasonably good health considering what I am fighting."

"Then, let's go fly," Gourgen said he turned to walk to his automobile. "We will go together."

The two pilots rode up the main highway without many words. They passed through the main gate of the Mil facility with the appropriate greetings to the guards and other personnel. The large snow-covered, grass area between the row of obscuring trees, scrubs and fence that marked the edge of the highway and the flight test buildings served as a parking area for many Mil helicopters. Some of them had been parked for years and did not have rotor blades. Only a handful of the two dozen aircraft had been flown, or at least cleared of snow and ice, in the last few days.

Fortunately, for the two culprits, there were only greetings for the Gromov pilot the ground crews had not seen in many months. They quickly, at Gourgen's urging to avoid too much friendly conversation, settled down to brief the first flight test points.

These flights would be part of a planned program to expand the normal flight envelope of the Mi-28 attack helicopter in preparation for the Paris Airshow in late spring. The aerobatic routine of the American AH-64A attack helicopter at Farnborough the previous year coaxed the engineering hierarchy to show the Mi-28 in an equally good light.

On these two flights, they would perform a series of rolling maneuvers. They would also have a chase aircraft, an Mi-17 medium transport helicopter, with photographic crew on-board to record the maneuvering on film. As in most situations in flight test, the film provided documentation in the even the test aircraft experienced any anomalies, but it also could easily be used to produce an exciting marketing film.

"Are you ready?" asked Gourgen, looking to Anatoly.

"This should be fun. I have never been upside down in a helicopter before."

"I have done it a few times, but if the American machine can do it, so can ours." Gourgen stood. They gathered their flight equipment bags and walked out of the building toward the waiting test aircraft. "With the Government decision pending on the future attack helicopter for the Air Force, we want to show the helicopter in the best light possible as well as generate some interest in the international aviation market. International sales potential would push us ahead of the Kamov competitor."

"What is that . . . the Kamov Five Zero, is it?"

"That is it. Coaxial main rotors. They built it off the Model Two Five . . . a radically modified fuselage and empennage, but essentially the same engines, transmission and rotors. They built it with a single seat only, as our answer to the American Army's new LHX competition. They wanted one seat."

"Why? Isn't it hard enough flying a helicopter? Do they have to make the poor pilot fly and operate all the weapons?"

"As you would expect, the Americans are using smaller and smaller computers to help the pilot. Apparently, they think this single seat stuff is possible, so we cannot let that pass."

"What will you do with the Mil Two Eight if the Government picks the Kamov machine?"

"We will try to sell it to our friends."

They reached the machine. The aircraft's crew chief, Viktor Zarmekov, came around from the other side to greet the crew.

"The bird is ready, Gourgen," Zarmekov reported.

"Excellent, as always, Viktor Petrovich. You remember Anatoly Demjanovich, don't you?"

"Yes, certainly," the crew chief extending his hand to the Gromov pilot.

"Anatoly Demjanovich has not flown the Two Eight before, would you be so kind to show him the important items in the front seat," Gourgen requested.

The two cockpits were completely separate and sealed with the front, copilot/weapons officer, seat substantially lower than the rear pilot's station. The only means of communication was a redundant intercom system. The front seat entered through a small door on the left side, while the pilot entered from the right side. As Zarmekov assisted Anatoly with getting everything hooked up and ready, Gourgen readied the helicopter for flight. He had the engines started, the heat on, and his door closed by the time Zarmekov finished with Anatoly in the front seat. As the front door closed and the crew chief saluted and retreated to the warmth of the test building, Gourgen radioed the flight test team.

Gourgen performed each of the prescribed maneuvers with the precision of a surgeon. The flight test supervisor on the ground reported nothing abnormal. Even the photographers in the chase aircraft indicated they obtained exceptional footage that would surely be of great value.

They returned to the test facility, debriefed the first flight, then briefed the second flight. They were back in the air to perform additional maneuvers, similar to the first flight. Again, everything happened exactly as planned.

"Mil Zero Four, this is Control. We have what we need. You can come home. That should be it for the day."

Without responding the radio, Gourgen keyed the intercom. "Tolya, you want to stay up a little more?"

"Yes, Gourgen, if you don't mind. I am not sure when I will get to fly again."

"Why don't we go make a low pass at Ramskoye."

"Sounds like a plan to me."

"Control, this is Mil Zero Four. We are going to stay up for a little while longer, perhaps 40 minutes. Chase . . . Zero Four . . . you can return."

"Zero Four, Chase, we will see you on the ground."

Gourgen looked out his right window to see the Mi-17 bank away from them, turning nearly a 180° for the short return flight. He keyed the intercom again. "Sorry you do not have a set of controls up there, Tolya."

"No problem. It is just a pleasure to look down on the Earth again. This is such a beautiful country. How could we let anyone foul the Motherland?"

"Indeed."

They flew silently for several kilometers, going nowhere in particular. Gourgen was certain he was thinking the same thing as Anatoly, returning to the spring and summer nearly three years earlier when science and engineering fell woefully short of the power of nature. Stories continued to come from the Ukraine, ByleoRussiya and Russia herself about the consequences of that grotesque nuclear contamination. All that damage for the sake of some electricity and the drive to be modern.

"How are you feeling?" asked Gourgen after several minutes.

"To be honest, I was feeling a little light in the stomach when you were throwing this machine around the sky, but I feel fine now. More importantly, I could not help but shed a few tears for what they have done to my birthplace. I am glad we were able to help seal that thing off for further damaging the Motherland."

"I thought you might be thinking the same thing I was." Gourgen banked the aircraft toward the south. "Let's go let Ramskoye and Zhukovsky know we are still here."

"Fine by me."

As they headed toward Flight City as they sometimes called it, Gourgen thought he would bring Anatoly up to date. "We have not finished our development flying, but it looks like we will soon be putting together an aerobatic airshow routine similar to what Anatoly Kovatchur told us about from Farnborough, and we saw on those films."

"Great."

"I think we will be ready for Paris in another month or two."

"Are you going?"

"It appears nearly certain."

"Good, Gourgen. I am happy for you."

"There is also talk about exchanging flights with the Americans. The Apache and its American test pilot, Cap Parlier, are supposed to be there. The managers are negotiating now to let me fly him, then he will fly me in the Apache."

"That should be fun."

"Yes. I am eager to see if that machine is as good as Anatoly has led us to believe."

"Hopefully, it will happen as you say."

"It will also give me the chance to get to know Cap Parlier, in case we really do need his help for your treatment."

"That would be good, too. Although, I hope we do not need his help."

Gourgen switched his radio over to the proper control zone frequency. He listened for a short time to make sure Ramskoye was not busy. No one seemed to be in the area. "Ramskoye Tower, Mil Zero Four," he radioed.

"Mil Zero Four, Ramskoye, go ahead."

"Mil Zero Four is ten kilometers to the northeast, request permission for a low pass."

"Mil Zero Four, Ramskoye, there is no traffic. Wind two one five at seven. You are cleared for a low pass."

"Cleared low pass," Gourgen radioed, then shifted his thumb to the intercom button. "Here we go."

Gourgen pulled the collective lever up to increase power to the main rotor right at the maximum continuous torque limit. He pushed the nose over to gain more speed. When he leveled out just a few meters above the tree tops, Gourgen checked his airspeed indicator. They were doing a respectable 250 kilometers per hour. There was no need to demand too much from the helicopter. As they approached the airfield boundary, Gourgen nudged the aircraft lower as there were no trees. He adjusted his flight path toward the tower and the row of hangars to the west. The tops of the apartment building could just barely be seen behind the buildings. As he neared the hangars, Gourgen adjusted his flight path to pass just to the right of the tower. At the right moment, he pulled up smoothly to about 20° nose up, waited until he had about 200 meters altitude and they were nearly over the apartment buildings, then rolled the helicopter through 540° to stop in the inverted position. Gourgen immediately pulled the nose down toward the earth below to gain speed, then rolled to the upright position. Although it certainly was not as elegant as the fighters could do, it was his form of a victory roll.

"Nice show," radioed the tower.

"Thanks. We are proceeding back to Mil."

"As requested," the Tower controller answered.

The short flight back up the highway to the Mil facility took only a few minutes. As they slowed for their approach to landing, Gourgen said, "How was that?"

"It could not be better, Gourgen. You have done well with this machine. I have been honored to fly with you. Thank you."

Gourgen felt the finality in Anatoly's words. He chose not to respond directly. "I am glad you enjoyed it."

They completed all their after mission tasks, then drove back to Zhukovsky. It had been a good day, and Anatoly was happy. There was true air of satisfaction and contentment. They both hoped the future days would go up from here.

# 30

*16:25, Tuesday, 6.June.1989*
*Le Bourget Airfield*
*Paris, France*

Gourgen Karapetyan acknowledged the distinctive features of the Paris skyline. The approach to Le Bourget Airport, northeast of the city, provided a perfect view of the Eiffel Tower, the spires of Notre Dame Cathedral, and the sprawling metropolis known around the world as an artistic and cultural well-spring — the City of Lights.

This was Karapetyan's first visit to the famous city. Kovatchur's pioneering and maybe even historic participation in the Farnborough Airshow the previous year enabled Karapetyan and many others to join in the 1989 Paris Airshow.

Gourgen developed the routine for the Mi-28 after watching video of the AH-64 Farnborough routine. The Mi-28 was designed to many similar specifications as its counterpart, the AH-64 Apache, and had numerous innovations to enhance operations in the field. Every time Karapetyan thought of the comparison, the effects of the Soviet Afghanistan experience boiled to the surface. The insanity of conventional warfare in the Afghan mountains influenced the Mi-28 design as much as the American counterpart. The thought of all those young pilots being lost in that terrible war never failed to depress him. He turned his awareness to the unprecedented maneuvering he expected to demonstrate in front of a world audience.

His arrival would be much less flamboyant than Anatoly Kovatchur's with the MiG-29, followed by Viktor Pugachov with the Su-27, an hour later. The fighter guys always liked to make a splashy entrance. Having watched Pugachov practice his most unusual routine at Zhukovsky, Gourgen knew the world would soon recognize his name and signature maneuvering.

"Le Bourget Tower, this is Mil Three Nine Zero calling," radioed Karapetyan in his halting English and using the words Anatoly had suggested.

"Mil Three Nine Zero, Le Bourget, go ahead."

"Mil Three Nine Zero is five miles to the east for landing."

"Roger, Three Nine Zero. Wind is two eight five at six knots, you are cleared to land."

"Mil Three Nine Zero cleared to land," he responded thankful the controller spoke slowly and distinctly so he could understand the heavily French accented English.

Gourgen recognized many of the world's aircraft parked in various spots all around the apron. The expanse of buildings, tents, people and vehicles of all kinds staggered the imagination. This was truly a major world aviation event. He was just one of those aircraft. He followed directions to his parking spot. They stepped through each event from Customs to basic orientation. The French authorities had a person who spoke perfect Russian like a schoolteacher as well as his native French. The formalities slipped by as smoothly as the interpreter's Russian.

His ground crew gave him a more practical orientation. They acted like young children given free reign in the most posh candy store. They were undeniably excited to be in Paris and in the midst of so many other professionals who only a few years ago had been forbidden to them – a faceless enemy.

The fighter guys, Kovatchur and Pugachov, arrived with characteristic flare separated by an hour. By late afternoon, the entire Soviet contingent met in the spacious cabin of the Il-96 wide-body airliner. The pilots were given their airshow slots as well as practice times while everyone was re-instructed on etiquette, procedures, transportation to the hotel and required coordination times, places and activities. The group resembled a summer camp in the forest, and yet remained professional and focused. They were given one hour before the buses would take them into the city and to the hotel. The time allowed the ground crews to complete their maintenance actions. A small group would remain with the aircraft since the government officials were still not entirely comfortable with the security arrangements.

"Have you found the American?" asked Anatoly once the crowd has dispersed.

"No. According to several of the Americans with McDonnell Douglas, Parlier is not scheduled to arrive until next weekend."

"He will miss the practice and certification process. Surely, he will fly the Apache again as he did at Farnborough."

"They say not."

"That must be wrong."

"They say the Apache is coming, and Parlier will be here, but not flying in the airshow."

"Why?"

"I could not determine the reason."

"We will talk to him when he gets here," said Anatoly waving his friend to follow him off the large Il-96.

They walked among the other aircraft and talked of things that fly until it was time to depart for the hotel. A partial respite in the rain or alternating mist allowed them to avoid being totally soaked. The weather forecast predicted another day or so of poor weather, but the forecasters thought the weather would clear toward the end of the week and for the airshow week proper.

Gourgen prepared for his practice routine with the Mi-28. He was the first of the Soviet pilots to fly. His routine was designed to answer the aerobatic routine performed the year prior by Parlier in the AH-64A Apache at Farnborough, England. Gourgen completed each maneuver just as he had developed it and practiced it at Zhukovsky during the winter and spring. In this session, he ran about ten seconds longer than his allotted four minute period. He would have to tighten up his sequence to save those few seconds.

"How did it go?" asked his chief mechanic when Gourgen

opened the cockpit door after shutdown his helicopter.

"She groaned a little, but it seemed to perform as we rehearsed it," answered Gourgen.

"Excellent. I will give her a good look see just to make sure."

Gourgen Karapetyan stowed his flight equipment in his locker in the trailer, then positioned himself at the nose of his aircraft. He watched Kovatchur make a lot of noise in full afterburner as he threw the MiG-29 around the sky. The nimble fighter displayed well as the pilots reflected on the agility, power and precision Anatoly demonstrated with the aircraft. His routine was not as dramatic as Pugachov's demonstration, but it was certainly equal to the other fighters in the show. Gourgen stood near his Mi-28 intently focused on the MiG-29.

Anatoly's practice routine was going quite well. His now trademark tail slide hushed the crowd, then produced the usual commotion. Even the sequence that worried Gourgen so much appeared near perfect. The nose of the agile MiG-29 hung 27° above the horizon leaving the aircraft standing on its tail just 200 meters above the ground and creeping along at a mere 140 kilometers per hour. As the fighter reached mid-field, Gourgen first saw then heard the afterburners light off. The aircraft began to climb out of its precarious slow flight attitude into a vertical climb.

Gourgen noticed the movement beside him. The ground crew was pulling the light blue, Sukhoi Su-27 out from its parking place next to Gourgen's Mi-28. Viktor Pugachov was already in the cockpit and ready to start his engines. This would be his first practice session and the first time the Western public would see the incredible maneuver he worked so hard to perfect.

Anatoly completed his practice routine and landed in front to small crowd of workers preparing the airfield for the big airshow that would begin the coming weekend. The larger Sukhoi fighter disappeared behind the row of buildings at the end of the flight line as he taxied for his takeoff slot. Anatoly brought the MiG-29 into the middle of the open ramp just vacated by Pugachov and shutdown his engines. His ground crew met him, secured the ladder for his egress and connected the tug to move the fighter back into the row of Soviet aircraft on display.

Within seconds, the even more powerful 27,500 pounds thrust from each of the two Lyulka AL-31F turbofan engines in full afterburner propelled Pugachov's Su-27 into a straight vertical climb right off the runway. The larger Su-27 looked just as graceful and agile as Kovatchur's MiG-29 and had similar aerodynamic characteristics. After a series of hard, high-energy maneuvers to show the excellent turning performance as well as the excess power of the engines, Viktor Pugachov leveled his airplane at about 700 meters altitude for what appeared to be rather mundane, quiet, relatively slow, straight pass, like he might have forgotten where he was in his routine and remembered he needed to be at the other end of the runway. Then, without any precursor indication, he pitched the large fighter's nose straight up passing the vertical. Gourgen saw the tailplanes move smoothly to the full, leading edge up position. Pugachov arrested the pitch rate, then managed to bring the nose right back down the way it had come up, all without appreciably changing the flight path of the aircraft.

Gourgen quickly scanned the people within his eyesight. Many pointed to the sky and jerked around as if to tell their colleagues they had just witnessed some incredible event. The animation of the small crowd told the story.

The maneuver Viktor Pugachov developed to show the awesome, low speed, maneuverability of the Su-27 fighter and the capabilities of its vectored thrust nozzles had been given the label most descriptive of its appearance – The Cobra – Pugachov's Cobra. Like the large, hooded, venomous snake raising its head slightly past the vertical, then striking forward, Pugachov made the machine resemble the snake's characteristic striking motion.

The rest of his routine seemed almost anti-climatic after the extraordinary Cobra maneuver, but the Su-27 performed an exceptional display routine. The place of many exceptional aviation events from Charles Lindbergh's landing after his historic trans-Atlantic flight to the first international public display of the American

SR-71 Blackbird, Mach 3, reconnaissance aircraft, Le Bourget Airfield now bore witness to yet another significant event. Viktor Pugachov made history.

Anatoly Kovatchur joined Gourgen Karapetyan near the nose of the Mi-28 before Pugachov came to a stop in front of them. "Looks like Viktor's Cobra had the desired effect," he said to Gourgen.

"I should say. People seemed to be shocked," answered Gourgen. "They will be talking about that maneuver for some time."

As Pugachov completed his engines and systems shutdown and climbed from the fighter, a small crowd gathered to see the man who had done such an amazing thing with a modern fighter airplane.

"It worked," shouted Kovatchur to their colleague.

The slightly smaller, more stocky, Pugachov smiled and walked smoothly through the growing crowd. "You think so?" he asked.

"Without question," Gourgen responded. "They pointed to the sky and acted as if they were awestruck by the maneuver."

"I would say you have made your mark, my friend."

"Good," said Pugachov, "then, all the work was worth it."

"I should say," added Anatoly. "I think they will remember your Cobra maneuver for years."

"Now the Americans can follow us," Viktor bellowed, more for the spectators within earshot who could speak Russian.

Anatoly leaned toward his friend. "You need to go easy with those thoughts, Viktor."

"Why? They have been dominating the international airshows. It is time they know there is another game in town."

"Yes, but Gourgen and I are going to meet with one of the American pilots to seek his help, and we do not want to offend the Americans."

"Why?" Pugachov asked simply as it applied to all the above.

"Gourgen," Anatoly said motioning with his head toward Gourgen, "has been working with Anatoly Demjanovich and his doctors. They think he needs special treatment in the United States to be cured of the illness from that disaster at Chernobyl."

"Is this correct?" asked Pugachov of Gourgen. He nodded his head in agreement. "Then, I shall tone down the rhetoric."

"Good," smiled Anatoly. "You have no reason to boast. Your maneuver speaks for itself."

"Then, so it shall be."

The three test pilots shook hands in the Western style then went their separate ways. Gourgen sat down in the Mil trailer. Various engineers and technicians moved into and out of the small travel trailer. Mark Vineberg sat down at the table across from him. The main topic, if not the sole topic, was the success of the Sukhoi test pilot's dramatic maneuver. It was as popular with the Soviets as it was with the attendant aviation community.

The chief mechanic entered the trailer. The black of oil stained his overalls and hands, and spotted his face. "Bad news."

"No, good news. Kovatchur and Pugachov have represented our country well today. This is a day to celebrate."

"Excellent, but that is not what I meant." Both men waited motionless and expressionless for the news. "The tail rotor intermediate gearbox has eaten itself. We found several broken gear teeth inside the casing."

"Do you have a spare?" asked Gourgen.

"No."

"Then, we must fly in a spare from Zhukovsky or Rostov," responded Karapetyan instinctively.

"Are there any other signs of damage?" Vineberg asked.

"Yes, some skin distortion on the aft tail."

Gourgen Karapetyan knew the next words to come from the head engineer.

"We must not fly until we can fully evaluate the aircraft."

"We are in front of the world, Mark."

"Precisely my concern. Do you want to end up in a pile of burning and crumpled metal?"

Gourgen refused to answer the last question. "We have also made overtures to the Americans to trade flights – a rare opportunity that may never return."

"I am aware of that, but my first concern is your safety and protection of the aircraft."

"We must fly," demanded Gourgen.

A professional disagreement, some might say argument, ensued. None of the Mil engineers including Vineberg supported the aerobatic maneuvers Gourgen put together for the airshow. They all said the aircraft had not been designed for high energy maneuvering. Gourgen knew the language of the aircraft. He agreed to the higher stresses, but he was convinced the machine to take the added burden.

The conclusion came when Vineberg agreed to ship in another gearbox, and Karapetyan agreed to defer to Marat Tishchenko, the General Designer of the Mil Bureau, for a decision on further airshow flights.

Practice and rehearsal progressed precisely as they developed their routines. The only exception was Gourgen's disabled Mi-28 attack helicopter which he hoped to get repaired in time. The near daily rain played havoc with the schedule, but did not deter the pilots.

Anatoly Kovatchur handled the wildly popular response to Viktor Pugachov's Cobra maneuver as he did most things, with professional admiration, appreciation and respect. There was little question what routine attracted the most attention. Everyone seemed to be talking about the dramatic maneuver. That is, up until the next to last day of qualification.

# 31

*14:10, Thursday, 8.June.1989*
*Le Bourget Airfield*
*Paris, France*

The smooth, blended body contours and sleek lines of the MiG-29 fighter with its distinctive underwing, canted, rectangular intakes and twin vertical tails offered elegance and grace in the skies immediately above the famous airfield. This was the fourth practice session for Anatoly Kovatchur. He had declared to the judging officials, this was his qualification routine to conclude the certification process for him and the MiG-29.

Anatoly waited at the takeoff end of the runway for his time slot to open. The tower controller gave him clearance to proceed. He checked his instrument panel one last time. Everything was as it should be. Anatoly pushed the throttle levers forward and held the brakes so he could watch the engines accelerate. The engines were matched and performing at the expected levels. Anatoly released the brakes and pushed the throttles through the resistance of the maximum continuous thrust detent. He held the fighter on the runway past the normal lift off airspeed to give himself some extra margin. As pulled back slightly on the stick between his legs, the fighter jumped into the air. He immediately retracted the landing gear and rolled into a climbing right turn. Anatoly performed a set of turns and turn reversals, then leveled his aircraft and rolled into a maximum rate, level turn producing 9 g's so every part of his body felt like it weighed nine times its normal weight. He adjusted his position over the airfield to roll out into a level straight-line pass offset parallel to the runway opposite from the main public area.

As Anatoly reached mid-field, he pulled the nose up sharply

as he glanced at his attitude indicator to verify the fighter was pointed precisely 90° straight up. With the afterburners lit and both engines developing their full, 18,250 pounds thrust each, the aircraft accelerated like a powerful rocket. As he passed 1,000 meters altitude, Anatoly throttled back to idle. The machine decelerated rapidly. When the needle of the airspeed indicator passed ninety kilometers per hour and the world outside hesitated just for a moment, he pulled the stick full aft. The airplane began to fall backward in what the pilots would call a classic hammerhead stall, a popular maneuver for the venerable propeller fighters of World War II but virtually unheard of among turbojet or turbofan aircraft.

Conventional jets did not appreciate the added backpressure on the exhaust from the reverse airflow of falling backward. Modern turbine engines usually coughed in protest. The Soviet designers were justly proud of the robust design of the Isotov RD-33, low-bypass, turbofan engines and automatic relight feature if the backpressure did cause a flameout of the engine. The hammerhead stall provided a very public demonstration of how rugged their engines were.

As the fighter fell on its tail, the force of the reverse airstream on the large tailplanes, now fully deflected, functioned in the opposite direction pushing the tail back and the nose down. The nose fell gracefully forward. Anatoly neutralized his control stick. He was now pointed 90° straight down. He quickly checked and adjusted his position on the far side of the show line and away from the myriad of blue and white stripped tents, or chalets as they called them, and the gathered crowd of professionals watching his qualification routine. Pulling back smoothly on the stick and feeling the g-forces build, cramming his entire body into the seat, Anatoly moved the throttles forward to the full throttle gate, actually a noticeable detent – a position of resistance – short of lighting the spray rings of the afterburners at the exhaust end of the engines. As the nose reached the horizon, he pushed the throttles through the detent, felt the kick of afterburners, rolled the airplane to 90° right and pulled smoothly to 9 g's, making him feel nine times his

93 kilogram mass. His visual field narrowed as he groaned against the crushing force. The aircraft turned through 450° in a level, high energy, short radius turn, so that he now had the orange glow of his engine exhausts pointed toward the crowd. He leveled the wings, released the stick pressure, then rolled back in the opposite direction and pulled hard again. This time, Anatoly pulled the throttles back to nearly the idle position.

The aircraft slowed. He adjusted his altitude, attitude and the tightness of his turn to place the fighter directly above the show line at 200 meters altitude. Anatoly allowed the nimble fighter to slow. To maintain his altitude as the airspeed decayed, he slowly brought the nose up and continued well past the landing attitude. He also continued to nudge the throttles forward. The aircraft soon stabilized at 27° nose up, in level flight with an airspeed just above 140 kilometers per hour. This was the segment of his routine the pilot's called a high alpha demonstration, to show the very slow speed handling qualities, clean aerodynamics and substantial excess power from the engines. Anatoly rapidly scanned his instruments to ensure the proper attitude and altitude as well as his checkpoints on either side of the aircraft since he could no longer see where he was going with the nose so high.

Anatoly Kovatchur smiled inside the oxygen mask strapped to his helmet and face underneath his dark visor. The aircraft settled perfectly into the abnormal but stable slow flight condition as he seemed to inch his way along the show line parallel to the main runway. He checked both sides of the canopy to ensure his flight path was as he desired since he could not longer see in front of him with the nose so high. In several hundred meters, at the intersection of the runways, he would firmly push the throttles through the gate detent, lighting both afterburners and climb like a missile with big wings. The impressive maneuver would not happen this day.

A small bird happened to be in the wrong place at precisely the wrong time as it was sucked down the long intake of the right engine and into the whirling blades of the first stage turbine disk. The impact caused several of the blades to break off and cascade through the subsequent turbine stages taking more blades with them.

Anatoly heard the bang – more like a sharp thud – behind him. He instinctively glanced at his instruments – nothing. He heard a low groan or rumble behind him as the nose began to slowly yaw – to slide – to the right. Anatoly added left rudder to hold the nose. Something was wrong. He glanced at the instruments, again. This time the situation was obvious. The right engine was losing power; the speed of the engine was rapidly decreasing. He tried to gently lower the nose to get out of the precarious attitude he was in. The engine was dying too quickly. He was at full left rudder and the nose was still moving to the right and gaining speed. The nose continued to move right and was not coming down fast enough. The control of the agile fighter was slipping from his hands. The people – the crowd – just to his right. The nose was now moving quickly toward the crowd. He was going to crash; he just could not let the machine go into the innocent crowd so close to his right.

Anatoly fought with the nose of the aircraft. In an instant, he knew he would not be able to fly the stricken fighter out of its fatal position. Instinctively, Anatoly shifted his purpose. He added some right stick to accelerate the right roll already induced by the yawing of the nose to the right. The nose fell sharply toward the ground. He pulled the throttles back to the idle stop as the nose passed the horizon. Anatoly continued to manipulate the controls until he had the nose pointed straight at the grass between the runway and the taxiway.

He reached for the red and white loops between his legs, and pulled them up. In an instant, he heard the bang of the canopy being blown away. The stiff board of the crotch protector rose from between his legs to nearly mid-chest level. He felt the hard surface of the plates holding his elbows against his torso, and his legs being drawn sharply away from the rudder pedals and against the seat base. The rocket motors under the seat fired, kicking him abruptly away from the mortally wounded and doomed fighter. The small, expanding sleeve rods with small drogue parachutes deployed from each shoulder of the seat. Anatoly felt the seat separate at the instant the rocket motors burned out.

The grass rushed toward him with shocking speed. He was going to hit very hard. As he closed his eyes for the impact, he felt the snap of the parachute canopy filling completely, just before he felt the crush of his impact with the soft, wet earth and the searing heat of the fireball that once was a graceful and powerful fighter airplane.

Anatoly felt his groan although he could not hear it, as he lay immobilized and half buried in the wet grass. He fought for air. He needed to breathe and yet he could not take a breath. He wanted to remove his oxygen mask, but neither of his arms could move. Anatoly opened his eyes, but could only see orange and white smears that were panels of his parachute canopy and the horrific black smoke interlaced with tongues of bright orange flame. He landed so close to the crashed fighter. He was alive, but for how much longer. Anatoly felt the blackness closing in on him. He was losing consciousness, or maybe he was dying. Just before the black took him, a vision – a human dressed in a blue, flight suit with his flight helmet on and visor down – appeared above him. Then, black.

# 32

*16:25, Saturday, 10.June.1989*
*Le Bourget Airfield*
*Paris, France*

"The Apache is arriving," announced one of the mechanics from outside the trailer.

Gourgen joined the others. The odd, angled lines of the McDonnell Douglas, formerly Hughes Helicopters, AH-64A Apache advanced attack helicopter – the American equivalent of the Mi-28 – flew down the long main runway. As Gourgen watched the aircraft land and taxi away from the array of show aircraft, he wondered whether Parlier was flying, and why was he going out to the east end of the airfield? At least, the American helicopter finally arrived on the last practice day before the start of the airshow.

Gourgen found Vineberg. "Any confirmation on the exhibition exchange with the Americans?"

Mark Vineberg diverted his attention from the discussion regarding the Mi-28 to his chief pilot. "In a manner of speaking, I suppose. They did confirm the aircraft would be here, and you have undoubtedly noticed, it has arrived. The information I was given indicates your man, Parlier, is supposed to arrive sometime in the next day or so. He is apparently carrying their instructions."

"So, he is not with the aircraft."

"Apparently not."

"Then, we shall wait for him," Gourgen said as he turned toward the trailer.

Viktor Pugachov stood waiting for him between the Mil trailer and the tail of the Su-27 several meters away. Gourgen sensed Pugachov had some additional news. The stoic expression gave nothing away.

"Anatoly Kovatchur has been released from the hospital. He

is walking, but still white as a sheet and still quite weak."

"Is he back at the hotel?"

"No. The ambassador invited him to stay at his residence, so the press does not hound him."

"That is a good sign."

"How is your machine?" asked Pugachov.

"I do not think they are interested in setting any records for shipment of the gearbox we need. Tishchenko, our general designer, is due here today or tomorrow. Mark told me they would decide tomorrow."

"You think you pushed the helicopter too far?"

"No more than you push your interceptor."

"But, it is a helicopter."

"All you noise makers are the same. You need to come fly with me to see what it is like to really fly."

Pugachov and Karapetyan laughed as they usually did over such conversations. Knowing Anatoly was out of danger brightened the day. Now, a positive decision from Tishchenko would complete the return to optimism.

The airshow began the next day without the Mi-28 or the MiG-29. Gourgen hoped to rejoin the airshow, so he could display for the world the abilities of his aircraft. They were already discussing using the two seat MiG-29UB in the airshow with one of Anatoly's back-up pilots. The debate still raged between Anatoly and the doctors. He wanted to fly, not rest.

With the day's show complete and the aircraft parked back in their display positions, Gourgen relaxed in the trailer waiting for the call to depart for the hotel. He was alone with his thoughts for several minutes as the crowds outside thinned. With Anatoly now safe, his thoughts found their way to Anatoly Grishchenko.

When they left Zhukovsky, Anatoly was once more in the All Union Center for Hematology in Moscow. His leukemia continued its inexorable progression. They told him his white cell counts had all fallen sharply. The cold he contracted had become life threatening. He could only hope for his recovery.

Mark Vineberg leaned into the trailer. "Gourgen, I have someone I think you want to meet."

"Parlier?"

"Yes. He is outside beyond the crowd barrier."

Gourgen nodded his head, stood and followed Mark into the cool, late afternoon air. The heavy overcast made it feel like early rather than late spring.

A tall, moderate built man wearing a blue, tailored flight suit and brown leather jacket with a dark brown fur collar stood beyond the security barricades. He kept his hands in his pockets. A broad smile grew across his face. He appeared to have an entourage, several other men gathered around him at various levels of pretended disinterest. Perhaps the American had his own governmental chaperons, the equivalent of the KGB, GRU, MVD or Foreign Office.

"Gourgen, this is Cap Parlier," said Vineberg in English as they approached the barrier.

Gourgen extended his right hand as Parlier did.

"Mister Parlier, this is our chief pilot, Gourgen Karapetyan."

Their handshake was firm, vigorous and friendly. Gourgen responded in Russian although he understood the English words.

"Mister Karapetyan says he is pleased to meet you. He has heard many good things from Anatoly Kovatchur," Vineberg translated.

"It is an honor for me to meet you." Parlier's expression turned serious. "I just arrived. I learned of Anatoly's accident in the press two days ago. The news reports indicate he is recovering. Is he OK?"

Mark continued to translate. Gourgen decided to communicate directly, but wanted Parlier away from the others beyond the barricade. He pulled the police barricade back just enough for one person to move through, then motioned for Parlier to enter. The American nodded and followed the instructions.

Once inside the perimeter they walked silently toward the tail of the Mil-28. His eyes focused on the machine he had never seen up close. Gourgen turned to his guest. "Anatoly Sergeiyevich is doing much better. Thank you," Karapetyan finally said in his halting English.

"He is a very good man."

"Yes, he is." Gourgen struggled with the English words. "Anatoly Sergeiyevich ask me to say hello." Parlier nodded with a broad smile. "He hopes to see you again later."

"Great. Great. I would very much like to see him again." Parlier's attention return to the Mi-28.

"Would you like close look?" asked Gourgen.

"Very much, if you don't mind."

The two pilots fell into a routine repeated millions of time since the birth of aviation — the mutual appreciation of an excellent flying machine. Parlier possessed a reasonable knowledge of the Mi-28 . . . maybe as a student, maybe from his intelligence community. They shared quite a bit as they compared the similarities and differences between the American AH-64A Apache and the Soviet Mi-28. The impromptu and informal tour was interrupted by Mark Vineberg summoning Gourgen to the waiting bus. The two pilots agreed to renew their discussions early the next day.

Over the following two days, as the airshow moved through the paces with professional ease, Karapetyan and Parlier continued their professional exchange. Gourgen enjoyed a reciprocal tour of the AH-64. The underlying topic remained an exchange of flights . . . *quid pro quo* . . . that had been discussed prior to the show. Government officials unknown to either pilot wrangled for several days over the terms and conditions of the exchange flights. The two pilots suggested with laughter they should ignore the bureaucrats and just go fly. However, the current impasse centered on the Mi-28. Unless they could both fly both aircraft, neither of them would fly. It was up to Tishchenko and the decision to repair the Mi-28 and return the helicopter to flight status. They all waited for the decision.

Midway through the airshow week at Paris Le Bourget, Gourgen decided he knew the American sufficiently. It was time to take their relationship to the next stage. He motioned for Parlier to follow. Once in the Mil travel trailer, Gourgen gestured to the left side bench seat across the table built into the wall. He retrieved the chilled bottle of vodka from the small French refrigerator and a loaf of traditional, Russian, black bread from the bin, then he sat down across the small table from Parlier.

"Russian tradition," Gourgen said. "Normal I do not drink when I fly," he added to dispel the popular and yet derogatory public image of Russians as drunkards. "Neither of us fly tomorrow, so we break bread together and toast future."

"I would be honored."

Gourgen found two small plates, a knife and two small glasses. He poured the vodka. The cold liquid quickly produced a frosty coating on the glass. He sliced a broad piece of the dark, richly aromatic bread for Cap, then sliced himself a piece.

Karapetyan held up the glass. Parlier joined him. "To our future in the air."

"To our future in the air," repeated Parlier.

Gourgen threw the contents of the glass down his throat and immediately bit off a large chunk of bread to absorb the alcohol in his mouth. Parlier followed exactly as he did, then the American lifted the bottle and poured another glass for each of them.

"Thank you Mister Gorbachev for *glasnost* and *peristroika*," Parlier toasted.

Gourgen was not exactly sure how to take the American's words, but he nodded his head and flashed a brief smile as he acknowledged the toast. Parlier must have sensed the question.

"A few years ago, this private meeting between Soviet and American experimental test pilots would have been impossible. The change in policy by your Mister Gorbachev has made this possible."

Karapetyan understood the meaning and smiled. "Yes, of course."

They talked about flying as pilots usually did. Parlier told him that he flew as an experimental test pilot for McDonnell Douglas Helicopter Company in the place called, Mesa, Arizona, flying both commercial and military programs, but mainly working on the Apache. Gourgen shared his work location flying at a Mil test site north of Zhukovsky and working at the design office in Moscow. Parlier had military experience like Kovatchur. Neither he nor Anatoly Grishchenko had military experience. They had been industry pilots from the early days.

"We heard in the news about helicopter pilots flying over Chernobyl," said Parlier. "Did you know any of the pilots."

Gourgen smiled at the American as if to say, how could you read my mind. "Yes, several of us did."

"You did? You flew at Chernobyl?"

"Military pilots did most of flying. Mil, Kamov and Gromov pilots did special flying."

"Incredible. Is everyone OK?" he asked tentatively.

"All pilots were sick from radiation. All have recovered except one," Gourgen answered thinking of Anatoly Demjanovich. Parlier shook his head with a grave expression on his face and in his eyes. "His recovery very slow."

"I hope he will be all right eventually."

"We hope, too."

Gourgen told Cap about the evening they flew out to the damaged reactor for the first time. The enormous and endless column of bluish-white light rising from the exposed core fascinated Parlier. He seemed enthralled by the preparations and precautions they took. Cap indicated several times that he had very little experience with external lifting and especially not extremely heavy loads as they had to lift at Chernobyl.

It was in that conversation Gourgen Karapetyan decided to take the next few steps. He was not quite ready to ask Parlier for assistance. The sensitive issue of the release for foreign travel, especially for medical treatment, required resolution before they could be assured the government would allow Anatoly to leave the Soviet Union.

A heavy fist on the trailer's metal skin near the door preceded Anatoly Kovatchur's entry. They instantly looked to the door. Parlier's curious expression transformed into his characteristic broad smile. The American stood. They embraced as old friends.

"How are you, my friend?" asked Anatoly in English.

"I'm fine, but more importantly, how are you? Have you recovered from your little ride?"

Anatoly laughed. "Ride. Yes. Interesting term – ride. I shall be fine. I am ready to fly, but the surgeons say no."

"It is not the same routine without you flying," Parlier said. He was correct. "It was a spectacular display," he added probably referring to Anatoly's ejection sequence having shown up in many aviation press journals.

"Good fortune blessed him," interjected Gourgen. "Several days of rain made the ground soft. They had to dig him from the ground."

"The ground was not so soft, as you say, Gourgen."

The three pilots laughed at the image as they might at a cartoon.

"How come you are not flying?" asked Anatoly as they sat at the table.

"The aircraft belongs to the Army. They tell me when I can fly."

"No airshow?"

"The French are not interested in the Apache. The British are."

"Ah, yes, business."

"We are still hoping you can repair the Mil Two Eight, so we can exchange flights."

"That is deal?"

"Yes," answered Parlier. "The Army wants me to fly with Gourgen, then he can fly with me."

"Maybe I can fly with you also?" asked Anatoly, a rather unusual request since he did not often fly a helicopter.

"I shall ask."

"Excellent."

Mark Vineberg joined. After more friendly discussion about Kovatchur's recovery, Vineberg indicated it was time to leave.

The remaining days of the airshow enjoyed better weather than the practice and qualification week. The pilots continued their exchange of stories. Marat Tishchenko, after consultation with government officials, decided not to return the Mi-28 to flight status. The exchange of flights did not occur to the dismay and regret of both helicopter pilots.

"There you have it, my friend," concluded Gourgen. "That is how we have arrived at this day."

"My God, you have been through a lot," Parlier responded.

"Yes, I suppose we have, but there is much work to be done."

"That is amazing that you were able to survive that disaster at Chernobyl. Are you really sure everyone is OK?" Parlier asked innocently, not to question the veracity of Gourgen's recounting of events across the preceding three years, but more to question the future.

"We think so. One pilot is still ill. He has not fully recovered, yet."

"I shall pray for his recovery, Gourgen. It sounds like all of the pilots who flew at Chernobyl have truly performed heroic feats."

"I do not know about heroic. We did what the Motherland needed us to do."

"Yes, but I am certain your efforts have also saved many more lives outside the Soviet Union as well."

"Perhaps, but our eyes are on the future. We shall place this nasty event in the history books and move on with our lives."

"If there is anything I can do to help," Parlier said in courteous form, "please let me know."

Gourgen nodded his head, not quite ready to share the rest of the story until he knew for certain the request would be warranted.

It was the day after the closing of the airshow they watched Anatoly Kovatchur depart, piloting the MiG-29UB on his first flight after his accident. The announcer even broadcast the departure to the cheers of numerous workers.

"Good bye, Cap."

"Good bye to you, Gourgen. I hope to see you soon."

"Sooner than you think," answered Gourgen with a smile and a wink.

Parlier nodded his head with a return smile. "Great."

The two men parted. Cap Parlier went to Charles de Gaulle Airport for a commercial flight to London. He had business there before returning to the United States.

Gourgen Karapetyan smiled to himself as he watched the American walk across the ramp. He was satisfied he would help when the time came. Anatoly would be pleased. Gourgen's only hope now was that they could move fast enough to help Anatoly. Time would tell.

# 33

*18:40, Tuesday, 20.June.1989*
*Building R5, Apartment 1*
*Zhukovsky, Russia, USSR*

"What did you learn at Paris?" asked Anatoly Grishchenko, as he sat in 'his chair,' a large, overstuffed chair in the living room. The white surgical mask covering his mouth and nose defined the seriousness of his condition.

"I learned that I do not want to see Kovatchur do that slow flight, high angle of attack maneuver again."

"We heard about the crash. Is he all right?"

"Yes, he actually flew the MiG-29UB from Paris on Sunday to some Air Force base near the Urals. He shall return from the East in a few days. He was very lucky."

"As many of us are in this profession. What else?"

Gourgen knew what his friend was searching for without asking directly. "We have found our man," he answered.

"Did you ask him?"

"No. Now that we know it is possible, I must make sure of our end. I will meet with Director Vorobiev. I want him to commit to help us. I do not want to waste time asking the American for assistance, only to find that our government intends to block this initiative. Vorobiev is the key. He has the influence in the Government to gain permission. There is still the helicopter airshow at Redhill in England in September."

"Are you going?"

"No, Alexei Ivanov is going, to represent Mil. We also know that Parlier is supposed to be there although he could not say whether he would have an aircraft or not. I must fly a special mission in the South of France, near Vichy . . . some heavy lift job the French want us to do for them. If I can obtain the commitment from

Vorobiev, I will ask Ivanov to approach Cap Parlier. We will get his help soon."

"I am not sure how much time I have, Gourgen."

"There is still much to arrange. We will get you to America for your bone marrow transplant. I will see to it. All I ask of you is, to take care of yourself, to make sure you are as healthy as can be for this difficult procedure."

"I will do my part."

Galina entered the living room with a tray of small sandwiches and glasses of orange juice. "So, did I hear correctly," she said, "the arrangements for Anatoly are nearly finished."

"Yes, Galya. We shall ask Parlier to help us. I am certain he will agree. But, first, we must have a sponsor to ensure approvals on this end."

"You are certain this is the correct path?"

"Yes, absolutely."

"Why must we wait until September?"

"I must make sure the government will not stop us."

Galina snorted. "The government makes my Tolya sick, and then the government will not help cure him."

"It serves no purpose to flail against that which cannot be changed. Gourgen is doing the best that can be done. We can have no better friend working for us."

Galina stared at her husband, at Gourgen and then back to her husband. "I just want you healthy, and this miserable episode behind us."

"As do all of us, including me," Anatoly responded.

They mapped out the actions for the next few weeks. Many of the important people they needed would be taking extended summer holidays away from the city. Since Gourgen's *dacha* was not far from Andrei Vorobiev's summer home, he decided to make a casual visit to the venerable physician among the sweet aroma of the pine trees.

Although Gourgen did not confide in his ill friend nor his wife, he was frustrated by the slowness of movement in making the next few critical steps before they asked the American for help. In addition to the scarcity of key people during those summer months, Gourgen had to fly numerous special missions in France and various parts of the Soviet Union. He kept telling himself he needed to get other pilots trained to do these jobs. However, the truth be known and admitted to himself, he enjoyed the challenges of the unique assignments. He also had to contend with a flare-up of his chronic hepatitis. Life was never easy, and this was no exception.

As September approached, the government made the crucial decisions. Vorobiev was successful in winning the final consent to move Anatoly to the United States, if he received an appropriate invitation. They also made the decision to take a Mi-24E, or Mi-25 as they sometimes called it – the newest export version of the famous attack helicopter – along with a Mi-26 and a Ka-25 to the Redhill Airshow. The stage was set. Alexei Ivanov would be the senior aviation leader for the contingent attending Redhill. Overtures had been made to the Americans in the hopes the AH-64A would return, and the exchange flights could be carried out as they had intended at Paris in the spring. Gourgen found Ivanov at the Mil Design Bureau, the week prior to their departure for England.

"So, you have an alternative mission for me," said Ivanov.

"Yes, as a matter of fact, I do." Gourgen smiled at his colleague. "As you know, I have been working on arrangements for Anatoly Grishchenko to receive special medical treatment in America."

"Yes."

"All is in order, here. The last of the government's conditions is a proper invitation from an American clinic."

"And?"

"It is my understanding that an American test pilot, Cap Parlier, will be at Redhill, as you will be. I want you to ask him for his help in gaining that invitation. You can remind him of our discussions at Paris. He was genuinely concerned and offered his help. It is time to ask him."

"So, I shall ensure he remembers your conversations in Paris, then ask him for medical assistance for Anatoly."

"That is correct."

"Does he know what type of medical treatment is needed?"

"No, not specifically," answered Gourgen. "The best thing to do, if he agrees, which I am certain he will, is to simply exchange telex and fax numbers, so we can begin communicating directly with him. The physicians tell me Anatoly needs a bone marrow transplant, and he can only obtain it in America, but I do not think we need to cloud the communications with that detail at the moment. The most important thing is to find someone in America with the passion to help us. Cap Parlier is the correct man."

"It should not be a problem. I will do as you ask and report back to you upon my return."

"Good luck, Alexei."

The next two weeks were long ones for Gourgen and Anatoly. Gourgen threw himself into the flying missions he had been asked to perform. Anatoly waited at his home, trying to preserve what strength he had. The Redhill contingent returned to Moscow before Karapetyan. Once he secured his aircraft, he had one of the engineers drive him up to Mil. He found Ivanov in a meeting. He signaled for him to step outside, but Ivanov shook his head that he could not separate himself. Gourgen waited not so patiently for the senior design engineer to finish his discussion.

"What did you find out?" asked Gourgen.

"I met with Parlier, asked him to help, and he said, yes."

"Excellent."

"The odd thing, Gourgen, he seemed to be so excited about the opportunity to help us, that he did not even ask what kind of medical treatment was needed."

"He will do whatever is asked."

"As we would."

"Yes, as we would."

"He said he would try to contact you at the numbers we agreed on here at the office, upon his return to Arizona. I suspect you will receive a call within the next few days, if it has not come already."

"Thank you, Alexei. You have helped us take an important step for Anatoly Demjanovich. Now, we just need to complete these last few tasks."

Gourgen went up to the top floor to check the various communications devices as well as his office. There were no messages from Parlier or for him. So, the wait continued.

He had faith in his American colleague. His faith was rewarded a week later.

"Gourgen," said the General Designer's secretary as she leaned in the door to his office, "you have an international telephone call on Tishchenko's open line."

"Who?"

"I could not understand his name, but I think he may be American."

Instinctively, Gourgen knew the caller. "Hello," he answered in English.

"Is this Gourgen Karapetyan?"

"Yes, and this is Cap Parlier."

"Thank, God, I finally got you. It has taken me many days."

"Sometimes it is difficult."

"I was asked by Mister Ivanov at Redhill to help obtain special medical treatment for your friend."

"Yes. I know. I was unable to attend Redhill, so I asked Alexei Ivanov to approach you."

"I have made some inquiries and now have a contact at our State Department. I think we may be able to help. There are many obstacles yet to be crossed, but I am encouraged."

"Thank you, Cap. What do you need from me?"

"I need to know Anatoly's diagnosis and prognosis . . . his medical condition . . . so, I can find the correct doctors and facilities."

"I will have that within a day."

"I should have asked Mister Ivanov, but do you know what type of illness Anatoly has?"

"Our doctors have told me it is a type of leukemia. They will not admit that it was caused by Chernobyl, but we all know it was. They say he can be cured by something called, a bone marrow transplant."

"Interesting. I have not heard of such a procedure. I guess I will learn something here."

"How shall I send Anatoly's medical information to you?"

"These telephone connections are very difficult. Can you send it to me by fax or telex?"

"Yes."

"Did you get my numbers from Ivanov?"

"Yes. Then, you can expect a message within the day."

"I don't know how long it will take me to make all the arrangements in this country, but I will work as fast as I possibly can. I will communicate with you by whatever means seems to work the best."

"I shall do the same."

"I hope we can help Anatoly."

"If it can be done, I know we can do it."

"Yes. I will stay in touch. Take care, Gourgen."

"You do the same, Cap."

Finally, some encouragement, Gourgen said to himself. He took advantage of the proximity to Marat Tishchenko's office to tell their leader the good news.

"That was Cap Parlier, the American test pilot I met at Paris. He has agreed to help Anatoly Grishchenko."

"Congratulations, Gourgen. Your hard work has been successful."

"Not until Anatoly Demjanovich is cured."

"As you say. You have my full support. We will do everything we can to assist you."

"Thank you."

He went down the hall telling his colleagues the good news. They were finally making progress. In his heart, he thanked many people. He actually found himself thanking President Gorbachev for *peristroika* and *glasnost*, which became the opportunities to contact other pilots in the West.  He had to admit to himself and others that it was this important change in policy that gave them the opportunity to help Anatoly in a manner that would not have been possible a few years earlier.

# 34

*17:10, Thursday, 28.September.1989*
*All Union Center for Hematology*
*Moscow, Russia, USSR*

"Anatoly," said Gourgen bringing the ill pilot out of a slumber. "I have good news."

Grishchenko nodded his head without enthusiasm. He did not move or speak otherwise.

"Ivanov met Cap Parlier at the Redhill Heliexpo in England. Parlier has agreed to try to make arrangements for your medical treatment in America."

"So, now I get to make another life or death decision," responded Anatoly.

Gourgen looked at his friend trying to find the edge to peel back the cover. Why had Anatoly turned so uncharacteristically melancholy? He decided to strike directly at the issue rather than ignore the depression.

"This is no different than the hundreds of times you have been in trouble in the air . . . we have been threatened. You have a choice, as we always do, you can sit in that bed, and your fate will be assured. Or, you can fight this as you did when you lost that chunk of your tail rotor. Your choice, my friend."

The two men stared at each other without observers as though they faced off in some contest. Karapetyan wondered what must be going through Anatoly's mind. Had he given up and resigned himself to his fate? They had seen or heard the moment so many times around aviation. Had the time come for Anatoly?

"That was just instinctive reaction, not a conscious decision," protested Anatoly.

"So."

Several deep, hard coughs rocked his body. He sounds like a perpetual cigarette smoker, but he did not smoke. The cough was new, perhaps another medical sign of his deterioration.

A smile eventually washed across his face.

"Just testing, Gourgen. Just testing. Of course, I will take the ticket. Doctor Vorobiev has been very candid with me. There is nothing more they can do for me here. It is either a bone marrow transplant in America, or the end will come within six months to a year, at most, if not much sooner. I have already lived longer than they expected."

"Let us not talk about death. We shall talk about life."

"So, then, tell me of Ivanov and his meeting with Parlier."

Karapetyan did not want to stay in the hospital room with the smell of antiseptic barely masking the odor of death and disease. He pushed himself to ignore his inner urges to leave. He looked around the room to find a chair and pulled it up to the bed.

"According to Ivanov, who is one of the top chief designers at Mil as you probably remember, near the last day, he asked one of the American people to find Parlier. A female interpreter with the American contingent ran around like an excited school girl until she found him." They laughed at the image. "Ivanov eventually met with Parlier and the interpreter. As I asked him to do, he recounted my conversation with Parlier in Paris. After confirmation of the connection, Ivanov asked Parlier if he would help obtain medical treatment for you in America."

"And, he said, yes, correct?"

"Again, according to Ivanov, he appeared surprised and rather struck by the request, but then he said he would be honored."

"So, we have a friend."

"It would appear so."

"What next?"

"Parlier has my telephone and facsimile numbers at Mil. I think, now, we wait for him to figure things out on his end. We will be ready when he is ready."

"I do not have much waiting left, my friend."

Once more, Karapetyan stared into the eyes of his friend. This time Anatoly averted his eyes. The now, nearly constant struggle against even minor infections was taking its toll. Anatoly had lost more weight and color. He aged substantially in the last few months of his battle. Gourgen reminded himself about the added burden of the fight with the government. Scores of firefighters and technicians at Chernobyl had given their lives, and yet the officials persisted in their denials of any loss of life. If, according to the government bureaucracy, the firefighters had not died due to extreme radiation exposure, then they surely could not accept Anatoly's leukemia as a direct result of his radiation exposure. Gourgen viewed the government's denials and obstruction as nothing more than another obstacle to be overcome to help his friend.

"I need to be at Mil," Gourgen said, not wanting to tell his friend he had a test flight to complete. "I want to stop on my way out to see Doctor Vorobiev," he added as he retrieved the gold, 5-point, star with its deep red ribbon and pinned it on his coat lapel. Anatoly recognized the determination in Gourgen's eyes and smiled in acknowledgment. "Take care of yourself, Tolya."

"I will and good luck."

Gourgen shook hands with his friend, then left the room. He knew the way to the Office of the Director General of the All Union Center for Hematology. Doctor Andrei Vorobiev held the respect of many Russians. He had personally saved many lives during the Great Patriotic War. Some said they might have lost the battle to defend Moscow if Vorobiev had not treated so many wounded and returned them to the fight. He was also unrelenting in his pursuit of excellence for his center. He proved himself numerous times to be an equally effective fighter within the government bureaucracy.

His walk through the poorly lit hallways and stairs to the fourth floor had a depressing element. Doctor Vorobiev's office was more brightly lit and appointed. His female assistant recognized the red ribbon and gold star instantly. Her perfunctory questions did not bother Gourgen, nor did the several minutes waiting in the outer office. The respected figure of the larger, trim and balding, Andrei Vorobiev appeared as the inner office door opened.

"Gourgen Rubenovich, it is a genuine pleasure to see you

again."

"Likewise, Doctor."

"What can I do for you?"

"May we speak in private?" asked Karapetyan ignoring the pained and slightly resentful expression of his assistant.

"By all means," he answered motioning toward his office. The door closed behind them. Both men sat in the comfortable leather chairs positioned around the circular conference table in his office. The view of the Moscow skyline was spectacular. "What troubles you?"

Gourgen poured himself some water from the pitcher on the table. He gestured to the Director General who held up his hand in refusal. He took several drinks of the lemon flavored water.

"My friend, Anatoly Demjanovich, is one of your patients."

"Yes, I know."

"As I understand from Anatoly, you agree there is not much that can be done for him here."

"Yes, correct again."

"Something called, a bone marrow transplant, is the only treatment that can save him."

"Yes."

"You may know, I have contacted a friend, an American test pilot like Anatoly and me, to help us get him such a treatment."

"Really."

"You do not think we can do it?" asked Gourgen sensing the pessimism in his simple response.

"Gourgen Rubenovich," he said, "let me see if I have this correct. You are proposing to move a Soviet State test pilot, one who possesses some of the State's most valuable aviation secrets, to an American hospital for an extraordinary treatment that we cannot perform in Russia. Further, Anatoly Demjanovich contends he has contracted his leukemia from his exposure to acute ionizing radiation at Chernobyl, a condition the State has not agreed to, I might add. And, you want all this exposed to the Western press?"

"First, Comrade Doctor, I have a great deal of respect for your contributions to the Motherland. I do not question your loyalty. I am a simple pilot trying to obtain a life-saving treatment for my friend . . . that is all."

"Then, what do you need of me?"

Gourgen considered whether it was worth any more time to seek the Director General's specific help with the final arrangements. The changes in the country and the Government encouraged him to continue. "General Secretary Gorbachev's initiatives for openness and reform present a different environment, one that makes this effort more possible. My colleagues and I have talked with the American pilots as friends, not as adversaries. I myself have met Cap Parlier, the American pilot, and have broken bread with him. He has contacted his Government and is making arrangements to receive Anatoly Demjanovich, as we speak."

"Then, I ask again, what do you need of me? I have given you my consent months ago."

"We need your help to ensure we can obtain the proper referrals, the correct permissions, and be able to move Anatoly as soon as the arrangements have been made."

"How do you propose to get him to America? Are you going to convince your aviation colleagues to fly him there . . . fly a Soviet aircraft into American airspace?"

"My friend, Cap Parlier, is making all the arrangements. All we need is, no government obstacles."

"A very tall order considering Anatoly's standing and his condition."

"That is why I have come to you, Director General."

Doctor Vorobiev considered the obstacles, consequences and what he might be able to do while he remained transfixed on Gourgen's unblinking eyes. Several minutes passed before Vorobiev averted his eyes and began shuffling papers around his large, hardwood desk. Gourgen continued to watch the Director General wondering whether he would get any help from the senior medical leader. Had he become too much a part of the government bureaucracy or would he remember the determined spirit of his war years?

Gourgen began to consider other options for getting Anatoly out of the country for his medical treatment as well as how to get him back into the country when he was cured. The latter portion did not bear the same importance for him. The return trip was just assumed. Neither of the pilots had any intention of leaving Mother Russia permanently. Although life was hard, they were very well taken care of by the State, and neither of them had any desire to give it up.

Vorobiev stopped shuffling his papers and returned his gaze to Gourgen. "You know what you are asking?"

"Of course I do, Comrade Doctor," he said with emphasis on the Soviet title as if to recognize the imposition of the State.

The Director General thought for a few moments more without moving. "I will see what I can do?"

"Excellent."

"I can make no promises."

"Agreed."

"There are a few conditions."

"Which are?"

"First, we must devise a reason why he must go to America without casting doubt on the Soviet medical establishment." Gourgen nodded his head without knowing how to do that. "Second, we cannot make any connection between his leukemia and the Chernobyl disaster."

Gourgen chuckled. "Doctor, the world knows."

"That is not my point. The State . . . ," he paused. Gourgen recognized the conflict within the accomplished medical expert. "The State will not acknowledge the linkage between the disaster and the injury."

"People have died," Gourgen spat. "Firemen who valiantly fought to contain the immediate fires died within days of their exposure to that open reactor, and we are going to maintain there is no connection? Are you serious?"

"Comrade Karapetyan." It was now Vorobiev's turn to invoke

the State. "I did not say I agreed with this position. I have simply stated, if we are to have any chance of being successful, for Anatoly's health, we must abide by the wishes of the State."

Gourgen Karapetyan stared intensely at the Director General. He was indeed correct. Politics had to be put aside for Anatoly's sake. "As you wish, then."

Vorobiev nodded his head. "Again, I can make no promises."

"I am asking for none. I only ask for your effort, for your attempt."

"Then, we are agreed?"

"Yes."

"You must give me a few days to make the proper inquiries."

"You can take all the time you need to be successful, Comrade Doctor. We are only talking about the life of a very good friend, a very good man, and a loyal servant of Mother Russia."

"You do not need to remind me," Vorobiev answered with a tinge of resentment in his voice.

"My apologies. I did not mean to offend," he said with a partial lie. "I just want to help Anatoly."

"As do I."

Karapetyan rose from his chair which in turn pulled Vorobiev to his feet. "I shall leave you to your task." He started to turn, then noticed the doctor's hand being extended to him. He turned to grasp the proffered hand and shook it firmly. "Thank you for your time."

"A pleasure to see you, Gourgen. We shall do our best for Anatoly."

"No doubt," said Gourgen as he turned to leave.

He walked down the dark hallway toward the stairs. While the meeting had not been enthusiastically successful, at least he had the agreement for assistance from a high ranking member of the medical establishment. He trusted Vorobiev despite his political position.

Should he stop to tell Anatoly of their meeting? He hesitated at the stair well. He looked at his watch. Although the crews would wait on him, he did have a test flight to fly. Even at this time, he would be late to the test site and more than a dozen technicians, engineers and support crew would be waiting on him. He needed to move along quickly. Gourgen decided to wait until he had news from Andrei Vorobiev or Cap Parlier.

He took the stairs two at time and walked briskly from the Institute to his tired automobile for the drive across town to the helicopter test site. He could only hope Vorobiev would be successful. The assistance of a senior doctor would make permission for Anatoly's treatment come much more easily. In his heart, despite Vorobiev's qualifying statements, he knew the medical hero would be successful. This was simply another battle to save one small part of the heart and soul of the Motherland.

# 35

*16:30, Thursday, 14.December.1989*
*Building R4, Apartment 44*
*Zhukovsky, Russia, USSR*

"Welcome home, Gourgen," said Ludmilla Karapetyan as her husband walked through the door and hug up his heavy winter coat. They embraced and kissed. "It is good to be home. These long assignments are even more difficult when winter comes early."

"Did you complete the task?"

"Yes. I forgot that winter comes even earlier in the Urals. The government needed me to do some special developmental flying on an experimental, one of a kind, helicopter," he said as his way of telling her he could not talk about his mission spanning the last two months.

"So, you do not have to go back?"

"No, fortunately. I am done."

Gourgen followed Ludmilla into the kitchen. She was making a large kettle of her special potato soup, one of his favorite dishes. She stirred the mixture as she told him, "Supper will be ready in an hour."

"Good," he answered as he grasped her from behind. "I need to talk to Anatoly Demjanovich for a short time." He released her and tore off a chuck of bread from a half eaten loaf. "While I was in the East, several messages came into the design office that I want him to see."

"Good news, I hope."

"I think so. It would appear the American pilot we have asked to help us – Cap Parlier – is making progress on the arrangements for Anatoly's treatment in the United States."

Ludmilla began chopping some green onions for inclusion as prescribed by her recipe. She kept her head down and spoke softly, giving her words a melancholy tone. "I hope you can get him the treatment he needs before it is too late."

"I know, Milla. The doctors think it may already be too late, but they have agreed to help us. We shall do our best."

"I know you will. Now, get on over to the Grishchenko's so you can pass your news and get home in time for supper."

Gourgen kissed his wife on the cheek from behind, then retrieved his coat and departed. The walk in the cold air with the sparse lights illuminating the path in the early dusk of near winter enabled him to compose his words for Anatoly.

He arrived at the Grishchenko apartment to be greeted by a solemn Galina. She was in the same process as Ludmilla although making some vegetable dish. She pointed to the living room without words, which seemed very odd for her. Something was on her mind or troubling her, but he did not want to ask.

Gourgen found Anatoly in their living room sitting by himself in a chair at the far end of the room. There were no lights, and the room was dark. He could see Anatoly but could not tell whether he was awake or napping.

"Good to see you, Gourgen," he said, answering the question.

"Why are you sitting in here in the dark?"

"It makes me feel better."

Anatoly wore his bedroom slippers over socks. He had what appeared to be pajamas on underneath a heavy bathroom robe. More significantly, he wore a large surgical mask over his lower face so that only his eyes could be seen.

"How are you feeling?"

"Not so good, if you must know. I am very weak. I have no energy to do anything, and the doctors have confined me to this apartment. I felt perfectly fine for the last month, then this."

"Do you have to wear the mask even inside here?"

"I must wear it all the time, now. They are worried about even the slightest infection."

Gourgen studied Anatoly. Even in the diminished light, he could see his friend's state was not good. Perhaps, this news would cheer him up. "I have been in the Urals for the last two months on a special project.  When I returned earlier today, there were two messages that arrived from Parlier while I was gone.  May I turn on a light so you can read them?"

"Yes, certainly."

As Gourgen's eyes adjusted to the sudden onslaught of light, he noticed Anatoly's eyes were shut.  He waited for his friend's eyes to adapt.  He opened the folder he carried with him, found the correct piece of paper, then handed it to Anatoly.

---

## McDONNELL DOUGLAS HELICOPTER COMPANY
### FACSIMILE TRANSMISSION

**Date:**      16.October.1989
**From:**      Cap Parlier
**To:**        Gourgen Karapetyan
**Subject:**   Medical Treatment for Anatoly
               Grishchenko

DEAR GOURGEN,

I RECEIVED YOUR FAX OF 10.OCTOBER.1989.  I HAVE MADE MOST OF THE ARRANGEMENTS FOR THE ENTRY VISA FOR ANATOLY AND GALINA GRISHCHENKO.  THERE ARE ONLY TWO ITEMS REMAINING WHICH I AM WORKING ON:

A.  WHICH MEDICAL FACILITY CAN PROVIDE THE CORRECT TREATMENT?

B.  HOW TO PAY FOR HIS TREATMENT?

I AM TALKING TO SEVERAL MEDICAL EXPERTS IN THE USA IN AN EFFORT TO FIND THE CORRECT HOSPITAL AND TO ARRANGE ADEQUATE FUNDING.  I HAVE BEEN ASKED SEVERAL QUESTIONS REGARDING ANATOLY'S MEDICAL CONDITION.  THE DOCTORS NEED TO KNOW MORE IN ORDER TO FIND THE CORRECT MEDICAL FACILITY.

1.  WHAT IS HIS DIAGNOSIS?

2.  DOES IT INVOLVE APLASTIC ANEMIA OR LEUKEMIA?

3.  WHAT ARE HIS BLOOD FINDINGS?

4.  WHAT TREATMENT HAS HE RECEIVED AND WHAT WERE THE RESULTS?

```
    WITH THE ANSWERS TO QUESTIONS 1 THROUGH 4, I
THINK WE SHOULD BE ABLE TO MAKE THE PROPER
ARRANGEMENTS.  IF I CAN ARRANGE THE CORRECT
MEDICAL FACILITY AND ADEQUATE FUNDING, I CAN
SEND THE INVITATION FOR HIS MEDICAL TREATMENT.
WILL YOU ARRANGE FOR THEIR TRANSPORTATION TO AND
FROM THE MEDICAL FACILITY?  WHAT OTHER
ASSISTANCE WILL THEY REQUIRE WHILE THEY ARE IN
THE UNITED STATES?
    I AM SORRY THAT IT IS TAKING SO LONG TO FIND
THE CORRECT MEDICAL FACILITY AND FUNDING.  I AM
TRYING EVERYTHING I KNOW OF TO FIND THE RIGHT
HELP.
WITH GREAT RESPECT,
CAP PARLIER
SENIOR EXPERIMENTAL TEST PILOT
MCDONNELL DOUGLAS HELICOPTER COMPANY
```

---

"Well, now," said Anatoly, "that explains why the doctors wanted to run some special tests in October. They would not tell me why. I thought they might have found something else wrong, but I guess they must have received a medical request even though you were not here."

"Perhaps. That would explain the next message as well. One of my compatriots must have done the work and responded to Parlier's message on our behalf."

"Yes, I suppose you are correct. You said you had another message."

Gourgen took the piece of paper from Anatoly and returned it to the folder. He leafed through the folder some more until he found the next item he wanted. "This is the message that started things moving for us. Parlier did a great deal of work with the medical specialists as well as the American Government to get this done."

## McDONNELL DOUGLAS HELICOPTER COMPANY
### FACSIMILE TRANSMISSION

**Date:** 2.November.1989
**From:** Cap Parlier
**To:** Gourgen Karapetyan
**Subject:** Decision

DEAR GOURGEN,
THANK YOU FOR ANATOLY'S MEDICAL INFORMATION.
BASED ON THE DATA PROVIDED, THE MEDICAL EXPERTS
IN MY COUNTRY RECOMMENDED THAT WE MAKE
ARRANGEMENTS WITH THE FRED HUTCHINSON CANCER
RESEARCH CENTER (FHCRC) IN SEATTLE, WASHINGTON.
I HAVE NOW CONTACTED DR. JOHN HANSEN AT
FHCRC, THE CHIEF OF THE BONE MARROW TRANSPLANT
UNIT. HE HAS AGREED TO WORK WITH US. THE FIRST
STEP NOW IS TO FIND A COMPATIBLE DONOR FOR
ANATOLY. DR. HANSEN HAS INITIATED THE DONOR
SEARCH WITH THE NATIONAL MARROW DONOR PROGRAM.
HE TELLS ME THE SEARCH PROCESS COULD TAKE WEEKS
OR MONTHS. HE ALSO SAYS THAT EVERY REGISTRY WE
KNOW OF IN THE WORLD WILL BE CHECKED TO FIND A
DONOR FOR ANATOLY. I HAVE BEEN TISSUE TYPED TO
SEE IF I COULD BE ANATOLY'S DONOR, BUT OUR HLA
TYPES ARE NOT THE SAME, MUCH TO MY REGRET. DR.
HANSEN CAUTIONS US THAT WE MAY NOT FIND A DONOR.
WE WILL DO OUR ABSOLUTE BEST.
I WILL KEEP YOU INFORMED OF OUR PROGRESS.
HOPEFULLY, WE WILL FIND A DONOR SOON. TAKE
CARE, MY BROTHER.
WITH GREAT RESPECT,
CAP PARLIER

Gourgen did not wait for Anatoly's response. "As it says, all we need now is a compatible donor.
"Yes."

"I am sorry I have been away so much and that I do not know the answer to this question, but . . . do you still have good days and bad days?

"Yes. Today has been a bad day."

"But, you still have good days, too."

"Yes, as I said earlier, although they seem to be less frequent."

Galina entered the room with her hands in the cloth of her apron. "Well, I see you were able to at least get him to turn the lights on," she said to Gourgen. "Are you staying for supper?"

"No, Galya. Milla should have our supper on the table about now, so I need to get home. I just wanted to show Anatoly the messages I received from Parlier while I was working in the East."

"Good news?"

"Would you like to read them?"

She nodded her head. Gourgen handed her the two relevant pieces of paper. She glanced at them. "I cannot read English. What do they say?"

"They say that Parlier is making good progress toward getting Anatoly to America for treatment. All we need now is a compatible donor."

"The doctors told us this treatment is fairly new, and there is a chance they may never find a donor."

"True enough, Galya, but there is also a chance they will, and we need to remain focused on the positive outcome."

Galina nodded her head again, then looked at her husband. "Supper is ready. Would you like me to bring it to you, or would you like to try to eat in the kitchen?"

"With Gourgen's good news, I feel better. I shall make the effort." Anatoly started to push himself up out of the chair very slowly.

Gourgen wanted to help him, but as soon as he moved, Anatoly shook his head rejecting any assistance. He walked behind his ailing friend to catch him if he should stumble or collapse. Gourgen waited for Anatoly to make it to the kitchen table chair.

"I am glad you are feeling better, Anatoly Demjanovich. Do

exactly what the doctors tell you to do." He looked to Galina. "Take good care of him."

She nodded her as she motioned toward the door. She followed him, and waited for him to don his coat before opening the door.

Gourgen embraced her and kissed both cheeks, then leaned near her ear and whispered, "We are going to save him, Galya, so take good care of him." As he pulled back, tears streamed from both eyes. He wiped them away then kissed her cheek again. "Be strong." Galina meekly nodded as she lowered her head to avoid his eyes. Gourgen touched her shoulder then departed, and heard to door close behind him.

# 36

*10:30, Wednesday, 28.March.1990*
*All Union Center for Hematology*
*Moscow, Russia, USSR*

The sense of urgency pushed Gourgen Karapetyan past his physical, or some might say, psychological, aversion. He now found his stomach turning every time he entered the medical establishment, and the reaction was getting worse. Anatoly had been in and out of various medical facilities in the years since the accident, but this time held the distinction of feeling more permanent. The doctors told Gourgen several days ago that his friend's latest bout with a simple, head cold, infection had taken his immune system precipitously near the edge of the abyss. They all knew there was not much time left. Even Anatoly knew, although we did not talk about it anymore.

Walking down the dark corridor of the third floor brought an anticipation to his meeting with Anatoly. The folder of papers in his hand made this visit much different and, from his perspective, more significant than all the previous visits.

"Comrade," called a rather large, matronly nurse Gourgen did not recognize. He turned to face the woman. "Comrade, I presume you are here to see Comrade Grishchenko, yes?"

"Correct."

"He had a very difficult night, comrade. He is finally resting, and you should not disturb him."

"Well, then, Comrade . . . ," he said motioning for her to fill in the blank with her name.

"Nagrovna. Comrade Nagrovna."

"Well, then, Comrade Nagrovna, let me see if I can help you understand." He held up the folder. "I have here Comrade

Grishchenko's salvation. I think he will be quite interested in seeing these messages."

"Then, it is my turn," she said with a measure of irritation. "What is your name?"

"Karapetyan."

Her expression conveyed the contemplative moment she experienced. "Karapetyan? Did I see something in the newspaper a few months ago? Are you . . . let me see . . . are you the Hero of the Soviet Union Karapetyan?"

"Yes, I suppose I am," he said with humility.

"An honor, Comrade Karapetyan," she said extending her right hand for a firm handshake. "My apologies," she said motioning past her toward Anatoly's room. "I just ask that you do not occupy him too much. He does need to rest."

"I shall do my best."

Gourgen left the nurse in the corridor to walk the remaining four doors. Anatoly's private room possessed a more amplified smell than the hospital in general. It was starkly appointed. The mechanical hospital bed, a single, straight back, wooden chair, and a small, white metal, two drawer, table that served as a multipurpose repository for things medical and personal.

Anatoly appeared to be sleeping peacefully. His gaunt and quite pale face behind the white surgical mask over his mouth and nose made him appear oddly more vulnerable. I only hope that this treatment comes in time, Gourgen told himself. He also questioned his insistence upon disturbing his friend. Maybe Nurse Nagrovna was correct. Then again, Anatoly was a fighter. Like most of their colleagues, they had survived by one predominant trait – never giving up, even in apparent helpless situations.

"Tolya," he said softly trying to wake his colleague. Not a twitch. "Tolya," he said a little louder. Still nothing. Maybe this was not such a good idea, he scolded himself. The ill man's eyes flickered then opened to an unseeing stare. Karapetyan did not know quite what to think. "Tolya," he called one more time.

Grishchenko's eyes blinked several more times before they

moved toward Karapetyan and focused. A weak smile bloomed on his tortured face behind the mask.

"Good to see, Gourgen," Grishchenko said weakly as though he was thankful his eyesight had not failed him.

"Sorry to disturb you, Anatoly Demjanovich. I just knew you would want to see the latest message from America."

"Yes, please."

Gourgen opened the folder, found the piece of paper he wanted, then handed it to Anatoly. "As you recall, the Americans have been looking for a bone marrow donor for you."

"Yes?"

Gourgen handed Anatoly the first message.

Anatoly held the paper at arm's length without trying to read it. "I remember you talking about this. I actually felt good when you told me the news, although it did not have all the answers for us."

"Yes, Anatoly Demjanovich. It gave me encouragement as well. Now, read this one," Gourgen said with mounting impatience.

Anatoly positioned the paper and read with earnest enthusiasm.

---

**McDONNELL DOUGLAS HELICOPTER COMPANY**
**FACSIMILE TRANSMISSION**

**Date:**      12.March.1990
**From:**      Cap Parlier
**To:**        Gourgen Karapetyan
**Subject**:

DEAR GOURGEN,
    WE HAVE GOOD NEWS ALTHOUGH WE STILL HAVE SOME DETAILED MEDICAL TESTS TO COMPLETE. THE HLA TYPING OF THE FRENCH DONOR HAS BEEN CONFIRMED. THE ADDITIONAL TESTS INVOLVE THE EVALUATION OF THE DONOR'S DNA WITH RESPECT TO ANATOLY'S DNA IN ORDER TO DETERMINE THE POTENTIAL FOR GRAFT REJECTION. DR. HANSEN INDICATES THAT WE NOW HAVE A 50 PERCENT CHANCE

SACRIFICE 331

```
THAT THE REMAINING TESTS WILL VALIDATE THE
DONOR.  WHILE THESE RESULTS ARE VERY
ENCOURAGING, IT IS IMPORTANT TO REMEMBER THAT
THESE DETAILED TECHNICAL TESTS MUST BE COMPLETED
BEFORE AN ACCEPTABLE DONOR MATCH CAN BE DECLARED
FOR ANATOLY.  I AM EXCITED THAT WE HAVE MOVED
CLOSER TO OUR OBJECTIVE.
   THE MONEY TRANSFER WILL BECOME INCREASINGLY
MORE IMPORTANT AS WE GET CLOSER TO A TRANSPLANT.
JUST A REMINDER: THE HUTCHINSON CENTER NEEDS THE
NEXT BLOCK OF US$15,000 AS SOON AS POSSIBLE.
YOU SHOULD BE PREPARED TO TRANSFER THE REMAINING
US$185,000 AS SOON AS WE HAVE FULL CONFIRMATION
THAT WE HAVE AN ACCEPTABLE MATCHED DONOR.
   GOURGEN, I RECEIVED YOUR FAX OF 12.MARCH.90.
I HAVE PASSED THE INFORMATION TO DR. HANSEN AT
THE HUTCHINSON CENTER.  I AM GOING TO TRY TO
SEND THIS MESSAGE BY FAX.  IF I AM UNSUCCESSFUL,
I WILL SEND IT BY TELEX.
WITH GREAT RESPECT
CAP
```

"You did not mention money," said Anatoly.

"Do not worry."

"Gourgen, that sounds like quite a bit of money. None of us have any money like that."

"I have worked with Doctor Vorobiev to get the Government to pay for the treatment. It is actually going to be paid by a government aviation export company. We do not pay in this country, right?"

"Certainly. So, they will give the money to the Americans?"

"The arrangements have been made."

"Excellent, my friend."

"That was two weeks ago," Gourgen said as he smiled and retrieved the last paper. "This is the very latest message from Parlier, I received this morning. I did not call you. I wanted you to read it for yourself."

## McDONNELL DOUGLAS HELICOPTER COMPANY
## FACSIMILE TRANSMISSION

**Date:** 26.March.1990
**From:** Cap Parlier
**To:** Gourgen Karapetyan
**Subject:** Medical Treatment for Anatoly Grishchenko

DEAR GOURGEN,

I HAVE VERY GOOD NEWS. THE HUTCHINSON CENTER HAS INFORMED ME THAT THE DONOR HAS BEEN CONFIRMED AS A MATCH FOR ANATOLY AND HAS CONSENTED TO DONATE HER MARROW FOR HIM. WE HAVE TAKEN A VERY BIG STEP FORWARD.

PLEASE TAKE STEPS TO IMMEDIATELY TRANSFER THE REMAINING US$185,000 TO THE HUTCHINSON CENTER AS INDICATED IN THE INSTRUCTIONS PROVIDED EARLIER.

THE HUTCHINSON CENTER HAS PROPOSED THE FOLLOWING SCHEDULE:

1. THE PHYSICAL EXAM OF THE DONOR HAS ALREADY BEEN ORDERED.

2. RECEIPT OF THE DONOR PHYSICAL EXAM - 30 MARCH.

3. RECEIPT OF US$185,000 IN FHCRC ACCOUNT BY - 4 APRIL.

4. LETTER OF INVITATION WILL BE SENT IMMEDIATELY UPON RECEIPT OF FUNDS AT FHCRC - 4 APRIL.

5. ENTRY VISAS ISSUED AT US EMBASSY MOSCOW ON OR ABOUT 6 APRIL.

6. TRANSPORT ANATOLY AND GALINA GRISHCHENKO (AND OTHERS) TO SEATTLE DURING WEEK OF 9 APRIL.

7. START PREPARATION FOR TRANSPLANT - 20 APRIL.

8. TRANSPLANT - 27 APRIL.

IT IS IMPORTANT TO NOTE THAT THE ABOVE DATES

ARE TENTATIVE AND MAY VARY SOMEWHAT. THEY ARE
SEQUENTIAL.

THE HUTCHINSON CENTER WOULD LIKE TO HAVE A
MEDICAL UPDATE ON ANATOLY'S CONDITION. IN
ADDITION, THE HUTCHINSON CENTER WOULD LIKE TO
KNOW:

A. SHOULD ANATOLY RECEIVE A PLATELET
TRANSFUSION ON THE DAY OF THE TRANSFER?

B. CAN HE TOLERATE A PROLONGED COMMERCIAL
AIRLINE FLIGHT WITH POSSIBLE ENROUTE DELAYS OR
MISSED CONNECTIONS?

C. WHAT IS YOUR PREFERRED METHOD OF
TRANSPORT FOR ANATOLY TO SEATTLE?

D. SHOULD A TRANSPLANT PHYSICIAN FROM THE
HUTCHINSON CENTER FLY TO MOSCOW TO ACCOMPANY
ANATOLY DURING HIS FLIGHT TO SEATTLE?

DOCTOR HANSEN INFORMS ME THAT INTERPRETERS
ARE AVAILABLE IN SEATTLE. CONSIDERING THE
IMPORTANCE OF THIS EFFORT, IT MAY BE BENEFICIAL
IF ONE OR MORE SOVIET INTERPRETERS CAN BE
AVAILABLE DURING HIS STAY IN SEATTLE. THE
HUTCHINSON CENTER INDICATES THAT YOU SHOULD
EXPECT A DURATION OF HIS TREATMENT TO BE ABOUT
120 DAYS UPON HIS ARRIVAL IN SEATTLE.

I HAVE ALSO BEEN INFORMED THAT THERE HAS
ALREADY BEEN MEDIA INTEREST IN OUR EFFORTS ON
BEHALF OF ANATOLY. WE SHOULD EXPECT
CONSIDERABLE NATIONAL AND INTERNATIONAL MEDIA
ATTENTION TO ANATOLY'S TREATMENT. A PUBLIC
ANNOUNCEMENT MAY BE ISSUED IN WASHINGTON DC ON
OR ABOUT THE COMPLETION OF STEP 4 ABOVE.

I AM VERY HAPPY THAT WE HAVE ARRIVED AT THIS
DAY. WE WILL ALL WORK AS FAST AS WE CAN TO MOVE
ANATOLY TO SEATTLE TO COMPLETE THE BONE MARROW
TRANSPLANT. THE OBJECTIVE NOW IS TO HELP
ANATOLY RECOVER TO GOOD HEALTH. I LOOK FORWARD
TO SEEING ANATOLY AND GALINA IN SEATTLE VERY
SOON. ANATOLY HAS A HARD FIGHT AHEAD OF HIM AND
I AM SURE HE IS READY. TAKE GREAT CARE, MY

WITH GREAT RESPECT,
CAP PARLIER

"You are not playing some grotesque practical joke on me, are you?"

A deep, heavy laugh burst from Karapetyan. "No, Anatoly Demjanovich. This is most genuine. It would appear our faith in Cap Parlier has yielded our desired objective."

"Did you notice the transplant date?"

Gourgen took the paper. "What about that! Four years from that damnable accident, almost to the day." Anatoly nodded his head with a smile, then turned serious.

"Once more, we managed to pull the rabbit from the hat." His expression compelled him to reveal the rest of the story. "Doctor Vorobiev, with some coaxing from me, has received a commitment from the Minister of Health that he will not stand in the way. Apparently, so I am told, the Central Committee has supported the decision. It is now up to us."

A broad smile grew on Anatoly's tired face. "It is good to have you as a friend."

"Nonsense. You would do it for me if our positions were reversed."

"I suppose." Anatoly looked out his window at the dreary, winter scene. "You really think this is the best thing to do?" he asked softly as he continued to stare out at some distant point.

Gourgen smiled. "Well, we shall see."

Anatoly looked his friend in the eye. "That is not a particularly resounding endorsement."

"I think he is going to make this work," answered Gourgen although thinking to himself – only when?

"Yes, but when?" Anatoly asked as if he was reading Karapetyan's mind. "The doctors will not tell me anything important." His eyes turned to some point far beyond his hospital room. "I do not think I have much time left."

"You cannot give up," Gourgen grunted.

Anatoly chuckled, then re-engaged Gourgen's eyes. "Who said anything about giving up? I was just talking about time. An airplane in a flat spin only has so much time before it meets the ground," he said with a laugh.

"Sorry, my friend. I supposed I have been doing too much thinking."

"Always a bad thing, Gourgen. You know that."

They both laughed – a good sign, Gourgen told himself.

"Now, let me see the last message from Parlier, again." The paper changed hands. "So, it is Seattle – the State of Washington – Northwest United States, if I remember my geography lessons."

"That is the one."

"What is so special about Seattle? Tell me again."

"As Parlier has told me, that is where the Fred Hutchinson Cancer Research Center is located," Gourgen said nearly choking on the word, cancer. He continued to have difficulty accepting that his friend's illness was a malignancy – mutated cells growing abnormally fast – that would most probably claim one of the country's pre-eminent experimental test pilots. Damn that reactor and that accident. They had taken so many good lives already, and they were about to claim another, more personal life.

"So?"

"Doctor Vorobiev says this Seattle clinic is the best in the world for your illness. He says the doctor who won the Nobel Prize for Medicine, a Doctor Thomas, as I recall, works there. He perfected this bone marrow transplantation procedure that you need, to be cured. He is more experienced than any other doctor, and the Doctor Hansen in Parlier's messages learned from Thomas and works with him. Parlier says this clinic is very highly regarded in America, as well."

"Now that the location is decided, how can I possibly get

there?"

"Well, my friend," Gourgen said with a broad smile, "that is the good part." He paused for some reaction. He received none. "Just this morning, I received a telephone call from an American female nurse who works at the American embassy. She has been talking to Cap Parlier. They have arranged for a series of flights on one of the American airlines to get you to Seattle and back."

"Is the government paying for these flights, also?"

"No. They are only allowing us to do this. No one has asked for travel money. I think this nurse – Susan Summers is her name – said she talked to some friends of hers here in Moscow, and Pan American Airways is donating the seats on their scheduled flight from Moscow to New York. Then, she told me that Cap Parlier has made arrangements for Trans World Airlines to donate a flight for you from New York to Seattle, since Pan American does not fly to Seattle. This is all quite magnificent."

"Does that sound right?"

"What do you mean?"

"Everybody giving us things."

"I do not know, and I do not really care. All I care about these days is getting your tired old body to Seattle, so you can be cured of this scourge."

"Then, we shall not look a gift horse in the mouth."

"A good idea."

"Does Galya know all this?"

"No. I came here first. It is probably better that you tell her."

"She does not like airplanes. In fact, she hates airplanes more than hospitals."

"She will like this one. She will be going with you and will help you be cured."

"Then, when do we leave?"

"As the message says, sometime during the week of the 9th of April. The tentative date discussed with Cap Parlier and Susan Summers is the 11th of April."

"Two weeks."

"Yes. An American doctor will come to examine you and fly with you to America."

"I shall be ready."

"Good."

"Do you know when Galya will come back to see you?" asked Gourgen.

"No. She was here yesterday. I imagine later today or tomorrow . . . perhaps, not until later in the week."

"She needs to know. She must prepare herself and your things."

"If you see her before I do, you should tell her. Help her, Gourgen."

"I will. Now, you rest. You must save your strength."

Anatoly nodded and closed his eyes.

# 37

*10:15, Wednesday, 4.April.1990*
*All Union Center for Hematology*
*Moscow, Russia, USSR*

The late winter storm so typical of Mother Russia in the early spring blew with all its ferocity outside the thick windows. The feeble attempt to heat the interior along with the howl of the cold wind dampened the depressing odors of the hospital. Anatoly slept peacefully and deeply. Gourgen and Galina sat in the room without words or even glances. Anatoly's illness and the struggle with the Government to recognize the cause continued to irritate and corrode Galina's tolerance of the official denials.

"Is this really a good idea?" asked Galina as she stared off vacantly into the white smears of frost beyond the window.

Gourgen turned his head from the window to study her face and eyes. There was no response. "Yes, Galya. I believe this is the only way."

"But, he will have to go away to America. They might capture him . . . keep him there and not let him return."

Karapetyan laughed hard breaking her distant concentration. "Galya, their Government is no different from ours."

"That is precisely why I am worried," she snapped.

"But, it is not the governments that are doing this. It is his fellow pilots. I trust Cap Parlier. Nothing is going to happen to Anatoly."

"How can you be so sure?"

"You have read the messages. Those are not messages from officials. They are messages from the heart . . . from the heart of a friend . . . a brother. Plus, you are going with him. Nothing is going to interfere with this effort."

A small, delicate smile brightened her otherwise worried face. "So you have told us, but I still worry. The government has told us all our lives that the Americans are our enemy – an enemy of the State."

"That is just so, Galya. The government has told us. Anatoly Kovatchur and I have both talked to Cap Parlier for nearly two years now. We know him. We know what he is about. I would trust my life to him."

"Should I really go with him, Gourgen?"

Again, he laughed. "Why do you have doubts?"

"Perhaps I should stay for the boys if something was to go wrong."

"They are grown young men. They will be strong no matter what happens. Yes, Galya, you should go with him. I think it will be important for Anatoly."

"Yes. I know."

"Then, let there be no more doubts."

Galina looked into Gourgen's unblinking eyes as if to search for some hidden clue. "Agreed."

They returned to the window and the blowing snow. The arrival of the American doctor marked a tangible milestone on the journey, but played to Galina's fears. Gourgen considered what could be done to ease her worry. Nothing popped out at him.

Heavy, quick footsteps in the hall broadcast some movement. One of the older, more round nurses leaned into the room. "Comrade Karapetyan, they are coming," she announced with respect.

Gourgen nodded his head.

Galina Grishchenko started to stand, then returned to her chair when Gourgen motioned to her. They waited a few long minutes. She watched Gourgen who could only alternate between Anatoly and her. Numerous footfalls – a some heavy, some light, some hard, some soft – approached down the hallway. Gourgen motioned again for Galina to remain seated and set an example for looking nonchalant.

The squeak of the door hinge gave Gourgen the cue he needed.

Turning to the sound, Gourgen saw the smiling face of Doctor Vorobiev leading a small contingent of maybe a half dozen people he did not recognize.

The taller man with thick, nicely trimmed, black hair and a heavy black mustache had to be the American. A shorter, round woman with a kindly face and much younger, and wearing a white doctor's coat was probably one of Vorobiev's specialists, and perhaps the interpreter. Two other older male doctors plus a rather stern looking senior nurse stood purposely back by the door. One or more of those three had to be the Center's security chief and principal conduit to the KGB.

"May I introduce our distinguished guest," Doctor Vorobiev began. The round woman leaned toward the dark haired man and spoke in English — she was the interpreter. "This is Doctor Pat Beatty from the Fred Hutchinson Cancer Research Center in Seattle, Washington, USA."

Before he could continue, Gourgen asked, "Who are the others?"

Motioning toward the interpreter, Vorobiev answered, "This is Doctor Zhenya Margulis, one of our bright young hematologists at the Institute who will also serve as our interpreter." Pointing toward the three in the back, "This is Doctor Kamarotzov and Doctor Professor Legonov as well as Nurse Nargonova, our senior nurse at this institute. Doctor Beatty, this is Gourgen Karapetyan, a Hero of the Soviet Union and famous test pilot." Gourgen lowered his head and shook it in humility. "This is Galina Grishchenko, wife of Anatoly, our renowned patient."

Everyone shook hands including Galina although she was quite reluctant and shy in the presence of all the doctors.

"Doctor Beatty is here to examine Anatoly and his medical file."

A long, awkward pause stopped everything. No one moved as if it was a contest to see who would flinch first. The American finally took the first move.

"As Doctor Vorobiev said," he paused for Margulis's

translation to Russian, "I am here to examine Mister Grishchenko for possible treatment in America." Another pause. "We have the collaboration of Mister Karapetyan," he said nodding toward Gourgen, "and Mister Parlier in America." He watched Margulis as if his words might not make it through the process. "Hopefully, we will find a way to help Mister Grishchenko."

"Can you cure him?" asked Galina.

"It is difficult to say. We must do a thorough examination and study the facts in order to make that determination."

"Then, we should get on with it," Gourgen added with impatience and caused a fumbling moment.

"Yes," the American said in Russian.

Everyone smiled and chuckled a little to ease the tension of first meeting. Galina turned to her husband to awaken him. A startled expression filled his eyes as he fought with his recollection and lack of awareness that all these people had gathered around him. Gourgen quickly moved to the foot of the bed, smiled and gave his friend a thumps up signal that everything was as it should be.

Doctor Vorobiev stepped closer to the bed. "Anatoly, the American doctor is here to examine you as we discussed yesterday." Anatoly nodded his head in recognition. Vorobiev turned to Beatty motioning him forward, then turned back to Anatoly. "This is Doctor Beatty from Seattle in America."

Anatoly extended his right hand across his chest. Beatty shook the proffered hand.

"I shall leave you to your duty," the chief of the institute said. Only Nurse Nargonova followed the venerable medical leader.

Beatty removed his overcoat and began to quietly take command of the moment. He asked for, received and then told Anatoly what he was doing with each instrument. Gourgen and Galina moved back to the interior wall along with the other two 'doctors' as they watched the American. He listened for the longest time to his lungs and heart, then checked his eyes, ears, mouth, reflexes and other routine elements. He also asked for numerous blood samples to be drawn. The examination took perhaps 30 minutes.

"Thank you," the American said in Russian, then indicated he had what he needed. He also explained through Margulis that he wanted to see the results of the tests before he could make a determination.

Gourgen knew what that meant and decided to follow the American. He nodded to Galina to stay with Anatoly. As Beatty and Margulis left the room, the two observer 'doctors' fell in behind them. Gourgen followed the four physicians by a few steps. They walked down the hallway, up the stairs to the top floor and into Doctor Vorobiev's corner office. No one seemed to notice nor object to Gourgen's presence in the large office.

The new arrivals waited for Vorobiev to complete an official telephone call.

"What have you found?"

Beatty responded through Margulis's interpretation. "We need the blood work to be completed to be certain, but my principal concern at this point is the spot on his upper left lung. The X-ray films are . . . shall we say . . . difficult to read." The American's way of saying poor quality. "Has he had any exposure to tuberculosis?"

"None that we know of."

"The spot could be just an old scar from tuberculosis or something else, but it could also be an active aspergillus infection or some other lung contamination."

"If it is aspergillus, then he is inoperable," observed Vorobiev.

"Correct."

A stone cold silence filled the room with only the minute hum of the wall clock to confirm their unimpaired hearing. Gourgen knew what that meant.

"Why?" Gourgen asked.

The doctors turned to capture Karapetyan's eyes like an impertinent student. He waited. They looked at each other, then back to him. Gourgen motioned with his hands and shoulders to say, I am waiting for an answer.

"Aspergillus is a very common fungus spore that we breath in every day," answered Doctor Vorobiev. "Normally, our immune system eliminates the intrusion almost instantly. It is only when the immune system is suppressed or compromised that it can make a hold in the lungs. Once rooted, it is very difficult to deal with and particularly virulent."

"Meaning?"

"In patients with leukemia, like Anatoly, it is nearly always fatal."

Again, the silence.

"So, what do we do?" asked Gourgen.

The real doctors looked to each other wondering who would explain the situation. The not-so-real doctors looked blankly out the window not wanting to participate. Beatty eventually took the moment. He turned and walked to within a few steps of Gourgen. Margulis stayed at his right shoulder, so she could perform the translations. Beatty looked directly into Gourgen's eyes.

"As Doctor Vorobiev stated, aspergillus is a simple, common but virulent fungus that is very serious in patients with depleted immune systems."

"How do we know if he does have this fungus?"

"The only positive method is surgical. However, please let me caution you, we cannot confirm that it is aspergillus either, without surgery."

Gourgen gestured his so-what-is-next signal.

"We need high resolution X-ray imagery."

Gourgen looked to Doctor Vorobiev. "Where do we get this?"

"America."

"So, the longer we wait, the worse he gets." Beatty and Vorobiev nodded their heads in agreement. "Then, we must move him to America as soon as possible."

"Again, I must caution you, if this spot is an active aspergillus infection, the risk of failure is substantially higher . . . near 100%, to be honest."

"And, if you don't take him to America, the risk is 100%," Gourgen pronounced sharply.

Everyone in the room was now looking at Gourgen Karapetyan. He was a force to be reckoned with, and everyone knew it. He waited stone faced and determined for a response. Andrei Vorobiev was the first to move.

"Gourgen, this is a delicate matter."

"Yes, it is . . . very delicate for Anatoly."

"What I mean is, we must make a proper medical judgment. If he does not have some reasonable chance for success, Anatoly is probably better off remaining here with family and friends."

"To die," said Gourgen with indignation.

"If you wish to be blunt, yes, to die. I believe it is better for him to die at home than in a strange country."

"Then, you have given up on him."

"No. We are simply trying to weigh all the factors, some of which are a bit misty. He is a man of some importance, and . . . ."

"He deserves whatever chance we can find. He is a fighter. He knows how to deal with long odds. He has lived his life dealing with long odds."

"Then, you think he should go?" interjected Beatty.

"If he has no chance here, and some chance in America – yes – damn you all – I think he should go to America as soon as possible. The longer we stand here talking, the worse his chances are."

"Given that I still need to see the latest blood chemistry results, if the tests confirm his Myelodysplasia and Multiple Myeloma, or Chronic Myelogenous Leukemia, as well as his advanced stage, then his only possibility for a cure is a bone marrow transplant." Beatty turned to Vorobiev. "We have the confirmed and qualified donor – a 42 year old, mother of three in France – whom I might add, donates blood regularly and has donated one of her kidneys to one of her children."

"And, she is still qualified as a donor with only one kidney?" asked Vorobiev.

"Yes. The loss of a kidney does not disqualify her. We asked for a thorough examination to ensure we would not put her at risk. We are satisfied. She has consented to be the donor, so everything is ready."

"Then, let us get on with this," Gourgen demanded.

"Mister Karapetyan," answered Beatty, "I appreciate your involvement, energy and drive to help your friend, but as physicians, we are governed by an oath to help cure the infirm, but first do no harm."

"What are you trying to say?"

"I am here, representing my institution and my profession, to make a judgment on Mister Grishchenko's suitability for this procedure and the risks associated with his specific treatment."

"As you say."

"If Mister Grishchenko has an active aspergillus infection, it will most likely be fatal. We would simply hasten his expiration. As such, I would have to recommend that we not do this procedure."

"As you stated, there is a possibility this is not an aspergillus infection."

"Yes, correct."

"Can you do the surgery, now, to deal with this possibility?" asked Gourgen.

Doctor Vorobiev immediately held up his hand. "That would not be advisable."

"Why?"

"First, a surgery of that nature would be very traumatic to a patient in Comrade Grishchenko's condition. Second, without the high resolution imagery that Doctor Beatty recommended, we would be flying blind as you pilots like to say. Third, and this is just for this room," he paused to look at the two 'pretend' doctors, "for an infection of this nature, his best chances for survival are in America. They have the medicines and equipment to handle such a surgery."

Gourgen stared at Vorobiev. Without showing any sign externally, he admired the courage of the venerable physician. His defiance of the State with the two, probable, KGB agents in the room ranked as high as any combat heroism although the American could not possibly have recognized it. "Then, he must go to America as soon as possible."

"So, we don't miss the point," Beatty added waiting for everyone's attention, "part of the transplant process totally eliminates his immune system. It is a necessary part of the procedure. If the aspergillus infection is indeed active, it will spread rapidly with no immune reaction to counter it. I have told you the consequences."

"If a pilot in a spin does not continue to try actions – even some that might seem illogical – when his first attempts at recovery fail, the result is given. You are telling us," Gourgen said motioning with his hands to all the doctors, "this bone marrow transplant is his only chance for recovery. If so, then we will take the chance, as we all would."

"We will need to explain this to Mister and Missus Grishchenko. We have informed consent rules we must adhere to in this circumstance."

"You will have no problem there," answered Gourgen. "He will give you whatever consent you desire. Trust me."

"We need to gather the remaining elements of information. It should take a day or so depending upon when we get the laboratory results back."

The group concluded the meeting with a series of actions. Vorobiev would ensure the laboratory moved as quickly as possible to obtain the necessary information. Beatty took the appropriate information to make several calls back to the United States. The final decision regarding the possibility of a bone marrow transplant rested with the chief of the center Beatty represented, Doctor John Hansen, the man Cap Parlier referred to in his messages. Gourgen planned to communicate with Parlier, as well, to make the final arrangements assuming everyone would soon agree to the transplant.

# 38

*18:40, Tuesday, 10.April.1990*
*Building R5, Apartment 1*
*Zhukovsky, Russia, USSR*

Gourgen knocked on the door of the Grishchenko apartment. The dark, cold landing provided access to three other apartments on the first floor of the ten story building. There certainly was not much to look at other than the metal number, 1, on the door. The door opened bathing him in bright light. The adjustment for his eyes hurt and took several seconds. Galina waited patiently. When Gourgen opened his eyes sufficiently to see her and smile, she motioned for him to enter.

"You have news?" she asked before they could leave the entryway.

"Yes, Galya. I do have good news. A message from Cap Parlier was waiting for me when I arrived at work this morning. The arrangements have been completed. I have talked with the American nurse at the US Embassy in Moscow – Susan Summers – and, she has worked with Cap over the last few days to get Anatoly to Seattle. You leave tomorrow afternoon. You will fly on Pan American Airways from Moscow to New York. There you will change airplanes to Trans World Airlines for the flight to Seattle. A representative of the American government's Department of Energy will meet you in New York to make sure you and Anatoly are given special treatment through customs. It will be tomorrow evening when you arrive in Seattle, and it will be a very long flight. Cap said he will be there to greet you when you arrive."

"This is so sudden."

"Perhaps, Galya, but it is very important that we get Anatoly to Seattle as soon as possible. His health is not getting better, and the American doctors tell us they need to move quickly."

"Does Anatoly know?"

"Yes. I saw him this afternoon. I told him to rest comfortably, and I would help you pack things."

"Thank you, Gourgen."

"It is nothing."

"Are you still certain this is the correct thing to do?"

"Yes. Without a sliver of doubt."

"Then, we should pack."

The process took most of the night. Galina felt compelled to take several breaks to inform her sons of their journey. The telephone connection required numerous attempts to complete, but eventually satisfied her need as a mother. Gourgen also made several trips to the Mil Design Bureau in Moscow as well as the Gromov Flight Research Center in Zhukovsky to gather appropriate objects as gifts to their hosts and those who would help them. Friends also brought treats and gifts of their own to Galina as word spread within the aviation community. The men of the aviation city – engineers, pilots and mechanics – were universally enthusiastic about the opportunity of the journey, while the women had nearly the opposite view, an apprehension for what lay ahead, although they were all supportive in the end.

Galina tried to get a few hours sleep just before dawn. Gourgen slept on the living room sofa until Galina's busy work in the kitchen woke him. They had several hours before they needed to cross the city to the Hematology Center to pick up Anatoly. Several telephone calls confirmed that he was ready to travel. Galina's nervous uncertainty began to wear on Gourgen although he remained determined to offer her his strength and support.

Nearly a dozen neighbors gathered in front of the apartment building as they loaded their suitcases and boxes in Gourgen's 15 year old, but still functional automobile. Galina's anxiety turned to somber resolution during the one hour drive to pick up Anatoly. She would not speak despite several attempts by Gourgen to find a neutral topic. Her expression gradually turned to worry by the time they reached the Center.

Doctor Vorobiev and many of the medical staff that treated Anatoly greeted them upon their arrival. The latest medical information was sealed in a large envelope to be given to the medical staff in Seattle. Doctor Zhenya Margulis would accompany them to Seattle and remain with them. She would act as their interpreter as well as use the opportunity to learn as much as she could about bone marrow transplantation. Margulis would also have to carry the additional responsibility of translating Anatoly's medical records from Russian to English, and vice versa. She mumbled numerous times, more to herself than for others to hear, about the nearly impossible burden she would carry. Her principal hope was, someone on the medical staff in Seattle could speak and write Russian to relieve her burden just a little.

The doctors instructed Anatoly that he must wear and maintain the surgical mask to avoid unnecessary exposure while enroute. His significantly depressed immune system could not handle many common contagions. As all the doctors had told him, he needed to be in the best health possible. A bone marrow transplant was a difficult, arduous procedure that required considerable will, endurance and focus.

A small caravan of automobiles carried Anatoly, Galina and Zhenya Margulis along with their rather extensive luggage to Sheremetyevo Airport. Several friends also met them at the airport to say good-bye. No one said the words, but everyone knew this might be the last time they would see Anatoly alive. The pilots joked about Anatoly running off to America for a vacation. The women tried to put on a brave face, but Galina's somber mood affected them. This journey was serious. They knew it, and there was some resentment of the rather cavalier attitude of the pilots.

The public address system announced the boarding of Pan American Airways flight to New York. As if on cue, the mood of the pilots changed. Everyone said their farewells. Gourgen waited to the last.

"You be careful, my friend."

"I will, Gourgen. I will see you in a few months when I have beaten this thing."

"Yes, you will."

The surgical mask did not interfere with their embrace of friendship and mutual respect.

"Thank you for making all these arrangements. I would not have this opportunity if it had not been for your efforts."

"Nonsense. It was nothing."

"No, Gourgen. It was life. I had no chance, and now you have given me a chance. I will get out of this as I have all the other times."

"Yes, you will, my friend. Yes, you will."

"Tolya," called Galina. "We must go, or we shall surely miss our flight."

"She is correct, Tolya. Safe journey."

The two veteran test pilots embraced again.

"I will see you in a few months."

"Yes, you will. I am counting on it."

Anatoly nodded his head, then turned to join his wife as they passed through the control point. Gourgen watched his friend disappear behind the partitions that separated the passengers from all others and led them to the boarding gates. Most of the well-wishers waited the nearly 45 minutes necessary to watch the large, blue and white, Boeing 747 leave the runway in graceful flight. When the aircraft disappeared into the overcast, several people left in silence.

Within a few minutes, only Gourgen Karapetyan and Anatoly Kovatchur remained. "Do you think he is going to come back to us cured, Gourgen?"

"It is difficult to say. I truly hope so. He has put up a valiant fight against this radiation induced blood disease."

"A shame such a good pilot must be sacrificed in this way."

"For Mother Russia."

"He is Ukrainian."

They laughed. "Yes, just as I am Armenian, but still it is Mother

Russia."

"As you say, but still a shame."

"Indeed."

Both pilots stood staring out the large window at the activity around the airport. Airplanes being loaded, moving, taking off and landing always attracted the attention of those who loved to fly. They both knew Anatoly Grishchenko was one of them – a man who loved to fly. They wanted their friend, neighbor and fellow aviator to come home cured and with a broad smile on his face.

"I had better return to Zhukovsky," said Kovatchur finally.

Gourgen nodded his head. "I shall go to Mil. I need to send a message to Cap Parlier. He is probably already in Seattle, but just in case, I should let him know Anatoly is on the way."

"Then, perhaps I shall see you tonight."

"I will let you know if there is any news."

"Thank you, my friend."

The two pilots separated. Gourgen proceeded directly to the Mil Design Bureau office building on the northside of Moscow. He updated those that were interested and found his favorite engineer to craft a quick message to his American counterpart.

Gourgen felt good about the situation, but also felt a certain nervousness. He concluded it had to be that he was no longer in control of events, that control passed to Cap Parlier and the doctors in Seattle. He had to trust them, that they would do everything he would do and more to help his life long friend.

"He has departed?" came the familiar voice of Vineberg, the deputy chief designer and his friend.

"Yes, Mark. He took off an hour ago with Galina and the doctor-interpreter. They are scheduled to arrive in Seattle, USA, about nine o'clock tomorrow morning, our time."

"I hear the Americans have perfected this bone marrow transplant procedure."

"So, I hear as well," answered Gourgen, not really thinking about the words.

"They shall take good care of him."

"As long as it not too late," he mumbled.

"What was that?"

"I am concerned that we may be too late for Anatoly."

"Why?"

"The doctors tell me he might have some kind of an infection that could make any treatment fatal."

The news produced a long pause as Vineberg considered the information. "So, you are telling me, he might not have any path out of the hole?"

"Correct."

Both men looked out the senior engineer's window across the roofs of the suburban buildings. Neither man shared his thoughts. Vineberg was the first to break the silence.

"Are you going to be able to fly the systems flight tomorrow on the Model Two Eight?"

Gourgen turned his head back to his friend. He stared at him as if he could not believe the question. Vineberg could only return his gaze not knowing quite what to say.

"Yes, I suppose," he answered, wanting to fly the test but not quite sure his mind would be completely on the flight.

"Excellent. We shall complete the final modifications tonight. The aircraft should be ready for test at about mid-morning."

"Then, I shall be there."

Gourgen stood, nodded to his friend and left his office. The lack of sleep the previous night and the tension of the quietly perceived finality of Anatoly's departure convinced him he needed an early night for a good long sleep. Flight test with a fatigue-clouded brain was never a good idea no matter how simple the flight might be planned. He could only manage a few smiles, gestures or retreating comments to colleagues asking about Anatoly. His patience with repetitive answers regardless of how well intentioned the questions, had worn thin with his fatigue.

His absent-minded drive to Zhukovsky caused several honks of protestation from other drivers as they avoided his complacent driving. He confided in Ludmilla although he knew she would not like what she heard. He felt compelled to share his concerns with someone. She handled the information with maturity and patience. Ludmilla also did what a good partner does in times of trouble, she fed him, made sure he took a long hot bath, then put him in bed at a very early hour to get a good night's sleep. The final release of self-imposed tension over the last few days brought a profound, deep and mind-numbing fatigue that claimed the last of his consciousness.

As he was so many times in his adult life, he was thankful for her care and concern for him. Whether many people knew or would admit it, Ludmilla had either directly or indirectly saved his life many times. This was yet another simple moment between two people who loved each other, protected each other and went the extra distance to help.

# 39

*14:30, Friday, 13.April.1990*
*Mil Flight Test Facility*
*30 kilometers north of Zhukovsky, Russia, USSR*

"What exactly do you expect to find with this test?" asked Gourgen Karapetyan.

The flight test engineers looked at one another, frustrated that they could not get their message through to Gourgen. The chief test pilot stared at them, willing to wait until they formulated a proper answer.

"What do you want us to say?"

"I want to you tell me why we are flying this flight? We have done these tests – I do not know how many times – and nothing has changed. Tell me what have you changed? What will I see that is different?"

"Let me see if I can explain this in a different way," said the engineer down from the design office. Gourgen turned his glare to the young man. He swallowed hard. "We have added some additional circuitry to the stabilization box. The new card should remove the last of the rotor and transmission vibration frequencies from the optical sight servo drive motors. Our calculations tell us you should gain several thousand meters of adequate optical resolution. You should be able to see the three stripes of the one meter target at nearly four point five kilometers."

"You are new out here, young man, so I shall be gentle. That is what the half dozen predecessors of yours have said as well. So, why should I waste my time?"

"Because we want you to check the sight performance," the chief flight test engineer stated.

"Not good enough," Gourgen barked, rose from the table and walked out of the room.

Gourgen Karapetyan left the building, walking several meters into the grass beyond the walkway. He turned toward the sun, closed his eyes and faced the warmth. The noise of the traffic on the main highway beyond the far treeline contaminated the chorus of birds singing in the morning air, a welcome respite from the odd storm the previous few days. He heard footsteps behind him, but he chose to ignore them. There was no movement for several minutes.

"What is wrong?" asked the chief flight test engineer.

"You know what is wrong."

"I have not seen you like this in quite some time. It is a simple test. Why are you chewing our heads off over a simple test."

"These damn optical tests are boring. I sit in a hover for hours, poking this and twisting that, and all we get is the same thing. At this pace, we will never get the machine ready for the Government tests. I want to see something change."

"The engineers are doing the best they can."

"It does not match the American Apache!"

"Gourgen, that is not fair. We do not have the computers and electronics the Americans do, and you know that perfectly well. So, you can dispense with that garbage."

"The specification states a five kilometer stable spot. We barely manage three kilometers. What am I supposed to think."

"It will not hurt you to evaluate the changes the design engineers have made."

"Perhaps." Gourgen returned his face to the sun, again.

There were several minutes of nature, and no words.

"Gourgen," shouted someone from the flight test building. Gourgen turned to see the voice. "Anatoly Grishchenko is on the telephone from America."

Gourgen ran to the building, through the door and into one of the small offices. "Hello."

"Gourgen, this is Anatoly."

"So, you made it there safely."

"Yes. The journey was long, but no problems other than one of our bags did not make it here. Most of our gifts were in that bag, but they are looking for it."

"Did you see Cap Parlier?"

"Yes. He was at the airport when we arrived in Seattle. I like him. I know why you asked him to help, and why you trust him. He is a good man."

"What is Seattle like?"

"A gorgeous city, a fantastic green city. Magnificent mountains with the forest all around and water everywhere. I am not sure if this is a lake or the sea, but it is beautiful nonetheless."

"What are they going to do with you?"

"They have many tests to perform in preparation for the transplant. I can tell they worry about this possible infection, but they will sort it out. These doctors are very professional. The people are very friendly."

"Is Parlier there now?"

"Yes. He is with Doctor Hansen. They are making the final plans for my treatment."

"Good."

"They tell me they want to fly me to a special government facility to do something they refer to as a full body scan. Apparently, they have sensitive instruments that can detect radiation in my body. They want to know how much damage was done at Chernobyl, and they say they need these measurements to define the proper preparatory actions."

"Too much, my friend, too much."

"Part of the transplant procedure involves more radiation to destroy the last of my damaged bone marrow, so the new marrow will have the best chance for success. They need to calculate the precise dosage for the procedure without doing more damage to other organs."

"More radiation!"

"Yes, but this is good."

"I hope so."

"I must tell you the Western press is going crazy. The hospital is keeping most of them away. They are very interested in what we did at Chernobyl. Galya says it is like we are some movie stars or something."

"So, they know what we did?"

"I have not discussed any details, but they seem to know quite a lot already."

"Good. The world should know what happened at that place."

"Galya is telling me I must hang up. Say hello to all our friends, and tell them I am doing fine. I feel good about this, Gourgen. I feel real good about this."

"Excellent. Is there anything else you need me to do for you?"

"Perhaps, a shipment of some gifts. These people are very nice to us. They deserve something from the Motherland to remember us by."

"I will see what I can do."

"As always, my friend."

"Do your best, Anatoly Demjanovich."

"I shall, Gourgen. I intend to get through this in good order and return home so we can go flying. You must take care of yourself."

"Good-bye."

Gourgen hung up the telephone and stared out the window. The building haze of spring did not lessen his sense of well being and the brightness he felt. The apprehension surrounding the decision to send Anatoly to the United States dissipated with the words spanning the globe. Today was a better day.

The Mil chief test pilot returned to the briefing room. The various people in the room stopped their conversation as Gourgen entered, as if he had called them to attention.

"Today is a good day. Let's go fly," he pronounced.

The engineers glanced at each other, then back to Gourgen. They did not want to question the change in mood. Gourgen grabbed his flight equipment bag and walked out the opposite side of the building toward the poised flight test machine.

Several weeks passed with no word from the United States.

Gourgen thirsted for information about his friend, but he also knew the preparations for the transplant had to consume considerable time. He also knew that Cap Parlier was deeply involved in the preparations as well as trying to do his own work. The fact that the American had to fly back and forth between Phoenix and Seattle, a thousand miles, added even more weight to his commitment. Patience was sometimes a scarce commodity, but he did not want to be a burden. Anatoly's fate now lay solely in the hands of the American doctors. Not even Cap Parlier would be able to do much for Anatoly until he came out the other side of the operation.

The scheduled day of Anatoly's transplant came and went, again without any information from the United States. Gourgen considered trying to call Galina in Seattle or maybe send a message to Cap Parlier, but in the end, he decided to find some more patience.

Early one morning, as he was preparing for a long test flight, a courier from Moscow arrived. He handed Gourgen a single sheet of flimsy facsimile paper.

---

## McDONNELL DOUGLAS HELICOPTER COMPANY
## FACSIMILE TRANSMISSION

**Date:** 4.May.1990
**From:** Cap Parlier
**To:** Gourgen Karapetyan
**Subject:** Anatoly Grishchenko

DEAR GOURGEN,

WE CONTINUE TO HAVE GOOD NEWS. ANATOLY HAD HIS BONE MARROW TRANSPLANT AS PLANNED ON THE EVENING OF 27.APRIL.1990. THE DOCTORS ARE QUITE PLEASED WITH THE IMMEDIATE RESULTS OF THE TRANSPLANT. YOU WILL BE INTERESTED TO KNOW THAT I HAD ARRANGED FOR A SWISS HELICOPTER PILOT TO FLY THE NEW MARROW FROM THE DONOR IN BESANCON, FRANCE TO GENEVA, SWITZERLAND. HE DID A VERY GOOD JOB. THE COURIER HAND CARRIED ANATOLY'S NEW MARROW THROUGH LONDON AND ARRIVED IN SEATTLE THE SAME DAY.

I HAD THE GOOD FORTUNE TO BE IN SEATTLE ON
1.MAY.1990.   I WAS ABLE TO SPEND 2 OR 3 HOURS
WITH ANATOLY.  HE IS EXPERIENCING SOME OF THE
EXPECTED SIDE EFFECTS OF THE TREATMENT.  HE
LOOKS GOOD, AND IS IN VERY GOOD SPIRITS.  HE
CONTINUES TO SURPRISE THE DOCTORS WITH HIS
POSITIVE ATTITUDE AND WILL TO SURVIVE.  ANATOLY
IS PERFORMING AS ANY GOOD TEST PILOT WOULD.  I
HAVE TOLD THE DOCTORS THAT HE WILL CONTINUE TO
SURPRISE THEM.  I ALSO TALKED TO ANATOLY TODAY.
HE CONTINUES TO MAKE GOOD PROGRESS.

DOCTOR MARGULIS IS PERFORMING HER DUTIES
EXCEPTIONALLY WELL.  SHE HAS ASKED THAT ANOTHER
INTERPRETER BE SENT TO SEATTLE AS SOON AS
POSSIBLE SO THAT SHE CAN DEVOTE MORE TIME TO HER
MEDICAL STUDIES WHILE SHE IS IN SEATTLE.  SHE
WOULD SHARE THE INTERPRETER DUTIES AS REQUIRED.
PLEASE ADVISE ME AS SOON AS YOU CAN ABOUT THESE
ARRANGEMENTS.

ANATOLY HAS ASKED ME TO HELP ARRANGE A VISIT
BY HIS YOUNGER SON, NICHOLAS ANATOLYEVICH
GRISHCHENKO, AND A COLLEAGUE & FRIEND, VLADIMIR
SEMENOV.  I NEED TO HAVE THEIR BIRTHDATES,
BIRTHPLACES, AND PASSPORT NUMBERS.  THE
INFORMATION PROVIDED BY ANATOLY & GALINA IS:
NICHOLAS BORN: 11.JULY.1972  PLACE:
ZHUKOVSKY, USSR.
SEMENOV BORN: 30.APRIL.1937     PLACE:   ?
I WILL FORWARD THE INFORMATION TO THE US
STATE DEPARTMENT AS SOON AS I RECEIVE IT.  HOW
WILL THEY TRAVEL TO SEATTLE?

WE ARE MAKING GOOD PROGRESS.  WE WILL KEEP
YOU INFORMED.  DOCTOR BEATTY WOULD LIKE TO KNOW
THE NAME AND TELEX OR FAX NUMBER FOR ANATOLY'S
PHYSICIAN IN MOSCOW SO THAT THE HUTCHINSON
CENTER CAN SEND MEDICAL UPDATES ON HIS PROGRESS
DIRECTLY TO HIM.  TAKE CARE, MY BROTHER.
WITH GREAT RESPECT,
CAP PARLIER

Gourgen took a deep breath of relief. "Thank you," he said to the courier who turned and departed.

The 4th of May, a week after his transplant procedure, everything is going perfectly. Anatoly is asking for his youngest son and one of his colleagues from Gromov. The signs are so good. He now had things he could do to help his friend, to feel a part of the effort to save a life.

Gourgen jumped into the task with vigor. He tracked down both of the Grishchenko's sons to tell them the good news. He had to make a special visit to the Ministry of Defense, using several specific contacts, to make arrangements for their youngest son, Nicholas, to be temporarily released from his military schooling for a journey to America.

Friends offered their assistance. Gourgen heard through some contacts at *Pravda* as well as *New Times*, the Soviet English news journal, about the reports in the Western press. The French seemed to be in a near frenzy trying to find any little tidbit of information that might enlighten their readers on events unfolding in a special hospital in Seattle, Washington, USA. The connection of the French people to these events through the extracted bone marrow of an anonymous French woman in Besançon made the global flavor of this valiant endeavor all the more poignant. It made Gourgen feel as if they were finally gaining the attention of the rest of the world about what had happened four years earlier in Northern Ukraine. The pilots would not go silently into the night.

The leaders of the Mil Design Bureau as well as the aviation community as a whole maintained a constant vigil. Gourgen used several full days to work the various tasks that needed to be done. He spent a significant amount of time answering questions for those who remained concerned. Information from America did not come as often as he wanted, but there were many sources to tap into for signs of progress.

Near the middle of May, Gourgen happened to be at the Mil

offices when a call from Anatoly came. He nearly knocked several people down as he ran to his office.

"How are you doing, Anatoly Demjanovich?"

"I feel like we just flew over that damnable reactor."

"That bad."

"Yes, but the doctors say this is normal, and I am making good progress."

"What do you need?"

"I just wanted to hear your voice. I miss home. I am too weak to want to talk, so I will ask Galya to talk to you."

"Get better, my friend."

"Yes. Here is Galya."

Gourgen waited as he listened to Russian and English in the background although the words were just beyond comprehensible. The loud bangs as the telephone handset was passed and bounced a few times on a desk or the floor marked the change in speaker. He could not imagine why it was so difficult to carry out such a simple task as passing the telephone.

"Gourgen?" came Galina's tentative and somewhat shaky voice.

"Yes, Galya. I am here."

She started sobbing softly, obviously trying to suppress her tears. It was the most emotional Gourgen had heard Anatoly's wife in many years. The pressure and tension of the Anatoly's treatment for what Galina was convinced was his exposure to radiation was taking its toll on her. He waited a little longer for her to gain control.

"Tolya is very sick," she choked out.

"Yes, I know, Galya. Unfortunately, it is the hardship of this medical procedure, but once he builds himself back up, he will be cured. The last message I received from Cap Parlier sounded very positive."

"I know what they tell me, but I also know my Tolya. He is in pain. He is always sick to his stomach, all his joints hurt him making any movement more painful, and he is so weak."

"It is as the doctors described, Galya."

"Yes, yes, but he wants Nicholas. I need Nicholas. I am so alone here."

"I will do what I can to speed things along, Galya."

"Thank you, Gourgen. It is so good to hear your voice. We miss all our friends back home."

"We miss you as well. Take care of Anatoly. If there are any problems, please call Cap Parlier. He will support you as I would. You can trust him."

"I know, but I just want to go home with Tolya."

"In time, Galya, in time. Help him fight through this. He will make it."

"Thank you," she choked back a sob. "Thank you."

"We will do our best to make everything all right."

"Thank you, Gourgen. It was good to talk to you."

As he had done so many times over the past few weeks, he hung up the telephone handset and stared out the window, any available window. Gourgen tried as hard as he could to image the hardships Anatoly and Galina were experiencing. He felt oddly impotent as if he was watching Anatoly Kovatchur's horrible accident at the 1989 Paris Airshow . . . there was little he could do.

Gourgen set himself upon the tasks to complete his unfinished business. He needed to send a summary fax to Parlier about the arrangements for the second interpreter, actually an additional physician from the All Union Center for Hematology. He also needed to ask some questions. Too many unknowns still crept into conversations both casual and official. Parlier could get more direct answers from the doctors in Seattle.

The fax was drafted and sent. Gourgen returned to his duties. The delayed response did not particularly concern him. After all, Cap Parlier was a busy person as well.

Two days later, the message from his counterpart sat squarely on his chair, so he would not miss it.

## McDONNELL DOUGLAS HELICOPTER COMPANY
### FACSIMILE TRANSMISSION

**Date:** 17.May.1990
**From:** Cap Parlier
**To:** Gourgen Karapetyan
**Subject:** Anatoly Grishchenko

DEAR GOURGEN,

I RECEIVED YOUR FAX OF 15.MAY.90. I WAS OUT
OF TOWN FOR TWO DAYS.

THANK YOU FOR YOUR EFFORTS ON THE SECOND
INTERPRETER. THE SECOND INTERPRETER WILL HELP A
GREAT DEAL.

MEDICAL UPDATES ARE BEING SENT TO THE ALL
UNION CENTER FOR HEMATOLOGY BY DOCTOR ZHENYA
MARGULIS FROM SEATTLE. DOCTOR HANSEN INDICATES
THAT THE MESSAGES ARE GOING TO DOCTOR SAVCHENKO.

ANATOLY IS DOING FAIRLY WELL CONSIDERING HIS
TIME IN RECOVERY. AS OF THIS MORNING, HE STILL
HAS NOT SHOWN ANY WHITE CELLS IN HIS BLOOD.
THERE ARE SOME SIGNS THAT HIS CONDITION MAY BE
IMPROVING THOUGH. THERE IS STILL A VERY SERIOUS
CONCERN ABOUT AN INFECTION FOUND IN HIS LUNGS
PRIOR TO THE TRANSPLANT. THE INFECTION IS
BELIEVED TO BE CAUSED BY A FUNGUS OF SOME TYPE.
THE DOCTORS HAVE BEEN WATCHING IT VERY
CAREFULLY. IT WAS STABLE FOR A TIME AND
UNFORTUNATELY IS GROWING NOW. THE DOCTORS ARE
BALANCING ANATOLY'S PROGRESS IN HIS TRANSPLANT
RECOVERY WITH THE NEED TO TREAT THE INFECTION.
HE MAY REQUIRE AN OPERATION AS EARLY AS TOMORROW
NIGHT (18.5.90) TO EXCISE THE INFECTED AREA. IT
IS IMPORTANT TO NOTE THAT THIS IS A VERY SERIOUS
OPERATION FOR ANATOLY SINCE HE DOES NOT HAVE ANY
WHITE BLOOD CELLS YET. DOCTOR HANSEN TOLD ME
THIS MORNING THAT ANATOLY IS FEELING BETTER
DESPITE THE INFECTION; THAT IS A GOOD SIGN.

I WOULD ADVISE THAT NICHOLAS GRISHCHENKO AND
VLADIMIR SEMENOV SHOULD APPLY FOR VISAS AT THE

US EMBASSY IN MOSCOW AS SOON AS POSSIBLE TO
ALLOW FOR PROCESSING TIME.  THIS SHOULD BE DONE
EVEN THOUGH THERE IS NO TRAVEL DATE OR
TRANSPORTATION ESTABLISHED.
    I AM TRYING TO GO UP TO SEATTLE TO SEE
ANATOLY VERY SOON.  I AM WORKING WITH DOCTOR
HANSEN ON THE BEST TIME TO GO UP THERE SO THAT I
CAN BE THE MOST HELP TO ANATOLY.
    ARE YOU GOING TO FARNBOROUGH IN SEPTEMBER?
I AM NOT SURE IF I WILL BE ABLE TO GO BUT I HOPE
SO.  IT WOULD BE NICE TO SEE YOU AGAIN.
    MY BEST REGARDS TO EVERYONE.  WE REMAIN
HOPEFUL THAT WE WILL SEND ANATOLY HOME TO HIS
FRIENDS IN GOOD HEALTH.
WITH GREAT RESPECT,
CAP PARLIER

---

The message clearly said Anatoly was doing fairly well considering . . . considering was a relative term. The positive aspect was he was doing well, period. The troubling part was the reference to the lung infection.

The meeting in Andrei Vorobiev's office came back to him. If the doctors were worried about a lung infection, then Doctor Beatty's concern and apprehension were coming to fruition. Gourgen also reminded himself what Doctor Vorobiev stated, the best place for his treatment, if it was an aspergillus infection, was in America. Again, he just had to trust that the Americans would do the best they could to save Anatoly's life.

Gourgen turned his attention to his flying. When he was not flying, he was making the arrangements for Nicholas to visit his parents in Seattle. He would also tell everyone that asked, Anatoly was doing as well as could be expected. His progress was good, as Parlier reported.

Based on the estimates provided by Parlier and confirmed by Beatty, Anatoly still had several months of recovery to complete in Seattle before he could return home. This was indeed a long journey. Gourgen wanted it to be over as much as Anatoly and Galina, although probably for different reasons.

# 40

*09:30, Monday, 25.June.1990*
*Mil Design Bureau*
*2 Sokolnichesky Street*
*Moscow, Russia, USSR*

Gourgen tried to listen. The skilled and experienced engineers presented the facts associated with a particular observed phenomenon he had detected in the Mi-28 helicopter. He wanted to participate, to contribute to the discussion, but his mind kept shifting to his friend, now critically ill and fighting for his very life. Gourgen wanted to be in Seattle to help Anatoly, to make sure his friend was receiving the very best attention and care possible. There was no doubt that Cap Parlier was doing the best he could and probably as good as Gourgen himself could do, but the concern remained.

The meeting adjourned with Gourgen still sitting in his chair staring out the window. The green leaves of the summer foliage did not register. He had never been to Seattle or any other city in the United States, and he probably would never actually see it, but Anatoly's description of the elegant city with all the water, mountains and evergreen forest seemed almost idyllic. A hand touched his shoulder.

Gourgen looked up in the direction of the hand to see Mark Vineberg's worried expression.

"It is Anatoly Demjanovich, isn't it?"

"Yes."

"What is his condition?"

"The last message, that I received this morning from Parlier, says he is critical but stable condition, whatever that means."

"It means he is in danger but not declining," answered Vineberg as if Gourgen really did not know what the medical term meant.

The senior engineer sat down next to Gourgen. "There is nothing we can do for him, now. He is in the hands of the American doctors, and from everything I have heard, he is probably getting the best medical care available."

Gourgen could only nod his head in response.

"What did this morning's message say?" asked Vineberg.

Without answering, Gourgen rose and walked in his contemplative daze to the office down the hall used by the pilots when they were in the city. He pulled the lowest drawer of a four-drawer file cabinet out. His fingers walked through the files until he found the correct one.

Gourgen pulled the file marked, ANATOLY. He opened it to find the message he wanted near the top of the rapidly growing accumulation of papers. "You should really read the previous two messages to understand the last," Gourgen said, then handed the single piece of paper to Mark.

---

## McDONNELL DOUGLAS HELICOPTER COMPANY
### FACSIMILE TRANSMISSION

**Date:**          12.June.1990
**From:**          Cap Parlier
**To:**            Gourgen Karapetyan
**Subject:**       Anatoly Grishchenko

DEAR GOURGEN,

ANATOLY IS MAKING GOOD PROGRESS ON HIS RECOVERY FROM THE BONE MARROW TRANSPLANT. HIS BLOOD COUNTS CONTINUE TO RISE. THE DETAIL MEDICAL DATA ARE BEING PROVIDED TO THE ALL UNION HEMATOLOGY CENTER.

I MUST INFORM YOU THAT THE DOCTORS ARE STILL CONCERNED ABOUT THE INFECTION IN HIS LEFT LUNG. THEY HAVE SCHEDULED ANATOLY FOR A SURGICAL OPERATION AT 15:30 12.6.90 TO REMOVE THE INFECTION. THE INFECTION MUST BE REMOVED TO AID HIS RECOVERY. I WILL SEND A MESSAGE TO YOU AFTER THE OPERATION.

I TALKED TO ANATOLY LAST NIGHT. HE IS IN

```
VERY GOOD SPIRITS AND IS READY FOR THE
OPERATION.  IT IS ALWAYS A PLEASURE TO TALK TO
MY BROTHER.  I TRY TO TALK TO HIM ON A REGULAR
BASIS.  THERE ARE SO MANY PEOPLE WHO CONVEY
THEIR BEST WISHES AND PRAYERS FOR ANATOLY'S
RECOVERY.
     MY BEST WISHES TO YOU AND ALL MY FRIENDS IN
THE SOVIET UNION.  TAKE CARE MY FRIEND.
WITH GREAT RESPECT,
CAP PARLIER
```

Vineberg handed the paper back to Gourgen. "What is this infection the message refers to?"

"When the American doctor was here to examine Anatoly, he said there may have been signs of an infection by some kind of mold stuff . . . he called it aspergillus, I think . . . that might have already been in his lungs."

"It sounds serious, if they must perform surgery to remove this infection."

"It is very serious, Mark . . . very serious," answered Gourgen as he stared out the small window at nothing.

"The good thing is, Parlier has talked to Anatoly, and as he says, Anatoly is in good spirits.  So, perhaps this is not as bad as you think."

Gourgen turned to look his colleague in the eyes.  "The American doctor told us before Anatoly left, that if the spot he saw on X-ray film was aspergillus, it would most likely be fatal in his weakened condition from the illness."

"Most likely, not absolutely."

Gourgen sneered at his friend, then turned his gaze outside again.  "A technicality."

Furrows creased Gourgen's brow. He tried to picture his friend in an American hospital room.  It must have been very hard for him, and yet having Galina with him must have made it a little easier.

That damn infection!  Gourgen tried to remember each word

exactly as they were spoken during the meeting in Vorobiev's office prior to Anatoly's departure. Had he pushed too hard? Had he compromised his friend's chances for survival? How much longer would he have lived without the bone marrow transplant? The questions plagued Gourgen.

"I may have forced this procedure to happen," whispered Gourgen, partially to himself, and perhaps a little for atonement in the presence of a friend.

"Nonsense," growled Mark. "You are not a medical doctor. The doctors make the decisions on medical treatment, not you." Gourgen waved his hand as if to shoo an annoying fly, Mark continued. "You did not do this, Gourgen. You did not damage that reactor. You did not force Anatoly to fly those missions with you. You did not send him to America."

"But, I did push, and push hard."

"To get him the treatment he needed."

"Perhaps, too late," Gourgen said softly.

"That is not what the message indicated."

Gourgen turned back to the desk and the ANATOLY file. He picked up the next message.

---

**McDONNELL DOUGLAS HELICOPTER COMPANY**
**FACSIMILE TRANSMISSION**

**Date:** 22.June.1990
**From:** Cap Parlier
**To:** Gourgen Karapetyan
**Subject:** Anatoly Grishchenko

DEAR GOURGEN,

ANATOLY IS STILL LISTED IN CRITICAL BUT STABLE CONDITION. HE IS STILL MAKING SLOW PROGRESS. HE REMAINS ON THE RESPIRATOR. THE DOCTORS FEEL THAT WITH CONTINUED PROGRESS HIS RECOVERY FROM THIS CRISIS WILL PROBABLY TAKE SEVERAL WEEKS. THE DIFFICULTY WITH HIS PRESENT SITUATION IS THAT IT CAN CHANGE QUICKLY. THE MEDICAL STAFF AT THE HUTCHINSON CENTER CONTINUE

```
TO PROVIDE 24 HOUR CARE AND ARE GIVING ANATOLY
THE BEST TREATMENT POSSIBLE.  DETAILED MEDICAL
UPDATES ARE BEING SENT TO DOCTORS VOROBIEV AND
SAVCHENKO AT THE ALL UNION CENTER FOR
HEMATOLOGY.
   HE IS A STRONG MAN WITH A RARE WILL TO
SURVIVE.  I REMAIN CONFIDENT THAT HE WILL MAKE
IT THROUGH THIS CRISIS EVEN IF THE DOCTORS ARE
MORE CONSERVATIVE WITH THEIR PROGNOSIS.  ANATOLY
CONTINUES TO NEED ALL THE PRAYERS AND BEST
WISHES WE CAN GIVE HIM.
   TAKE CARE, MY FRIEND.  MY BROTHER, ANATOLY,
IS IN GOOD HANDS.  YOU MUST TAKE CARE OF YOUR
HEALTH AS WELL.
WITH GREAT RESPECT,
CAP PARLIER
```

"Gourgen, it still does not say he is in trouble. It says," Mark paused to reread the desire portion of the message, "making progress."

"Slow . . . progress."

"Nonetheless, progress means improvement. Anatoly Demjanovich is also getting constant medical care, and Galina is with him. He is not alone in some buried clinic in Moscow."

"True enough."

"Parlier also recognizes what we all know. He is a fighter."

"Yes, he is a fighter," Gourgen said aloud to the window.

# 41

*08:00, Monday, 2.July.1990*
*Mil Design Bureau*
*2 Sokolnichesky Street*
*Moscow, Russia, USSR*

Gourgen instinctively knew he had to be in Moscow first thing Monday morning. The last message from Parlier said, Anatoly's medical condition could change quickly, either way. The building was slow to get started on the summer morning. Gourgen recognized the guards at the entrance and greeted various people he knew as he ascended the stairs to the fourth floor and walked down the long hallway toward the General Designer's office.

General Designer Tishchenko's assistant was already at her desk.

"Good morning, Svetlana."

"Good morning to you, Gourgen. Another message arrived over the weekend," she said, as she stood and went to the file tray next to the international fax machine. She found the paper and handed it to Gourgen.

---

### McDONNELL DOUGLAS HELICOPTER COMPANY
### FACSIMILE TRANSMISSION

**Date:**      29.June.1990
**From:**      Cap Parlier
**To:**        Gourgen Karapetyan
**Subject:**   Medical Condition of Anatoly
               Grishchenko

DEAR GOURGEN,

ANATOLY REMAINS IN CRITICAL BUT STABLE CONDITION.  HE HAS A FEW GOOD DAYS AND A FEW BAD DAYS.  I TOLD THE DOCTORS AT THE HUTCHINSON CENTER YOUR MESSAGE.  I ALSO AGREE THAT THE

MEDICAL TEAM IS DOING EVERYTHING HUMANLY
POSSIBLE. ANATOLY IS STILL FIGHTING HARD. IT
IS IMPORTANT THAT ALL OF US REMAIN POSITIVE IN
ORDER TO HELP ANATOLY THE MOST. HE NEEDS ALL
THE HELP WE CAN GIVE HIM.
I TALKED TO ADMIRAL ZUMWALT YESTERDAY. HE
AND HIS FAMILY ARE LOOKING FORWARD TO THEIR TRIP
TO THE SOVIET UNION. I UNDERSTAND YOU ARE
HELPING THEM. THE ADMIRAL ASKED ME TO PASS THE
ADDRESS WHERE THEY WILL STAY IN MOSCOW. THE
ZUMWALTS WILL BE WITH:
      SVETLANA LEVNOKOVA
      MARCHLEVSKOHO 50
      APARTMENT NUMBER 213
      MOSCOW 101000 USSR
      THEY WILL BE IN MOSCOW FROM 12 TO
16.JULY.1990. THE ADMIRAL HAS BEEN FOLLOWING
ALL THE EVENTS SURROUNDING ANATOLY'S TREATMENT.
AS I TOLD YOU EARLIER, HE IS CHAIRMAN OF THE
NATIONAL MARROW DONOR PROGRAM HERE IN THE UNITED
STATES, AND THE FORMER CHIEF OF NAVAL
OPERATIONS, THE MOST SENIOR POSITION IN THE US
NAVY. HE WOULD VERY MUCH LIKE TO MEET YOU IN
MOSCOW.
WE MUST KEEP THE FAITH MY FRIEND. ANATOLY
HAS MORE FIGHT IN HIM. I KNOW HE IS WORKING
HARD. ALL OF THOSE AROUND HIM MUST BE THE MOST
POSITIVE FOR HIM. PLEASE TAKE CARE OF YOURSELF,
GOURGEN. MY BEST WISHES TO ALL OF YOU.
WITH GREAT RESPECT,
CAP PARLIER

---

"It does not sound like Mister Grishchenko is doing so well," she said.

"Indeed," answered Gourgen as he turned to leave the office.

"Gourgen," she called to stop him. He turned to look at her. "If I may be so bold, who is this Admiral Zumwalt?"

Gourgen did not appreciate the intrusion but accepted her

curiosity. She was an important ally in the communications linkage with Seattle. "As the message says, he is an important person in America . . . a very high ranking naval officer."

"And, he is coming to this country?"

"It would appear so. I have learned about him from the American . . . Parlier. He has helped Parlier. He is a friend. We will be honored to have him."

"Will he come here . . . to Mil?"

"I doubt it. He will be on holiday travel with his wife, who is Russian by the way."

"If he is coming while Anatoly Demjanovich is in the hospital, then it must mean he thinks it is all right."

"This visit has been planned for many months, probably before Anatoly went to America. He has met Anatoly Demjanovich in Seattle, perhaps not recently, but he will not likely have the current information when he arrives."

"Good luck, Gourgen, and best wishes to Anatoly Demjanovich."

"Thank you, Svetlana," he responded and left the office.

Gourgen walked down the hallway to the pilot's office. He sat down in the chair and turned it to look out the window. Gourgen stared at nothing in particular as his mind returned to his hospitalized friend. His thoughts considered the sequences of events as seen through Cap Parlier's messages to him. The last message . . . did it have some forecast of impending doom, buried in the words? There was no question of honesty, candor and forthrightness in Parlier's communications. Everything had always been from the heart. It was obvious his American brother held onto an aviator's hope for Anatoly's recovery. Gourgen was confident that everything that could be done, had been done.

Svetlana knocked on the door jam, then entered the small office. "Excuse me, Gourgen. I should have asked you earlier . . . did you tell General Designer Tishchenko about the visit of this American admiral?"

"No."

"Should you?"

"I suppose. I don't think he will be coming out here during his visit, and other than my time with him, I do not think his visit will affect Mil."

"Does the Government know, just out of curiosity?" she asked.

Gourgen stared into her eyes. Those questions always made him uneasy. It reminded him of the Stalin days when everyone seemed to be informing on everyone else just to stay on the good side of the KGB or MVD agents. Gourgen had known Svetlana for many years and never had a reason to suspect her loyalties. The question probably was as she indicated, just curiosity, but it still make him feel uncomfortable. He had nothing to hide, and he had done everything just as it should be done.

"Yes, Svetlana," he said with just a touch of disrespect. "I have informed the Ministries of Health, Defense and Interior of the famous man's visit. Interior knew about the visit before I called. Everything is as it should be."

She held her arms out, palms up, as if to gesture that her question was innocent. "I meant no harm, Gourgen."

"I am sorry. I still remember those crazy days when Stalin suspected everyone of conspiracy. None of us want to go back there."

She smiled. "You are most assuredly correct. Thank you," she added then walked out, only to return an instant later. "One more thing, excuse me. Should we make a copy of that message for Tishchenko?"

"If you think he might be interested, no problem," he said as he retrieved the last message from his file folder. "Here," he said as he handed her the paper.

Svetlana took the message, walked down the hallway to her office, presumably made a copy of it for the General Designer, then returned it to Gourgen.

Gourgen reread the message one more time before returning it to the file. All the arrangements were complete. Alone once again in the office, his mind returned to Anatoly and his struggle for life. He sensed the worst and prayed for the best.

# 42

The flight took the better part of the afternoon. Several European companies wanted to utilize the expanded lift capacity of the huge Mi-26 heavy lift helicopter. The testing to expand the envelope of lift limits took many careful steps from the technical tethered hover to the restricted slow flight moving and positioning of excessive loads. To Gourgen, it seemed the more lift they provided, the more people demanded, just as they found with the cover plate at Chernobyl. All the work they had done several years earlier to lift the 35 metric ton plate was now being translated into modifications to expand the operational external lift limit beyond the current 20 ton limit.

There were always limits, and today they found some of them. The debriefing would take longer than normal. It would probably be near dusk when they finished.

"You look like you took a bath," said one of the younger flight test engineers as Gourgen walked into the building.

"It is summer. You bastards tell me I cannot use the air conditioner, plus you keep me in a hover for hours with those big engines running at maximum power, and you think it is funny that I am all soaked in my own sweat."

"No offense."

"None taken. I just need some water."

"You look like you need some vodka instead," someone else interjected.

"No vodka, just water."

The young engineer fetched a large, unopened bottle of water. Gourgen sat in one of the chairs at the middle of the large, rectangular table. He used a screwdriver to open the cap on the bottle, tilted it up and took a long drink. He waited for the remainder of the ground and flight test crew to gather around the table.

Each step and segment of the flight were examined including the preliminary assessment of the instrumentation data. They tried to reach 25 tons on the standard hook. Parts of the very restricted flight envelope were acceptable, not great, but acceptable. The data showed that as soon as they started to move and reach the translational lift vibration boundary, the loads at numerous sites throughout the aircraft exceeded the allowable limits. The aircraft needed to be thoroughly inspected. The debriefing was spilling over into its second hour when the grim face of Deputy Chief Designer Mark Vineberg entered the room. While it was not unusual for the senior engineers from the design bureau to come all the way out of the city to the test site, such a visit so late in the day did have an air of urgency to it. When Vineberg found Gourgen's eyes, the grim expression conveyed the message. It was not good news.

Gourgen returned to the debriefing as the others did. The mood of the meeting changed. Everyone sensed the moment. Another 20 minutes were needed to close the flight debriefing.

"Unusual to see you out here so late in the day, Mark."

"Yes, well, I am afraid I bear bad news," he said as he handed Gourgen the single piece facsimile paper.

---

### McDONNELL DOUGLAS HELICOPTER COMPANY
### FACSIMILE TRANSMISSION

**Date:**        2.July.1990
**From:**        Cap Parlier
**To:**          Gourgen Karapetyan
**Subject:**     Anatoly Grishchenko

DEAR GOURGEN,

I JUST RECEIVED A TELEPHONE CALL FROM DR. HANSEN AT FHCRC IN SEATTLE. I AM TERRIBLY SORRY, GOURGEN, BUT ANATOLY DIED THIS EVENING AT 22:20 LOCAL TIME. HE APPARENTLY TOOK A VERY SERIOUS TURN FOR THE WORSE LATE THAT AFTERNOON.

I WILL LEAVE FIRST THING IN THE MORNING FOR

SEATTLE. I WILL DO MY BEST TO HELP GALINA
THROUGH HER TIME OF SORROW. WHEN I HAVE SOME
INFORMATION ON ANATOLY'S RETURN TO RUSSIA, I
WILL IMMEDIATELY PASS IT ALONG TO YOU.
    DURING MY MANY VISITS TO SEATTLE, I CAN TELL
YOU, ANATOLY PUT UP THE MOST TENACIOUS FIGHT
AGAINST HIS ILLNESS. THE DOCTORS WILL PERFORM A
THOROUGH POST-MORTEM EXAMINATION, AS IS USUAL IN
CASES SUCH AS THIS, SO THE PRECISE CAUSE OF
DEATH WILL NOT BE KNOWN FOR SEVERAL DAYS.
HOWEVER, THE DOCTORS ARE QUITE CERTAIN IT WAS
THE ASPERGILLUS INFECTION THAT ULTIMATELY
CLAIMED HIS LIFE.
    ALTHOUGH IT IS NOT MUCH SOLACE, HIS BONE
MARROW TRANSPLANT WAS PROGRESSING IN NEAR
PERFECT MANNER. THE DOCTORS FEEL PROFOUND
REGRET. THEY TOLD ME THAT HE MOST LIKELY WOULD
HAVE BEEN CURED IF WE COULD HAVE DONE THE
TRANSPLANT SIX OR MORE MONTHS EARLIER.
    AGAIN, I AM TERRIBLY SORRY, MY BROTHER. I
WILL CONTACT YOU AS SOON AS I HAVE MORE
INFORMATION.
WITH GREAT RESPECT,
CAP PARLIER

---

"I am terribly sorry, Gourgen."

Gourgen swallowed hard struggling to choke back the tears welling in his eyes and the nauseating ripples in his fatigued body. "Yes . . . well . . . he put up a good fight."

"He did."

"They did their best for him."

"Certainly."

The tears could no longer be contained. His friend embraced him as if to support him. He could feel other hands touch his shoulders, back and head. The others knew. Gourgen allowed himself a moment of grief before pushing his emotions back behind the wall. He straightened his back and pulled away from Vineberg.

"Have we heard from Galya?"

"Not that we know."

"How about the boys?"

"They are being notified by the Ministry of Defense."

"Then, we must make arrangements for his final resting place."

"Tomorrow, Gourgen, tomorrow."

"Yes, yes, of course. It is late."

"Go home. You have done enough and all that can be done. Go home."

"Yes, you are right, Mark."

Gourgen did not turn to acknowledge his friends and colleagues. To do so would only bring on more grief that he would never see Anatoly standing again. He raised his right hand as he left the building. The veteran pilot went directly to his car. As he drove through the gate, he did not acknowledge the guards who waved to him. Instead of turning left to head south toward Zhukovsky and home, Gourgen turned right toward Moscow. An urge compelled him to the design office, perhaps to find any further messages from Cap Parlier, or maybe just to review the last few messages. For a reason he could not identify nor did he really care about, Gourgen needed the solitude of his thoughts. He would call Ludmilla from the office.

A few lights in the building marked the locations of a dozen engineers and specialists who remained at work for one reason or another. Gourgen took the stairs to the fourth floor. His office was halfway down the hallway toward the General Designer's corner office and opposite from Mark Vineberg's office. He opened the door and switched on the light. He hesitated at the threshold, then turned to walk further down the hall. Marat Tishchenko, the Mil General Designer, kept his outer office unlocked. The facsimile machines connecting them to the outside world sat on the table behind his secretary's desk. He checked all three. Gourgen had to search through a dozen pieces of paper. There was nothing new from Parlier or any other message pertaining to Anatoly.

Although Gourgen was alone, a more determined unemotional persona took over his actions. His mind ran through the steps he had to take in preparation for Anatoly's return. Possibilities and variations occupied his attention as he returned to his office.

What was he going to tell Galina? Would she blame him for the loss of her husband and the father of their two sons? She had never accepted the Government's explanation for his illness. Galina knew Anatoly's medical condition was a direct result of his flights over Chernobyl. She said many times that Anatoly had been in near perfect health prior to April 1986. Gourgen knew she was right. Anatoly rarely contracted a cold in the years prior. He might have one day of flu or something in every other year or some such. The four years since Chernobyl marked the progressive deterioration of his health. If it was coincidence as the Government contended, then it was a most profound and ironic coincidence.

The infection that claimed his life had only been allowed to start because of the damage done to his immune system by the Chernobyl radiation. Everything the medical experts said pointed toward the reality than Anatoly was now recognized as the first pilot victim of Chernobyl. Others would surely follow including possibly himself. They would all need special treatment in the West. The Soviet Union, or at least the most senior medical specialist in the country, reluctantly acknowledged their limited ability to help the future victims.

Footsteps in the darkened hallway drew his attention from the papers. Gourgen looked up waiting for the person to appear, fully expecting a security guard. It was Mark Vineberg.

"I suspected this is where you would come," he said.

"I needed to see the last few messages. He tried to present the positive element of what was already a grave situation for Anatoly." Mark sat in a chair opposite Gourgen. He just looked at his friend choosing not to speak. "Perhaps he never had a chance."

"Gourgen," Mark shouted. "Anatoly had the best chance possible thanks to your efforts. He may have had the infection before he left, but you did everything that could be done."

"We have been through so much together. We have survived so many close calls. Why now? Why did he have to be the one?

So many of us were down there. The Air Force pilots had higher exposures than Anatoly. Why, why, why?"

Mark paused to let the rhetorical questions pass into silence beyond the electric hum of the wall clock. They sat there for several minutes. Gourgen stared at the messages from Parlier on his desk. Mark watched his friend and colleague. Gourgen gained no satisfaction from the fact his thoughts were common to all humankind when a friend and lifelong compatriot passed away.

"Nothing will be solved here, tonight," whispered Mark. "You need to go home."

"I know," Gourgen answered. "I just wanted to know I had not missed something."

Vineberg snorted a couple of times halfway between a chuckle and a snarl. "Gourgen, everyone did the best they could do including Anatoly Demjanovich."

"Tomorrow I shall make arrangements for him in Zhukovsky along with the other heroes of the air. He shall be remembered as a true hero who sacrificed his life to protect thousands of others and to save the Motherland. The real hero . . . ," he said allowing his voice to tail off.

"Indeed."

Gourgen Karapetyan stood, arranged the paper neatly in the folder and returned it to the drawer. "Let's go home, then. Tomorrow is another day."

Vineberg finally chuckled in relief. "As you say, my friend."

The drive south in the dark to Zhukovsky with only the spot of his headlights and the occasional glare of an oncoming automobile left him with his thoughts. Many arrangements needed to be made. Perhaps, the American Navy admiral would have some information for him after he arrived. The timing of the visit was unfortunate, but beyond the realm of control for any of them. The message indicated that he was affiliated with the same organization that Cap Parlier referred to many times in his messages. With the usual medical procedures, it would most likely be a few days before the Grishchenko's returned home. Would Galina arrive at the same time as the admiral and his wife? Had they already met? Too many questions for a late night drive. Gourgen turned his thoughts to the more pragmatic elements. He knew exactly where he wanted Anatoly's memorial to be placed. Tomorrow, he would make it so.

# 43

*08:40, Monday, 9.July.1990*
*Sheremetyevo Airport*
*Moscow, Russia, USSR*

The hazy sky and heavy air of summer befit the return of
Anatoly Grishchenko and his wife, Galina. The main terminal
shielded most of the waiting citizens from the heat. The stale air
reeked of old sweat. For the majority, the approaching moment
would be a happy time. Gourgen could not find anything happy.
Galina would be grieving, and Anatoly would be in a box.

Gourgen waited with Anatoly Kovatchur and a few others.
There were no smiles although there was laughter echoing in the
cavernous terminal. The hum and rattle of people gathered and
intermixed with others who remained strangers offered a background
of white noise that made the wait slightly more tolerable. Life
remained. The people filling the terminal were alive. Gourgen
found a slight smile with the thought that Anatoly and many of the
helicopter pilots, including himself helped to repair a grievous
wound just four years earlier that enabled many people of live.
None of them regretted their efforts, nor the contribution of so many
special people to the safety of the world.

"There it is," someone said.

Gourgen instinctively turned his attention to the large windows
in front of him to see the graceful lines of the huge Pan American
Airways, Boeing 747 race past with its spoilers fully deployed and
engines in full reverse. The aircraft disappeared behind the arrival
portion of the building. Several minutes passed before the aircraft
taxied to its parking space, and passengers began disembarking.
Gourgen wanted to be in two places. He knew he had to be where
he was to greet Galina. She would need the reassurance. However,
he also worried about Anatoly and wanted to be in the cargo area to

make absolutely certain his casket was handled with respect and care. He chose the living. The arrangements would be adequate.

Without words, the small group awaiting the return of the Grishchenko's moved to the exit area from Customs. People crowded so tightly, it was impossible for arriving passengers to join them.

Gourgen wanted to take control and disperse the eager, waiting throng to make a proper passage for the arrivals. He led the group toward the back of the crowd intending to make room, but also fighting the attraction to move closer so Galina could see a friendly face when she emerged.

"She is not going to be able to see us back here," said Anatoly.

"I know, but if we all keep pushing forward, no one will be able to get out."

Anatoly Kovatchur was the same medium height as Gourgen, but he was also thinking beyond the immediate. Gourgen felt a hand on his shoulder, turned and saw Anatoly with a broad smile on his face standing on a crate of some sort. With the acknowledgment, the fighter pilot turned his attention to the passengers struggling to make way through the welcoming crowd. Some stopped to greet friends or family making the process all the more difficult. Gourgen caught the sight of several Western businessmen dressed in their suits, and expressions of frustration and annoyance with the obstacles to their progress. He continued to scan every face he could see. The message had said, Galina would be alone since the physician-interpreter, Zhenya Margulis, stayed in Seattle to complete her medical exchange with her American counterparts.

"There she is," announced Anatoly, then jumped down off the crate. He pushed his way through the crowd without much concern for those in his way. He was like a powerful bull shrugging a shoulder, waving his head and strong neck, and stroking with each hand like a swimmer.

Gourgen remained behind with the others. He took advantage of Anatoly's crate to watch his friend reach Galina, give her a hug and a kiss on each cheek. Anatoly led her back out through the crowd that had collapsed behind him. As they approached, Gourgen stepped down off the crate and backed up several steps to give her room. She saw his eyes and could only nod her head. Her face was drawn and dark. Her skin nearly translucent and devoid of color. Gourgen could tell she had suffered in the last weeks and probably long before as Anatoly's life washed away from her.

Galina nearly leapt the last few steps between them. She wrapped her arms around his chest pulling him tight and burying her face in his chest. Gourgen could feel the convulsions of her sobbing and the growing wetness on his shirt. He held her gently, patting and stroking her back. The others touched her shoulders, head and arms. She felt tired and nearly limp as Gourgen supported her until her weeping tapered off.

She drew back just enough to reach her eyes with a handkerchief. She did not have to wipe away much since most of her tears wet Gourgen's shirt.

"It is good to have you home."

"Anatoly?"

"Do not worry. All the arrangements have been made. We have special transport for him, and it shall be waiting for us to follow to Zhukovsky."

"Thank you, Gourgen."

"It is nothing. Now, let us gather up your baggage, so we do not keep Anatoly waiting."

The others offered words of condolence, grief and support as they waited, then collected her bags. The design center's Zil limousine waited for them directly in front of the terminal exit. Galina and Gourgen would ride in the limousine. The covered truck was indeed waiting for them. Anatoly's casket was respectfully covered and out of view. The others piled into the remaining automobiles for a caravan following Anatoly across the city and down to the aviation community of Zhukovsky.

The sun shown bright and hot on the summer days that passed so fast as the aviation community mourned the loss of one of its notable citizens. Family and friends made the journey to cry, wail and commiserate. Anatoly was remembered as a strong but gentle man, a devout father loved by his wife and sons, a pre-eminent aviator of laudable accomplishments, and lastly, a selfless man with a willingness to sacrifice his health for the good of humanity. The mourning culminated with the interment of Anatoly just inside the main gate at the head of the row of the most prominent of the aviation community who have gone before them.

The grave side ceremony concluded with the typical aviation tribute recognized world wide. A flight of four fighters in the most common formation, known as the right hand, finger four, with a venerable MiG-21 leading the formation of a MiG-29 on the left wing, an Su-27 on the right wing and an Su-7 on the far right. As they passed overhead, Victor Pugachov, flying the Su-27 pulled up out of formation as the others continued straight ahead with the missing man slot. Pugachov lit the afterburners to full thrust climbing straight up toward the heavens until he was nearly out of sight, and then rolled the fighter through two full rolls. The aircraft continued to climb until only two orange dots could be seen through the shroud of heat. Not a dry eye remained.

The pilots waited the several weeks for Anatoly's monument to be completed and installed before they returned for the more personal tribute to their brother, one of their own. They gathered in the late afternoon light before the large, dark marble, obelisk engraved with his likeness, the expanse of his life and the significance of his contribution. Each of the pilots stood before Anatoly's monument, bowed his head and silently conveyed his thoughts. They waited without words for a group of nearly two dozen, some of the Soviet Union's most famous pilots, before Gourgen Karapetyan began handing out the glasses. Anatoly Kovatchur followed him pouring several fingers of vodka. This was one of those occasions when the need to celebrate their friend with the warm embrace of alcohol overrode all other considerations.

"Friends," Gourgen said hesitating for every set of eyes to turn to him, "we toast our brother who gave his life for the Motherland."

Several affirmative sounds interspersed the downing of the liquor. Anatoly poured another round.

"He was a good man and a great friend," said Kovatchur.

More comments and swallows. The animation of the group began slowly as the liberation of the alcohol took effect.

"Do you remember the time he had to jump from that broken helicopter?"

Laughter finally came to the somber place.

"Yes. The damn machine is burning in a pile in the middle of a field. He is marching back dragging his parachute behind him still harnessed, and he was yelling at the engineers for not listening to him."

"It was the ground crew tripping and stumbling next to him trying to figure out if he was injured that seem the funniest."

"We have all been there."

"Yes, indeed."

"And, some of us did not walk away."

The mood darkened quickly. Gourgen did not want this time to be sad. He glanced to several others. His eyes spoke the message.

"Never a prouder father."

"Hell, he practically broke my back with his embrace when Nicholas was born."

"Where did he get those cigars?"

"A friend traded something with one of the Cubans," answered Gourgen.

"They do make the best cigars."

"As we make the best vodka."

"And airplanes."

"And airplanes," someone repeated.

"You have done well, Gourgen," said Valery Menitsky, the chief pilot for Mikoyan.

"Thank you."

"But, aren't we missing someone?"

"Yes, indeed, Cap Parlier."

"He was crucial in the attempt to save Anatoly. He should be here."

"So, where is he?"

"In America."

"He said he would come," Gourgen added. "I will try to get him here as soon as possible, but it is difficult to say, when."

Anatoly instinctively knew they needed more vodka. With the glasses finally ready, Anatoly said, "Here is to our brother, Cap Parlier. May he keep his ball centered, air under his wings and come to us soon."

"As you say," Gourgen shouted as he bolted his entire glass of vodka.

"If we are not careful, we are going to get drunk."

"What better excuse can we have. Our dear friend has passed, and we are celebrating his freedom, and none of us has to fly tomorrow."

"Hey, that is it, then. Another toast to Anatoly."

The sky darkened as the pilots continued their traditional celebration. There were many other pilots lying next to Anatoly Grishchenko, some were heroes, some were legends, but this evening belonged to Anatoly. The cemetery had no lights, and the pilots needed none.

"Why couldn't they have protected him?" one of the younger pilots asked.

"There was nothing that could protect him from that place," answered Gourgen as he remembered his feelings upon seeing that luminescent, blue-white, column of light rising from the destroyed remains of Reactor No. 4 at Chernobyl.

"Why did you do it?"

Gourgen chuckled. "There was no other choice, Peter. There was no other choice."

"Remotely piloted vehicles?"

"There was no time. There was no such vehicle in existence anywhere. There was simply no time, and there was no one else. Either we did it, or it could not have been done. The damage has been great. We probably do not even know how great, and it would have been infinitely greater if we had not flown those missions."

"There was no choice," added Anatoly as if to speak for Anatoly.

"Still, it seems like such an enormous waste of such a good pilot."

"We must all make sacrifices for the Motherland. This was Anatoly's," said Gourgen.

Then, youth spoke the unspeakable. "Are not all the pilots going to suffer the same fate?"

There was no gasp or sigh, just a shuffling of feet in the pea-gravel, and mumbled, unintelligible sounds. They had all avoided that question for the years since the accident although it sat like a cooling ingot of freshly poured lead in their thoughts. They all knew the answer, but it was not something any of them wanted to talk about, especially Gourgen.

"Perhaps," was all Gourgen could calmly offer.

"You do not ask such things," admonished Anatoly.

"Why not? I need to understand. Someday I may be asked to do a similar thing."

"Then, you shall do your duty, to serve the Motherland, to save lives," Gourgen answered.

"One last toast to our brother," announced Anatoly in a strong, commanding voice, "before we all must go home to our families."

"Before we do," Gourgen said holding his left hand up high signaling, stop, "we all know, those of us exposed at Chernobyl will experience the long term effects of radiation poisoning. That is why we must redouble our efforts to raise awareness, and whatever support we can in this country and all over the world. We are all going to need help someday."

Heads nodded, but no one wanted to speak.

The vodka was poured. They gathered a little closer together in the cooling air of the night and the diminished light from distant electric light bulbs. Several of the pilots held their glasses up waiting for someone to offer the toast. Anatoly and a few others looked to Gourgen, Anatoly's closest friend.

Gourgen Karapetyan did not want to make the final toast. He could not imagine why, but he knew he did not want to do it. Anatoly nodded several times trying to coax his colleague. Gourgen finally gave in.

He held up his glass. "Here is to our brother, Anatoly . . . a true son of the earth, brother of the sky, one of the best among us, a good father to his sons and our future, and my . . . our friend." The darkness masked the tears streaming down his face as the others acknowledged the tribute and drank.

Gourgen waited for the others to leave before he wiped the dampness from his cheeks.

"It was the same for me," said Anatoly as he placed a heavy arm around Gourgen's shoulders.

"I miss him."

"He will always be here for us, Gourgen."

"Thanks."

The two veteran pilots walked slowly, heads bowed, and silently toward the apartment buildings. Another day would bring new challenges. They intended to rejoice the passing of a celebrated aviator, and yet, in the end, they mourned the loss of a friend. Gourgen silently feared this would not be the only such event in the Soviet Union over the next few years, as the damage of Chernobyl claimed more precious lives. They had to make sure this never happened again. With their memory and determination, they would be successful.

# 44

*09:30, Friday, 13.July.1990*
*Apartment No. 213*
*50 Marchlevskoho Street*
*Moscow, Russia, USSR*

The sting of Anatoly's funeral remained with Gourgen Karapetyan. His monument was not complete nor installed, and the loose ends continued to plague Gourgen. He avoided flying and stayed to himself. He had even sent his family to their *dacha* so he would not have any distractions. Gourgen needed to be alone with his thoughts.

The visit of the American Navy admiral less than a week after Anatoly's funeral did not strike Gourgen as a good thing to do. He was enough of a realist to recognize that journey's such as this one for a man so important took many months to arrange. If he asked the question, he would probably learn that the Zumwalt family journey to the Soviet Union had been set up prior to Anatoly's journey to the United States. Cap Parlier obviously thought a great deal of the man, and somehow, Gourgen sensed that Admiral Zumwalt had been a part of helping Anatoly Grishchenko. So, his mood had little significance for an important meeting such as this.

The call had come into the office late the previous day. The Zumwalts had arrived in Moscow. They wanted a day to visit with their hostess. Gourgen went back through his message file to find her name, Svetlana Levnokova, and her address. Their scheduled meeting time was mid-morning the following day.

Gourgen took the time to gather up whatever information he could without drawing attention to Admiral Zumwalt's visit. He suspected the Ministry of Defense and the KGB were well aware of the admiral's presence. For all he knew, the admiral had schedule visits with his counterparts in the Soviet Navy, but there was no purpose in attracting more attention.

He found the address. It was a very nice section of the city. The apartment building was very well kept. The interior corridors were well lighted and clean. This building housed important people. Gourgen found the correct apartment, checked his note one more time to make sure he had the correct place, then knocked.

A petite woman, distantly attractive, and perhaps 10-15 years older than himself answered the door. "You must be Gourgen Karapetyan."

"Yes, I am, and you must be Svetlana Levnokova."

"You are correct. Please come in. I have some family here who desperately want to meet you."

Gourgen felt slightly self-conscious as he followed her into the apartment. The aroma of freshly baked, sweet pastry filled the air of the apartment. Artwork, some of it quite impressive, along with framed photographs covered the walls. This was a happy place, he could just feel it.

As he entered her living room, their guests were standing. Svetlana motioned to a woman who resembled her although appeared to be slightly younger. "This is my sister, Mouza Zumwalt," she said in Russian which seemed odd to Gourgen, then gestured to a much larger man with a barrel chest, thinning gray hair and thick gray eyebrows, "and her husband Admiral Elmo Elmovich Zumwalt of the US Navy. This is Gourgen Karapetyan."

"It is honor to meet you," Mrs. Zumwalt said in perfect Russian, startling Gourgen somewhat.

"The honor is mine," Gourgen answered tentatively as he shook their hands.

The admiral's handshake was strong in the Russian style. "Good morning, Gourgen," he said, also in Russian.

"Do you both speak Russian?" he asked to their guests.

"I do," she answered. "My husband understands more than he speaks."

"I can speak English," Gourgen said, "if you are more comfortable."

"Not necessary," Admiral Zumwalt said in Russian, then switched to English. "Between Mouza and Svetlana, they can translate for us if we get stuck on words."

"How did you come to speak Russian?" he asked, although he really wanted to know how a Russian woman came to marry an American Navy admiral.

They all chuckled. It was obviously a question, in one form or another, that had been asked many times.

"I am Russian," answered Mouza. "My family was in China when the war started. I met Bud in Shanghai at the end of the war. We were married in 1945."

"I am sure there is much more to that story, but it is good to have you in our country, and as I said, it is an honor to meet you. Cap Parlier has told me so much about you."

"Cap, has also told us much about you especially about your extraordinary friendship," the admiral said. "I must tell you how terribly sorry we are for your tragic loss. Many people in several countries worked very hard to help Anatoly Grishchenko. It is most unfortunate that we could not treat him sooner."

"Do you think the outcome would have been different if he had gone to America sooner?"

"The doctors who treated Anatoly have told me that his bone marrow transplant was progressing very well, but it was a fungus infection that spread rapidly through his lungs and compromised his respiratory system."

"Sooner," Gourgen said pensively.

"Yes," answered Zumwalt. "We must not let that happen again."

"What did you learn from Anatoly Demjanovich?"

"One thing we do know is, the specialists at Hanford Nuclear Research Center in Washington State detected abnormally high concentrations of radiation in his thyroid, liver, bones and other organs. The nature of his leukemia, as indicated by those findings, suggests quite strongly that he contracted his malignancy from his exposure to ionizing radiation. According to the specialists, the clinical manifestations are consistent and virtually textbook examples of delayed and chronic radiation poisoning."

"Chernobyl."

"Yes, and I understand you flew with him at Chernobyl as well as other helicopter pilots."

"Air Force," Gourgen said with his thoughts on other things.

"Are any of the other pilots ill?"

"We were all sick from the radiation, but so far, only Anatoly did not recover."

"What you and Anatoly, and your fellow pilots did to contain the horrific damage at Chernobyl, is truly heroic. You all deserve the recognition of heroes."

"Thank you."

"Is there anything we can do?" Zumwalt asked.

"Since you are probably familiar with the nature of radiation exposure, the specialists tell me we are not likely to see the worst of the human injury until 20 years after the accident. So, we have more pilots to worry about."

"I know Cap is working to find ways to help the other pilots."

"We also want the world to know what happened at Chernobyl. We do not want it to happen again anywhere in the world."

"I can tell you, we will do everything we can to do just that. A number of key scientists and physicians in Ukraine, ByeloRussiya, Russia, Israel and the United States have formed a partnership to learn as much as we can about the medical consequences of that tragedy as well as make recommendations regarding prevention and ways to treat those who have been exposed."

"You are most generous."

"I have followed most of the events surrounding Anatoly Grishchenko and the work that you and Cap Parlier did on his behalf. I want to tell you from my heart, you have done a truly heroic act in helping Anatoly the way that you did. You should be proud."

Gourgen obtained a clarification of a few words. "I would be much more proud if Anatoly was here to talk to you as well."

"I know Cap feels the same, but no one could have done better.

We must find ways to treat the other pilots before they deteriorate too far as was the case with Anatoly."

"Other pilots, most in the Air Force, were exposed to the same if not greater radiation levels. They were sick, but the doctors say they have recovered."

"That is the nature of radiation exposure. Everyone reacts to it differently, but for those exposed to the levels Anatoly was exposed to or greater, they will most likely develop malignancies of one form or another in the years to come."

"Then, that is my fate as well."

"We must do whatever we can to help you and the others, but it is very expensive and overwhelming even for the American medical system. As I said, Cap Parlier is doing what he can. I know there are many others who will do the same."

"Too much seriousness," said Svetlana. "Who would like some tea and biscuits?"

Gourgen nodded his head. Both Mouza and Bud agreed. The conversation shifted to the kitchen as the steam kettle whistled, and the sweet fragrance of fresh tea mixed with the rich smell of the tray of cookies.

The Zumwalts had been to Moscow several times. This was to be the longest trip with no official duties or impositions. Gourgen wanted some of the other pilots to meet Admiral Zumwalt. Many would not believe his tale of meeting the retired chief of the American Navy; these things just did not happen in the Soviet Union.

They had a full schedule with many historic places to go. Some adjustments were made, but the demands on their time proved too great. Gourgen understood. This was a holiday journey for the Zumwalts to fully appreciate the Motherland.

"It has been a genuine honor to meet you, Admiral Zumwalt, and you, Mouza Zumwalt. I truly appreciate the time you have given me."

"You have blessed us, Gourgen. We shall cherish this moment in history."

"Would you be so kind, upon your return to America, to tell

my brother, Cap Parlier, that we are joined for life, and we eagerly await the time when he can come to visit us."

"Yes, absolutely," said Bud Zumwalt. "I know he regrets the conflicts that prevented him from returning with Galina to bring Anatoly home. I will mention our meeting to him. Perhaps, he can find a way to pay his respects to Anatoly. He feels very strongly about what you have done for all of us, as does the rest of the world."

"The press is not something we are used to in the Soviet Union. It has been overwhelming for us. Galina Grishchenko could not believe the attention the Western press showed to Anatoly."

"It is the way things are in the West. However, I can tell you all the press I have seen or am aware of has been the most positive for what you and the other pilots did to cover the damaged reactor and prevent further contamination."

"Then, it was worth it."

"Yes, I think so."

"Well," Gourgen said shaking hands with the two women first, then with Admiral Zumwalt, "thank you once again for this delightful time."

"We shall wait until our next meeting."

"Enjoy your visit to the Motherland."

"We shall."

Gourgen returned to his automobile. Although he had not looked forward to the meeting so soon after Anatoly's death and funeral, he was now very glad he overcame his reluctance. In his heart, he knew this had been a historic meeting. One of those rare moments in time when the course is changed.

As he drove through the city, a recurring thought kept coming to him. If someone as important as a former chief of the American Navy knew what happened at Chernobyl, and what the helicopter pilots did at that place, then their efforts would not be forgotten.

All the pilots wanted to be proud of what they had done to seal the wound. They did not want their efforts to be buried in the obscurity of bureaucratic self-preservation. For the first time, since this whole tragic episode began more than four years earlier, Gourgen felt they might gain the recognition they deserved.

As Gourgen suspected from the earliest discussions among the pilots, the affinity among those who manipulate the controls of flying machines transcended borders and languages. Anatoly Kovatchur's first public flight demonstrations outside the Soviet Union in 1988 began the process of exchange. Anatoly's trials and passing enhanced that process. The interest in what happened at Chernobyl would not overwhelm, diminish or dilute the accomplishments of the pilots who had been asked to help.

The two ensuing weeks began the process of recovery for everyone — returning to normalcy. Galina continued to grieve with the support of her family, neighbors and friends. That element of the recovery would probably take the longest time to complete. For the aviators, returning to flight established their supremacy over the loss they all suffered.

There was work to do. The participation of Soviet aviation continued to expand in the world arena. Their work was recognized by the community of flight. Inquiries about their machines filled them with optimism.

The message Gourgen received from Cap Parlier on Monday, the 30th of July, accentuated the thirst of the public world-wide for more information as well as the desire to recognize the contributions of the pilots by many people both within and outside the aviation community.

---

**McDONNELL DOUGLAS HELICOPTER COMPANY**
**FACSIMILE TRANSMISSION**

**Date:**    30.July.1990
**From:**    Cap Parlier
**To:**    Gourgen Karapetyan
**Subject:**    Anatoly Grishchenko
DEAR GOURGEN,
    I RECEIVED YOUR FAX OF 27.07.90.  IT IS

UNFORTUNATE THAT YOU WILL NOT BE ABLE TO ATTEND
THE CEREMONY HONORING ANATOLY AT THE GOODWILL
GAMES.  I PASSED THE MESSAGE TO DOCTOR HANSEN.
WE SHALL MEET, AGAIN, ANOTHER TIME, I KNOW.
 I APPRECIATE YOUR RECOGNITION OF MY EFFORTS.
FORTUNATELY, ANATOLY TOLD ME MANY STORIES, WHILE
HE WAS HERE, OF YOUR EFFORTS.  HE SAID HE KNEW
HOW HARD YOU WORKED ON HIS BEHALF AND THAT WAY
HE KNEW HOW HARD I MUST HAVE WORKED.  I AGREE
WITH ANATOLY'S STATEMENT.  YOU DESERVE GREAT
RECOGNITION FOR YOUR EFFORTS.  I MAY NOT HAVE
KNOWN ANATOLY WHEN WE STARTED OUR EFFORTS.  I
THINK OF HIM AS MY BROTHER.  I WAS HONORED FOR
THE FAITH YOU HAD IN ME, AND THE OPPORTUNITY TO
PERFORM MY SMALL PART IN HELPING ANATOLY.
 I HAVE TALKED TO THE EXECUTIVE DIRECTOR OF
THE SOCIETY OF EXPERIMENTAL TEST PILOTS.  HE
WILL FORWARD A PACKAGE OF APPLICATIONS FOR YOU
AND THE OTHER MIL DESIGN BUREAU PILOTS.  YOU
SHOULD BE AWARE THAT A SIMILAR PACKAGE HAS BEEN
SENT TO THE MIKOYAN AND SUKOI DESIGN BUREAU
PILOTS.  IN FACT, VALERY MENITSKY OF MIKOYAN IS
SCHEDULED TO SPEAK AT THIS YEAR'S INTERNATIONAL
SYMPOSIUM IN LOS ANGELES, 27.09.90.  I WILL SEND
YOU A MESSAGE WHEN THE APPLICATION PACKAGE IS
ENROUTE.  SEVERAL COSMONAUTS ARE ALREADY
MEMBERS.  THE ONLY ONE I KNOW IS IGOR VOLK.
THERE IS NO PROBLEM WITH THE SOVIET PILOTS
JOINING THE SOCIETY.  I WILL HELP YOU IN THIS
EFFORT.
 I WOULD LIKE TO TELL YOU THAT A GOOD FRIEND,
JOHN PEKKANEN, IS PLANNING TO VISIT MOSCOW FROM
ABOUT 10.09.90 TO 20.09.90.  HE IS WRITING AN
ARTICLE ABOUT ANATOLY AND OUR EFFORTS TO HELP
HIM.  HE WROTE A BOOK ABOUT ADMIRAL ZUMWALT AND
HIS SON'S FIGHT AGAINST LEUKEMIA.  GALINA AND
ZHENYA HAVE BOTH MET HIM IN SEATTLE.  I WOULD
ALSO LIKE TO SAY THAT I AM TRYING VERY HARD TO
BE ABLE TO COME TO MOSCOW AT ABOUT THAT TIME.

```
MY VISIT IS NOT POSITIVE YET.  I HAVE ALREADY
APPLIED FOR MY ENTRY VISA.  I WILL KEEP YOU
INFORMED AS PLANS BECOME FIRM.
     PLEASE PASS MY WARMEST GREETINGS TO ALL OUR
FRIENDS IN THE SOVIET UNION.  ALSO, PLEASE
CONVEY MY GREETINGS TO MARAT TISHCHENKO WHOM I
HAVE MET SEVERAL TIMES.
WITH GREAT RESPECT,
CAP PARLIER
```

Gourgen continued undaunted to mix his work as a professional aviator and his enthusiasm to strengthen the connection with pilots in the West. As in virtually every situation, there were always constraints. Cap Parlier could not come to the Soviet Union when he wanted to, and Gourgen Karapetyan could not go to the United States when he wanted to go.

At least, he was able to help Galina and Nicholas Grishchenko return to Seattle to be honored by the host community that worked so hard to welcome them and repair the damage to her husband. It was emotional for Galina, but she handled it extremely well.

The attention of the aviation community continued long after Anatoly's passing. It was good.

"You would think Anatoly Demjanovich is still alive," observed Anatoly Kovatchur as they gathered at Anatoly Grishchenko's final resting place one month after his burial.

"Yes," answered Gourgen as he looked at the black obelisk with its commemorative engraving. "If we had only known this a few years earlier, Anatoly, and probably many others, would still be alive today."

"You cannot think that way, Gourgen. The past is now history. Anatoly has taken his rightful place in that history. It is up to us, now, to expand and make permanent what has happened."

"Correct, as always, my friend."

"How are your talks with the American journalist going?" Anatoly asked.

"He is an interesting man. He has gone to Chernobyl for a

few days of research."

"Why would anyone want to go there?"

"Perhaps, it is because he can," Gourgen said and smiled at his friend. "This man, Pekkanen . . . ."

"Must be Finnish."

"Yes, certainly a Finnish name, but he is an American, there is no doubt."

The two pilots stared at Anatoly's monument. The chirping of birds filled the background as a gentle breeze moved through the trees.

"They care about us," Gourgen added. "At first, I was not sure what Cap Parlier was trying to do when he referred to Anatoly and me as brothers. He has told many other people the same thing including this fellow, Pekkanen. At first, I thought it was just a phrase. But, now, I truly feel like he is my brother . . . connected by blood of some sort."

"I know what you mean. I have always liked him from the very first moment I met him in England. Hopefully, he can join us here, one day, to pay tribute to our friend."

"Yes."

The two pilots threw the contents of the small glasses of vodka down their throats and held their empty glasses to their fallen colleague. They both instinctively knew there would be more.

# 45

*15:35, Wednesday, 30.July.1991*
*Sheremetyevo Airport*
*Moscow, Russia, USSR*

The tall American had a smile that stretched from ear to ear when he finally saw Gourgen Karapetyan outside the customs area. He walked with confidence carrying one large bag and one small business case. Gourgen walked toward him. Cap Parlier dropped his bags, and they embraced. The American's visit was now a reality just over a year after Anatoly's passing. The moment marked the beginning of a promise fulfillment the two pilots made at the conclusion of Anatoly's struggle.

"It is great to have you with us," Gourgen said in his best English.

"Great to see you, Gourgen, and an honor to finally be here."

"Do you have all your bags?"

"Yes."

"Then, we should be off."

Parlier followed Gourgen as they made their way out of the terminal and to his car. They headed into Moscow down the wide boulevard. Gourgen pointed out several landmarks including the large sculpture monument on the right side of the road. He slowed the car as they approached.

"This is the monument for the defenders of Moscow in the Great Patriotic War. Many gave their lives to stop the German tanks. This site marks the closest the Germans advanced to the capital."

Cap looked at the buildings of central Moscow in the distance ahead, then back to the monument. "That's pretty close."

"Yes. Much too close. It reminds us of the patriots and how close we came to losing. It tells us to never let this happen again to the Motherland."

"I should say."

"The young Doctor Vorobiev served here. He was a true hero that day. He patched the wounded, but he also stopped several tanks by himself."

"Our Doctor Vorobiev?"

Gourgen nodded his head.

"I didn't know."

"Yes, well, we remember."

Cap kept his eye on the monument to see the back side until it disappeared from view. He sat quietly as Gourgen drove. Cap Parlier had served in the American military, so his mind was probably imagining the heroic struggle that occurred several kilometers behind them, 50 years ago. Gourgen waited until Cap began looking around again.

"I shall take you to your hotel. It is probably best that you rest. Tomorrow morning, we begin a very full week of special meetings and activities. As you requested, I have arranged for us to fly together. We shall fly the Mil Two Six later in the week."

"The same machine you and Anatoly flew over Chernobyl?" asked Parlier.

"No, not the same aircraft. That bird is permanently quarantined in the support city of Pripyat . . . too much radiation."

"I meant the same type of machine."

"Yes, yes, the exact same type."

"Great. I'm really looking forward to it. The Mil Two Six will make an extraordinary connection between you, Anatoly and me."

Gourgen nodded his head in agreement and drove along silently for several more miles. As they weaved through the city traffic, Gourgen outlined the agenda in broad terms as they bobbed and weaved their way through the streets to the Friendship Hotel, the favorite of Western businessmen, on the banks of the Moscow River, just upstream from the Russian White House, the government office building of the Russian Federated Republic. Gourgen helped Cap check into the hotel as well as settle into his room even though the hotel staff spoke fairly good English, and Gourgen was not needed, but it was a perfect time for the two pilots to fill in the gaps of the last year. When Cap's eye lids became heavy, Gourgen excused himself after setting the time for them to meet in the morning. It would be a full week and a half.

The next day began early, at a full sprint, and did not falter. The first chunk of time other than transport was occupied by the leaders of TsAGI — the Central Aerohydrodynamic Research Institute — on the west side of the main roadway across from the Gromov Flight Research Center and the main part of the Ramskoye Aerodrome at Zhukovsky. Gourgen dropped Cap off at the main entrance to the Administration building, stayed for the introductions, then departed to return for a luncheon and retrieve their guest. Parlier would see the range of research wind tunnels, big and small, fast and slow, vertical and horizontal. *Glasnost* and *peristroika* enabled this unprecedented opening of the formerly closed city.

By the time Gourgen returned, Cap and his TsAGI hosts were in the Director's conference room with an ample spread of food and drink. The pleasant meal in the Russian style for an important guest and friend paid tribute to the efforts of Cap Parlier on behalf of one of their own.

Next stop, the Gromov Flight Research Center. Anatoly's colleagues gathered in the small auditorium to listen to Parlier and ask questions. The laughter among the pilots and engineers signaled their acceptance. The American quickly seemed at ease among his colleagues despite the language differences. Cap's face lit up like a beacon when Anatoly Kovatchur entered the back of the room.

After the nearly two hour exchange, the session broke up. Some remained behind, but it was clearly the reunion of Anatoly and Cap that captured the moment.

"It has been too long," Anatoly said in English.

"Indeed. Are you in good health?"

"Like the ox he usually is," interjected Gourgen.

The three men laughed which quickly spread to the few

listeners.

"And you?" asked Anatoly.

"Great. Everything is perfect, and I am honored to be here."

"It is our honor to have you. We are . . . ," he hesitated to ask the interpreter the correct word, "most grateful for what you did for Anatoly."

Cap Parlier bowed his head and nodded several times. "For a brother," was all he said.

"We have much planned," announced Gourgen. "Now, we go to visit Anatoly. Then, tonight we go to Galina. We have a meal and celebration with Galina and friends."

After a few remaining questions about his work and life in America, Cap followed Gourgen to the car. They drove the several kilometers distance to the cemetery behind the cluster of apartment buildings. Only a handful of pilots joined them for Cap's indoctrination in the traditional Russian tribute to fallen heroes. Cap recognized Anatoly's monument the instant they walked through the gate. His awareness impressed them all. He knelt on one knee in the gravel before Anatoly's grave and bowed his head. Cap remained silent and motionless for several minutes before he stood.

As he had done so many times before, Gourgen handed out the glasses. Cap's puzzled expression was allowed to remain. Several of the others tried to tell him the purpose. The confusion of the interpreter, unaccustomed in the ways of the pilots, could not translate the words adequately. It was left to Gourgen.

"We honor those who have gone before us," Gourgen said in English.

As the others raised their glasses, Parlier joined them and said, "To those who have gone before us." He watched his fellow pilots down their drink, then followed step for step. Cap nodded his head for another. He wanted to make his own tribute. "To Anatoly," he said motioning toward the monument, "and to all those who have sacrificed to save others." The words were translated into Russian although most of the pilots understood the English. Everyone nodded their heads toward Anatoly before tossing down the vodka.

The pilots walked slowly, almost meandered, down the central, wide, gravel patch. They stopped at the graves of famous or highly regarded Soviet pilots to repeat the acknowledgment. The last vestiges of any barriers fell rapidly. Russian mixed with English as the interpreter found her services not particularly in demand. Parlier tried to answer simple questions in Russian while the others made every attempt to communicate in English. Laughter among these comrades cemented the moments of solemnity as they moved through the cemetery.

They were nearly two thirds down the length of the path when Gourgen stopped and pointed down the remaining path. A jet aircraft approached at high speed and treetop level across the airfield directly toward them. As the airplane neared the trees of the cemetery, the pilot pulled up sharply causing an enormous condensation cloud above his wings. It was an Su-7 fighter with its centerline inlet, swept wings and afterburner in full light. He pulled straight up so they were looking into the bright orange glow of the exhaust. The aircraft rolled three times before pulling out of the climb and disappeared behind the trees.

Gourgen waved his hand toward the retreating sound of the jet. "Anatoly."

"Kovatchur?" asked Parlier.

Gourgen smiled broadly and nodded in his head.

"He is flying a Sukhoi Seven."

Gourgen looked at Parlier with an odd expression, not really understanding the questioning tone of his words. "He flies anything they will let him. That machine belongs to Gromov. It was the most convenient for today, and it serves our purpose well."

"Indeed it does."

Parlier enjoyed the demonstration as any pilot or aviation enthusiast would.

"For Anatoly." Gourgen hesitated. "For you." Various pilots repeated the words.

Parlier held his glass for another pass. Once ready, he said,

"To good friends."

Everyone drank quickly. Each of the Soviet pilots patted Parlier on the back or hugged him in Russian style. The bond among the pilots transcended language and nationality.

Dusk came, telling the pilots they needed to move on. They were due at Galina Grishchenko's apartment. Many of the pilots would attend. Some would even bring their wives and children.

Her apartment was already crowded when Gourgen and Cap arrived. Several of the wives had been feverishly preparing the food and drink for their important visitor. The reunion with Galina was emotional and personal for Cap as they embraced.

"Thank you, Cap," Galina said in English with some embarrassment, for her pronunciation, but genuine gratitude.

"It is an honor to be here, Galya." The words were translated into Russian for her.

"The honor is mine," she returned.

Introductions were completed including Galina and Anatoly's two sons, Boris and Nicholas, home on leave for Parlier's visit. Food and drink filled the apartment. They laughed and told stories as all pilots do. A few of the women joined in the occasion. They passed gifts among them. Parlier was inundated with them. Anatoly Kovatchur joined them and presented a highly polished, inlayed plaque of the Su-27 with a special message on the back. Boris contributed his flight helmet and oxygen mask, but the most poignant moment came when he asked Parlier to be the godfather to his yet unborn child. Tears of joy and pride flowed, and bonded these people. It was Gourgen Karapetyan who drew an end to the party in the small hours of the morning. He had to drive Cap back into Moscow. They had several long days of special events to complete.

The next several days were spent touring Moscow with various people. Most of the famous and notable sites were visited from the Kremlin and St. Basil's Cathedral to the University of Moscow and the state radio broadcast tower with its rotating restaurant high above the city. They also visited the Mil Design Bureau and spent a short time with General Designer Marat Tishchenko and the other Chief Designers who knew Parlier, Mark Vineberg and Alexei Ivanov.

The big day came five days into Parlier's visit. Gourgen drove him to a large open park on the Northwest outskirts of the city. A medium green, Army Mi-26 heavy lift helicopter had been staged at the small airfield at the edge of the park. This would be the flight Gourgen and Cap would fly together.

Gourgen completed the introductions quickly, then took the left seat. Cap was pointed toward the right seat, normally the aircraft commander's station. The remainder of the crew, the navigator and communicator, the flight engineer and the crew chief were in the military assigned to the aircraft. Gourgen did not take time to explain the procedures necessary to get the world's largest helicopter running. Since they had a rather narrow window to pass through the air defense network surrounding Moscow, he did not want to take any risks of missing their schedule. Cap listened and watched intently, to absorb most of what was happening since helicopters were helicopters and air traffic control instructions were the same regardless of the language.

Gourgen flew the pre-briefed route listening to the times associated with each checkpoint. Once the apartment buildings and other urban buildings of Moscow fell behind them, he gave Cap the aircraft. Being an accomplished test pilot himself, the American began a series of small inputs to develop a sense of feel for the large aircraft. Gourgen could not relax knowing that most, if not all, of Cap's experience was in relatively small, agile machines, not the big, lumbering lift types. Fortunately, Cap was respectful of the new aircraft for him, and appropriately gentle.

The bright, clear day accentuated the colors of summer. Green dominated the world around them. Gourgen pointed out several key features as they flew. Nearly 90 minutes later, the buildings of the old, waystation, community of Torzhuk appeared beyond the windscreen. The substantial elements of a Frontal Aviation Regimental airfield on the eastern edge of the city were unmistakable. Cap instinctively adjusted his flight path to approach the airfield. Landing instructions in Russian were conveyed to the American by hand signals that he followed naturally. He landed the Mi-26 in the designated spot with the touch of a veteran pilot.

After completing the shutdown procedures, they extricated themselves from the cockpit. A small crowd of military uniforms, mostly senior officers, waited outside.

"Cap Parlier, this is Colonel Dimitri Kalashnikov," Gourgen announced.

"Like the rifle?" asked Cap with a smile.

"My uncle," answered the distinctive, fine, rugged featured colonel in English and with a broad smile of someone proud of his white teeth. He shook hands firmly. "Pleased to meet you, Mister Parlier."

"It is an honor to meet you and to visit your base."

"Colonel Kalashnikov is the commander of this regiment," explained Gourgen.

"Gourgen has told me of your heroic work at Chernobyl."

"And he has told us of your generous efforts for Anatoly Grishchenko."

"It was nothing."

"Perhaps to you, Comrade Parlier, but to us, your work has been like a miracle on earth, so it is much more than nothing."

"I didn't mean . . . ."

Kalashnikov held up his hand to stop the embarrassed American. "No need." He smiled. "I was just, as you say, kidding."

They laughed. Kalashnikov embraced Cap, then introduced him to the other senior officers of the regiment. Parlier handled the onslaught in admirable fashion. He could not possibly remember all the names that came at him, but he tried as he repeated each name with rather good pronunciation for a non-Russian speaker.

As an honored guest, they wanted him to see their museum of the aircraft used by the regiment over time — from the venerable Mi-2 to the gangly Mi-10 crane configuration. They even showed him the relatively new, still experimental version of the coaxial rotor, commonly naval helicopter, Kamov Ka-25 combat search and rescue helicopter they were still testing. He asked many questions only a knowledgeable, informed pilot could ask. They enjoyed their guest.

Gourgen Karapetyan smiled in the background as several of the senior officers wanted to take Cap to their regimental cemetery for the requisite tribute to their honored predecessors. A small caravan of three large, Air Force sedans took the group to the cemetery first. They also took the opportunity to show him some of the landmarks of the old waystation community. The orthodox church converted to a jail, and now in the process of restoration to its original grandeur and purpose. Several public houses used by travelers from St. Petersburg to Moscow for a night's rest on their journey. Cap seemed to have a connection with the community, the history and the aviators that impressed even these seasoned and sometimes cynical officers.

"Now, with all our obligations done," announced Colonel Kalashnikov, "we have a late luncheon planned for you, Comrade Parlier. We want to feed you well before your scheduled return to Moscow."

"Great."

"Then, we shall be off."

They returned to the base and the main mess hall. It was the only room large enough. The stark interior was well kept in true military fashion. The large square room had been rearranged with the tables forming a broad 'U' that filled the room. Cap was directed to the center of the head table with the most senior officers on either side. The two interpreters sat directly in front of Cap, so they could help him understand the words. The seats filled completely. Gourgen sat at the very end of the left leg.

Kalashnikov clapped his hands several times for attention, then spoke in Russian. "Comrades, we have as our honored guest, Comrade Cap Parlier, an American Marine, a brother in arms," he paused for the applause, "who has joined us here in our home, Torzhuk." More applause. "We must eat before we toast our guest, but first, I must recognize our famous test pilot and a Hero of the

Soviet Union, Gourgen Rubenovich Karapetyan."

They stood and turned toward him clapping vigorously as well as adding a few cheers. Gourgen stood briefly, bowed his head several times to acknowledge the recognition, then sat back down. He lifted his right hand toward Cap in a way signaling the honors should be directed to the American.

"It is Comrade Karapetyan who has brought Comrade Parlier to us." More clapping. "Between these two men," he said motioning to both Gourgen and Cap, "they have done more for the Chernobyl pilots than the entire government." Cap could almost hear a gasp at the courageous criticism that would not have been so well received a few years earlier. "They will do more for us. Now, it is time to eat."

The sumptuous meal occupied the better part of an hour as the pilots traded stories of their flying exploits. The interpreters remained so busy, they hardly took a bite to eat. While the lone American among all these Soviet pilots and crewmen did not share common events, they had the commonness of flight. Laughter and chatter filled the room with life.

A junior officer entered the room, walked briskly toward his commanding officer, then leaned down to whisper a message in his ear. Colonel Kalashnikov stood.

"Our guest's return window is rapidly approaching," he announced. He reached for his glass. Everyone in the room joined him. "I ask that we raise a glass in tribute to our honored guest, Comrade Parlier." Kalashnikov bolted the small glass of vodka as the others followed. Another few centimeters were poured.

Gourgen leaned toward Parlier and whispered, "We make an exception to drink a tribute to our fallen comrades."

Parlier nodded his head in recognition of the suspension of no mixing of drinking and flying rule they both lived by. This was a unique occasion, and an exception could be tolerated by both pilots.

When the vodka was poured, Kalashnikov continued, "I want to thank Comrade Parlier of behalf of the Regiment for coming to Torzhuk to visit the pilots, officers and men of what has become known as the Chernobyl Regiment. We flew more missions over that hell hole than any other unit, a dubious honor, I am sure." Several officers nodded their heads. "As most of you know, Comrade Parlier helped one of our Gromov test pilots, Anatoly Demjanovich Grishchenko, receive specialized medical treatment in America." The audience clapped. "He has graciously agreed to continue his efforts along with Gourgen Rubenovich," he said motioning toward Gourgen, "to assist the other Chernobyl pilots, many of whom are in this room, as they need medical attention in the years to come." They again downed their drinks.

Parlier waited until his glass was filled, then he held it up to make his own toast. "It is a humbling honor," he waited for the translation into Russian, "to be among such heroes." He paused. "While the world knows the name, Chernobyl, as a great disaster of unprecedented proportion, the world does not yet know of these heroes that flew over Chernobyl," he said, moving his glass and looking to each face in the room. "I promise you, the world will know what you have done for all humanity." He paused, again. "We will do our part to help you as you have helped us."

Several of the officers moved to embrace Cap and kiss each cheek. They responded to him as a long absent brother returning home. Tears could be seen in the eyes of many of them. They just wanted to be remembered, appreciated for what they had done.

Kalashnikov motioned across the room. A young, female captain with short, dark hair and pilot's wings at the far right side of the table turned behind her to retrieve a painting, then walked behind the others toward the head of the table. The respected leader held up his hand for everyone's attention.

"I want to introduce to all of you and especially our guest, Comrade Parlier, Captain Valerie Shmakova, one of the Regiment's exceptional navigators, and I must add with some pride, our resident artist. She has painted an image," he paused to take the painting from her and hold it high over his head. The characteristic mumbled conversations of three dozen people turned to stone-cold silence. "Many of us have this picture etched permanently in our memory."

The distinctive elements leapt from the canvas. The red and white stripes of the exhaust tower, the bluish-white light among the rubble of a tortured and broken building and the diminutive image of an Air Force Mi-8 helicopter with a sack suspended beneath the aircraft on a long line reaching toward the bright light. There was no question what the painting was — Chernobyl Unit No. 4 Nuclear Power Station, or more appropriately what was left of it. "I am certain there is no person in this room who does not recognize this painting. This was hell on earth. The world must never forget what has happened here," he said shaking the painting. It was not clear whether he was referring to the disaster or the heroism after the accident, or perhaps both. He lowered the painting.

"Now, I must tell you, when Comrade Karapetyan first told us Comrade Parlier would visit our Motherland and he asked if he could bring Comrade Parlier to us here in Torzhuk, there was no question. I asked Captain Shmakova to paint something from her heart that we could give to Comrade Parlier as a permanent link between our lives. I think she has done that." He held the painting up one more time. He turned to Cap. "This painting by Comrade Captain Valerie Shmakova is entrusted to your safekeeping, Comrade Parlier. Do not let the world forget what happened there."

Cap took the painting in one hand as he quickly wiped tears from his eyes. He coughed several times to clear his throat. This moment joined these pilots together forever. "I am humbled to be among such heroes," he said motioning to the entire group. "I am not worthy of such an honor."

"Yes, you are," Kalashnikov injected in English.

"I shall strive to be worthy. I promise you I will do whatever must be done to ensure the world knows what you have done. You will not be forgotten. We will do our best to help you as you have saved us."

"We can ask no more."

"Thank you. Thank you. Thank you so very much."

"I have the signal. All cherished moments must come to an end, for they pass into memory. Comrade Parlier must go, or he will not make it back to Moscow, today."

Emotional good-byes were passed from the Soviet Air Force pilots to the former American Marine pilot who had joined their ranks. It would be a long relationship. They all knew the reality yet to happen, but they saw it as clearly as the present. Their sacrifice would not be forgotten.

# Epilogue

The historic facts of this story remain as macabre reminders of the power of modern technology but more importantly the heroic sacrifices made by the firefighters and technicians during those fateful early morning hours of 26.April.1986, and by the pilots, construction crews and military personnel of the Soviet Union who struggled to contain the disaster. They succeeded in containing the damage of the worst nuclear disaster in history. We can only pray that it remains the worst and is not replaced some day by an even more tragic disaster.

The experts remind us that the physiological damage caused by ionizing radiation poisoning is cumulative. The acute effects are dramatic and relatively short lived. The chronic effects take much longer to manifest themselves but are just as deadly. For a population, the peak of chronic disease occurs at around the 20 year post-exposure point – the year 2006.

While Anatoly Demjanovich Grishchenko is the most publically visible of the Chernobyl heroes, the majority of those whose quiet sacrifice saved the Earth from far more damage have yet to face their greatest personal challenge. The medical professionals offer dire predictions of what the Chernobyl veterans will face – leukemia, thyroid cancer, liver cancer, cataracts, and host of other serious diseases. The heroes of Chernobyl deserve the remembrance of mankind as well as the assistance from all us who benefited from their sacrifice. Please consider contribution to the Grishchenko Fund to enable the deployment of Western medical technology to save those heroes.

## About the Author

# Cap Parlier

Cap Parlier is a former Marine aviator and experimental test pilot who currently is serving as the Chancellor of Embry-Riddle Aeronautical University, Prescott, Arizona campus. where he lives with his wife Jeanne. He has served in several aviation executive positions and is currently a director of the Boards of the National Marrow Donation Program and the Marrow Foundation. He is an avid aviator and enthusisatic proponent of space exploration. He has co-authored TWA 800: Accident or Incident? and authored The Phoenix Seduction, a science fiction novel. He has also written a forthcoming fictional saga of aviation and war in the 20th century.